The
FAMILY GUIDE
to
SEX
and
RELATIONSHIPS

AUTHOR'S ACKNOWLEDGMENTS

The author would like to thank the many people who made this book possible: Dr. Kenneth Fox for writing the Foreword; Dr. Neil Frude for writing the chapter on Sexual Offenses and Counseling; the distinguished medical consultants whose detailed and constructive scrutiny of the text improved it immeasurably; the editors and designers at De Agostini Editions whose high standards and hard work are evident in the pages that follow; Frances Gertler, Publishing Director at De Agostini Editions, whose enthusiasm, vision and, above all, extraordinary patience, brought the book to fruition; Tim Foster and David Robinson for their painstaking care over the design; Anne Johnson for her contributions to the chapters on Sex and Relationships and The Family and Sexuality; Mark Noble FRCOG, for his helpful advice and comments; and last, but not least, my family for their constant support and encouragement.

MACMILLAN
A Simon & Schuster Macmillan Company
1633 Broadway
New York, NY 10019-6785

Created by De Agostini Editions Ltd

Publishing Director: Frances Gertler
Art Director: Tim Foster
Editors: Michele Byam, Erica Marcus, Catherine Rubinstein
Senior Art Editor: David Robinson
Designer: Martin Hendry
Editorial Assistant: Philippa Cooper
Illustrations: Siena Artworks

Library of Congress Cataloging–in–Publication Data

Walker, Richard, 1951–
    The family guide to sex and relationships / Richard Walker.
        p.   cm.
    Includes bibiliographical references and index.
    ISBN 0–02–861433–X
    1. Sex.   2. Sex (Biology).   3. Hygiene, Sexual.
    4. Man–woman relationships.   I. Title.
    HQ21.W273   1996
    306.7--dc20   96-20660
                                            CIP
                                            REV

Printed in Italy

10 9 8 7 6 5 4 3 2 1

by Lego spa - Vicenza

The
FAMILY GUIDE
to
SEX
and
RELATIONSHIPS

RICHARD WALKER, Ph.D.

MACMILLAN • USA

Contents

About the consultants   6

Foreword   7

Introduction   8

1 The Reproductive Body   12

The female reproductive system   14
Menstrual and ovarian cycles   20
The male reproductive system   23
Sperm and hormone production   27
Conception   30

2 Baby to Child   32

Sex determination   34
Sex and gender   37
Developing sexuality: from birth to puberty   41
Sexual development and parental influence   43

3 Adolescence   46

What is puberty?   48
Changes common to girls and boys   50
Puberty in girls   54
Puberty in boys   63
Emotions and relationships   68
Becoming a sexual being   72
Teenage pregnancy and parenthood   78
Adolescent health   82

4 A Healthy Body   86

Diet and exercise   88
Personal hygiene   90
Emotional health   91
Female health   93
Male health   110
Nonsexually transmitted diseases   114
Sexually transmitted diseases   117
Drugs, addictions, and sex   126

5 Contraception   128

Using and choosing contraception   130
Barrier methods   132
Hormonal methods   142
The IUD   152
Natural methods   156
Sterilization   164
Emergency contraception   167

6 Sex and Relationships   170

Sexual desire   172
Sexual pleasure   174
Sexual attraction and body language   181
Sexual fantasy and variance   186
Communication between sexual partners   188
Sexual difficulties   190
Maintaining a long-term relationship   197
Sex and illness   199

7 Pregnancy and Parenthood   202

Physical aspects of pregnancy   204
Emotional aspects of pregnancy   211
Pregnancy and sex   214
New baby, new relationships   217
Sex and contraception after birth   222
Infertility   224
Ending a pregnancy   230

8 The Family and Sexuality   232

Family dynamics   234
Separation and divorce   241
New families   243
Being a single parent   245
Gay and lesbian parents   247

9 Middle Years   248

Forward planning for a longer life   250
Feeling good and looking good   251
Sexual relationships and the
   middle years   256
Midlife crisis—myth or reality?   258
Contraception in the middle years   259
Parenting   260

10 Menopause   262

What is menopause?   264
Menopausal changes and symptoms   266
Managing menopausal symptoms   271
Complementary therapies   275
Diet, exercise, and a healthy lifestyle 278
Relationships during menopause   280
Sex and menopause   281

11 The Later Years   284

A new lease on life   285
Retirement   287
Looking good and feeling good   288
Sex in the later years   290
Maintaining relationships   295
A changing family role   297

12 Sexual Offenses and
       Counseling   298

Sexual harassment   299
Rape   300
Voyeurism and Exhibitionism   303
Pedophilia   304
Child sexual abuse   306
Incest and pornography   309
Prositution   310
Help for victims of sex offenses   311

Glossary   **312**
Further reading   **315**
Helplines   **315**
Index   **316**
Acknowledgments   **320**

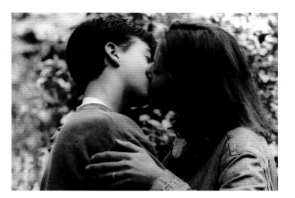

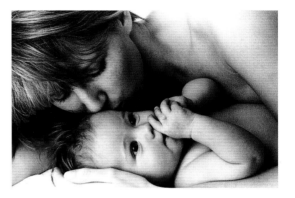

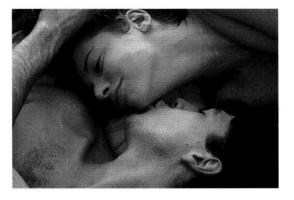

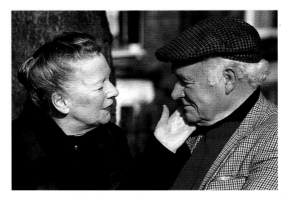

About the Consultants

The author and publishers are very grateful to all our consultants, listed below, for their expertise and advice, which were invaluable in the preparation of this book.

Agnes Begg, MBChB
Senior Chemical Medical Officer, Edinburgh Healthcare NHS Trust, Family Planning and Well Woman Services (Emeritus).

Gary Brook, MD, MRCP, DipGUM, DRCOG
Senior Registrar, Department of Genitourinary Medicine, Mortimer Market Centre, London.

Kenneth L. Fox, MD
Instructor, Department of Social Medicine, Harvard Medical School, Cambridge, Massachusetts; Member of the American Academy of Pediatrics and the American Anthropological Association.

Neil Frude, PhD
Professor, School of Psychology, University of Wales, Cardiff.

Robert A. Hatcher, MD
Professor of Gynecology and Obstetrics, Emory University School of Medicine; Director, Emory University Family Planning Program, Atlanta; Consultant to the World Health Organization; co-author of Contraceptive Technology.

The Terrence Higgins Trust
London-based AIDS charity.

Charles Kawada, MD
Chairman, Department of OB/GYN, Mount Auburn Hospital, Cambridge, Massachusetts; Assistant Clinical Professor of OB/GYN, Harvard Medical School.

Richard Kogan, MD
Psychiatrist and Associate, the Helen S. Kaplan Group for Medical Sex Therapy, New York City; Senior Supervisor, Human Sexuality Training Program, New York Hospital-Cornell Medical Center.

Patricia Last, FRCS, FRCOG
The London Women's Clinic; formerly of St. Bartholomew's Hospital, London, and Director of Women's Screening for BUPA; now a medical journalist and lecturer specializing in the health aspects of retirement.

Diana Mansour, MRCOG, MFFP
Deputy Medical Director and Medical Advisor/Lecturer in Family Planning and Reproductive Health Care, Margaret Pyke Memorial Trust, London; Advisory Doctor, the Brook Advisory Centre, London.

Nicholas Pannay, BSc, MRCOG
Research Fellow, Chelsea and Westminster Hospital, London.

Angela Robinson, MBBS, MRCP
Consultant Physician, Department of Genitourinary Medicine, Mortimer Market Centre, London.

Sylvia Rosenfeld, CSW, ACSW
New York-based psychotherapist specializing in couples counseling, sex therapy, and childhood sexual abuse.

Camille San Lazaro, MD
Consultant Pediatrician, The Lindisfarne Centre, Royal Victoria Infirmary, Newcastle upon Tyne, England.

John Studd, DSc, MD, FRCOG
Director of Menopause and Osteoporosis Clinic and Consultant Gynecologist, Chelsea and Westminster Hospital, London.

Foreword

Kenneth L. Fox, MD

Once upon a time the world was safe and simple and quiet. Male and female identities and the sharp gender divison of labor in family life were experienced as expressions of a natural order. The sexual lives of adults were entirely private matters, shrouded in silence, bound by laws of God and nature. A child, by definition, was innocent of and unmoved by sexual impulses and messages. Common sense organized family and society in fair and immutable ways…. Or was it ever really like this?

Nostalgic yearning is often most powerful for worlds that never actually existed. Ties imagined to bind were also forces that distorted and knotted lives in ways that were less than happy, healthy, or romantic. Silence about gender and sexual identity and roles hurt many people. Rules of order often muted human experiences in destructive ways. Apparently, the opposite applies today. We seem able to enjoy unfettered freedom to voice our sexual and relational needs.

But our times of broken silences are also full of hazards. The deafening noise over issues like gender roles and "family values" can drive us to withdrawal, paralysis, or confusion. However, adopting an ostrich position and hiding our heads in the sand is inadvisable in times of pervasive family disruption, child abuse, teenage pregnancy, and AIDS. Families are bombarded with countless images of sex. Talk shows, "how-to" books, and other forms of "infotainment" make matters of sexuality and intimate relationships seem like public utilities, to be made merely more efficient by

information and technique. In consumer cultures, sexuality is treated as a way to sell products rather than as a sacred aspect of full and healthy family lives.

Who needs another book about sex? In short, we do. Clear words and images make this book a useful map by which to move safely through the highly charged world of sexuality. There is great emphasis here on developmental issues—how families grow in relation to the social contexts in which they exist. The book is serious about and respectful of our minds and bodies as it celebrates sexuality within family life over time.

This book belongs on the family bookshelf. It is not a "sex guide" to be hidden away at the back of Dad's sock-and-underwear drawer for curious and naughty children to find. It is not a book that a mother would be worried to find in the bedroom of a teenage daughter or son. Everyone in the family can use it openly. This guide is for adults in the family who want to understand their own bodies and relationships more clearly or need to talk to their children about such matters. Older children and adolescents can use the book to explore questions on their own. Younger children can appreciate the pictures of loving families as they process basic matters like nudity and privacy as well as other issues such as pregnancy and birth. Open and accessible at home over the years, this resource will create a space of helpful talk about a dynamic realm of family life. This book is just what the modern family—and the primary care doctor—ordered.

Introduction

Sex, it has been said, may not be the most important thing in life, but there is nothing else quite like it. College, work, looking after children, shopping at the supermarket, watching TV, practicing the piano, or surfing the Internet may all be key points of reference in our daily lives; sex is not. Most of us think about sex sometimes—be it hourly, daily, or weekly; make new relationships or maintain old ones; and enjoy, even relish, the pleasures of sexual arousal and orgasm. But many of us feel this sexual side of our nature to be intrinsically private and personal, hidden and mysterious, to be shared only with our lovers and intimates, or perhaps just with ourselves.

Although sex can be a source of great happiness and fulfillment, it can also be an area of insecurity and worry in our daily lives. Misinformation, ignorance, or embarrassment can blight what should be as natural a part of existence as eating and sleeping. Whatever inhibitions, fears, or anxieties we have about sex are not unique to us as individuals. They develop as a result of the influence of parents, friends, and society in general. Increasingly liberal attitudes toward sex since the 1960s have produced a climate in which many men and women have found themselves fulfilled both sexually and in their relationships. But others, perhaps dazzled by images of sex in the media, have questioned their sex lives and found themselves unable to come to terms with their sexuality and relationships.

However, there is no great mystery about sex, and no reason why we should not make the most of this aspect of our lives. We need, however, to contextualize it by understanding the nature of sex, and by unburdening ourselves of the baggage of sexual myths, prejudices, and inhibitions passed down to us by previous generations.

Reproduction or pleasure?

Humans are no different from all other species of living things on this planet in our need to reproduce. The unavoidable fact is that if it does not reproduce itself a species will die out. Like most animals, we humans reproduce sexually. This involves two individuals—a male and a female—and the fusion of sex cells (sperm and egg) produced by them, in order to generate offspring that share the basic features of but are not identical to their parents. Built into these sexually reproducing creatures is an instinctive motive or drive to have sex. Without such motivation, sex and reproduction would simply not happen.

Should we view ourselves, therefore, with other animals as no more than "breeding machines"? Are sexual pleasures merely an enticement to do our biological duty by getting out there and reproducing to pass on our genes to another generation? At a basic biological level, the answer must be yes. On the other hand, humans differ from all other animals in the extraordinary degree to which our intelligence and social organization have developed. We are also the only species that can use spoken and written language to pass on cultural memories from one generation to the next. True, we retain our motivational desire to reproduce. But this instinctive drive has become integrated into the more complex arena of sexual desire. And while we all have sexual desires, their precise nature varies from one person to the next for the simple reason that they are shaped by what we as individuals observe, learn, and experience from infancy onward.

The pattern of our sexual activities also reveals a difference between the nature of sex in humans and that in our closest animal relatives. Most animals have restricted periods of sexual activity, known as a breeding season, while for the rest of the year they are not "interested" in sex. Adult humans, in contrast —both men and women—are potentially sexual at any time of year, whatever the season; nor is this just in those brief intervals each month midway between a woman's periods when she can conceive. Such constant readiness indicates that sex in humans is not just about procreation.

Further evidence of the pleasurable function of sex is provided by our sexual behavior. We characteristically pursue a comparatively long period of courtship, allowing us to bond with our potential mate with a view to a long-term relationship by seeing if we are mutually attracted and compatible, and to develop a romantic and sexual attachment—more familiarly known as falling in love—that will usually culminate in having sex. As a typical prelude to making love we devote time to mutual pleasuring and arousal (foreplay), a phenomenon unique to humans. Sexual intercourse itself is generally prolonged, lasting for several or many minutes; it is not over in seconds like the copulatory acts of our nearest relatives, the apes. Our sex organs themselves are also testament to our inherent eroticism. A woman's clitoris has just one function—to be stimulated in order to provide sexual pleasure, often resulting in an intense orgasm unique to female humans. The human penis is comparatively much longer and wider than apes', reflecting the part it plays in sexual pleasuring during prolonged intercourse. Furthermore, sexual behavior does not cease if conception is impossible: a couple that uses contraception to prevent pregnancy, for example, does not in general lose interest in sex; most women continue to enjoy sex after menopause when they are no longer fertile; and homosexual couples—be they gay men or lesbians—have sexual desires as potent as those experienced by heterosexual couples.

So why do we humans show these elaborate and unique patterns of courtship and sexuality? The answer must be in order to create close, long-term relationships. Such relationships evolved over hundreds of thousands of years of human history to enable us to provide continuity of parental care to nurture the intelligent but demanding creature that is the human child. Relationships between sexual partners, between parents and children within a family, and between relatives in extended families also form part of the human social infrastructure, creating a frame of reference within which we can feel secure and content, and develop our potential to the full.

Sex through history

Sexuality is not just a matter of inner drives — it is shaped by the customs and practices of the society we live in, which themselves have been influenced by the mores of preceding generations. That in the past two centuries Western societies have witnessed dramatic and, recently, rapid changes in attitudes toward sex may help to explain our often ambivalent feelings about sex today: our sexual heritage is confused and ambiguous.

While sexual restrictions have always existed, their extent has changed constantly throughout time. We can, by analogy, appreciate such changes by considering moral codes in different parts of the world today: it is possible, for example, to buy a wide variety of sex aids and magazines quite openly in a sex store in Amsterdam, while it would be impossible, and illegal, to do the same in Riyadh, Saudi Arabia. Although a detailed account of the history of sex is not within the scope of this book, a few historical snapshots can provide some explanation for our perception of ourselves as sexual beings.

How did our ancient ancestors behave sexually? Although their lives were shorter and harder than ours, we should not presume that they were any less capable of love and tenderness. But it is unlikely that they recognized that pregnancy was a direct consequence of intercourse: sex was probably a pleasurable interlude in a life of hardship rather than a specifically procreative act. Recognition of the link between sex and procreation is thought to have occurred around the time that humans first settled into agricultural communities, some ten thousand years ago. Becoming aware of the significance of sexual intercourse gave people greater control over their lives, and is likely to have changed the criteria employed in choosing sexual partners, laying the foundations of today's courtship and relationship patterns. But this era probably also saw the origins of the suppression of women that has continued in most societies up to and including the present century.

The accounts that we have of human history over the past four or five thousand years record great fluctuations in sexual tolerance. In ancient Israel, for example, adultery, homosexuality, and masturbation were forbidden and punishable. In ancient Greece, at least for a while, homosexuality in both men and women was tolerated and even venerated, and sexual freedom extended to ready acceptance of prostitution and group sex. As Greece went into decline, the mantle of sexual freedom and experimentation passed to Rome. Both cultures, however, witnessed sudden about-faces, when the state punished sexual freedom. And in both, the position of women was often subordinate to that of men, although this was challenged by women at various times who took on positions of power.

The coming of Christianity brought widespread condemnation of earlier "excesses" and sexual freedoms, at least in theory. The "party line" stipulated adherence to monogamous relationships, sex for procreative purposes only, and a ban on homosexual and other "unnatural" practices. Human nature being what it is, the Church's teachings on sexual restraint were often ignored. But sex was established in Western thinking as something essentially sinful, a legacy that has passed down to the 20th century. If things went wrong—failed crops or an outbreak of the plague, for example—sexual excesses could be blamed and the perpetrators punished. Such use of scapegoats was most evident between the 15th and 17th centuries, when women were blamed for arousing "lowest" need—lust—in men, and some were burned as witches for their sins. These customs died out with scientific advances from the 16th century onward that demythologized many aspects of sex by revealing how the human body works, but the view of sex as sinful endured.

The 16th century was also the era that reintroduced the biblical idea of romantic love. Under the romantic schema, there is only one man for each woman; the virginal lovers fight through adversity to make their match and stay together forevermore. The concept has survived to the present day, especially in romantic fiction, although few couples today fit such an idealized description.

Romantic ideals were far from universal, however. Puritan settlers of the 17th and 18th century in New England considered having and talking about sex to be perfectly natural, and premarital intercourse was positively encouraged as a "test drive" to see if partners were suited to each other. Consequently the majority of brides went to the altar pregnant. Liberal attitudes toward sexuality were also found on the other side of the Atlantic.

This situation was not to last. The 19th century brought with it an increasingly prudish attitude. Not only was sex regarded as essentially depraved and disgusting—apart from procreative sex, which was, of course, not to be enjoyed—but the same anxieties applied to language referring to anything sexual or any body parts. Even words seen as alluding to sex because part of them had a sexual connotation were banned, especially in the United States. This explains why today the British refer to cockerels and titbits, whereas Americans say roosters and tidbits. Most appalling of all sexual practices to the Victorians was probably masturbation. This practice of "self-abuse," a "crime against nature," was believed to lead to insanity, weakness, consumption and finally death. Some children—both boys and girls—were subjected to unspeakable cruelties to prevent them from masturbating. Repression of sexuality reached new heights and yet, paradoxically, men could still find sexual expression by visiting prostitutes: there were, for example, at least 8,000 prostitutes in London in 1850, and some 12,000 in Philadelphia by 1870.

This, therefore, was the confused and ambiguous legacy passed down to the inhabitants of the Western world in the 20th century. But gradually the sexually repressed fortress constructed by the Victorians has been chipped away. Sigmund Freud and Havelock Ellis wrote the first studies of sexuality. The work of Alfred Kinsey, and later researchers including William Masters and Virginia Johnson, revealed for the first time how people actually behaved sexually, exploding Victorian myths about "depravity." The pioneering work of Margaret Sanger and Marie Stopes, often against stiff resistance from the establishment, gave women and men ready access to birth control. Access to contraception, as well as other social change in this century, has also empowered women to achieve more and aspire to an equal role with men, a struggle which still continues. Further liberalization of attitudes about sex has come with the legalization of abortion and homosexuality in most Western countries in the past 30 years. From the 1940s and 1950s on, premarital sex was widely considered unacceptable, adolescent sex was thought to be nonexistent, and homosexual sex was illegal and seen as depraved. Now at the end of the 20th century, we find ourselves experiencing the fallout from a sexual revolution that should have made sex much more natural, acceptable, and easy to talk about. Or is it? Do attitudes about sex in the media reflect the way we feel today?

Sex and the media

We have access to an array of communications media that our ancestors could not have dreamed of. Sex, sexuality, and relationships are reported, described, explored and exploited quite openly—within the bounds of "decency" imposed by the laws of individual countries—in the form of books, newspapers, magazines, photographs, art, movies, videos, TV programs, and CD-ROMs, and on the Internet. But all too often sexual imagery is idealistic. We are presented with images of people with "beautiful" bodies, having sex frequently as and when they please, always achieving earth-shattering orgasms; the inevitable conclusion is that people who are not having lots of passionate sex are leading miserable lives. But the visual and print media can be deceptive when it comes to sex. First, they may present a one-sided, often male,

view of sex, typically overinfluenced by Western male stereotypes of beauty and sexual attractiveness, and a male concept of sex as involving domination of women. Second, media views of sex are often one-dimensional: they display the physical side without exploring the sensual, emotional, and relationship aspects of sexual love. It is hardly surprising, therefore, that some of us find media representation of sex disturbing because it makes our own sex lives appear inadequate; myths and false expectations engendered by media images can destroy self-esteem and, by affecting people's sex lives, destabilize relationships. For what else can we compare our sex lives with? People are likely to feel inhibited when it comes to discussing sexual matters with friends if they imagine they lack sexual competence.

But each of us has our own complex sexual feelings and desires; we cannot conform to an impossible sexual "norm" created by the media. To make the most of our individual sexuality and relationships, we need to discover and understand our sexuality.

Understanding ourselves as sexual beings

Sex is not just the sexual act. To understand ourselves fully as sexual beings we need to take a holistic approach. We are not sexual machines, but individuals each with our own sexual agenda, experiences, and expectations. Our sexuality is affected by our childhood, our parents, our friends, our health, and our lifestyle. Knowledge about the body and how it works, an understanding of what happens during sex, how pregnancy occurs, and how sexuality can change as we pass through the various phases of life can add an extra dimension to our appreciation of sex. The act of sex between two individuals may be a private affair, and rightly so, but a clear understanding of all aspects of sex and relationships should be in the public domain. Sex is a natural part of life, and knowledge about it can only serve to empower people in their relationships with partners and families. The aim of this book is to do just that: to present a comprehensive and accessible account of sex and relationships.

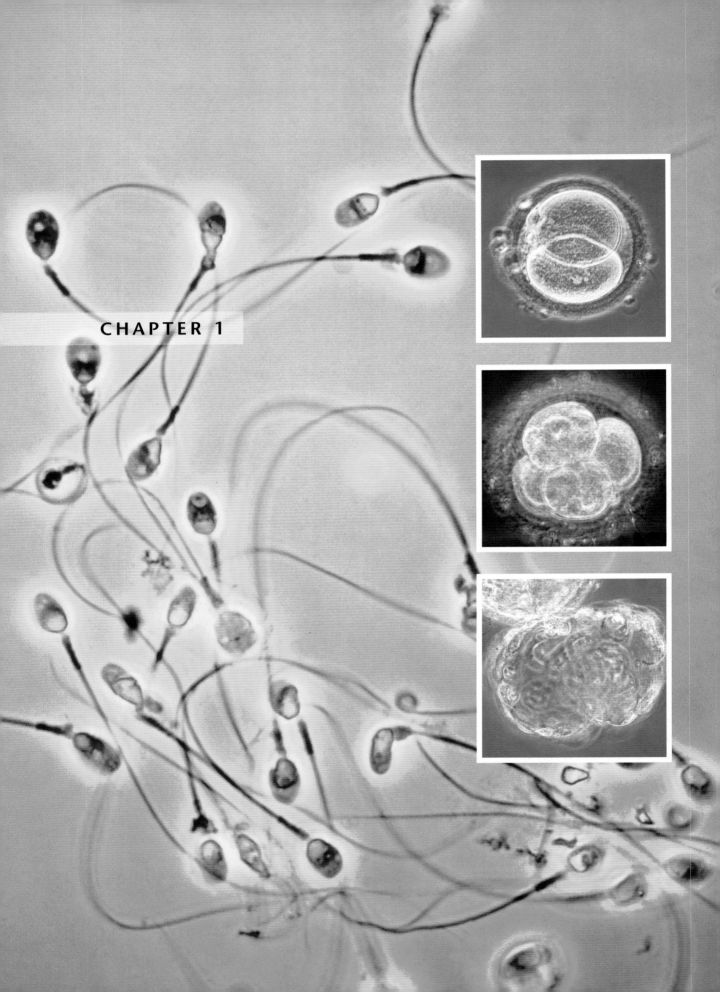

CHAPTER 1

The Reproductive Body

A characteristic of all living organisms, from the tiniest bacteria to the biggest whales, is their ability to reproduce, in order to carry on the species. Human beings are no exception.

The human body's reproductive system comprises the organs that produce and facilitate the union of sex cells, whose combined genetic material provides the blueprint for new life. The reproductive systems of males and females differ, each having its own role.

Reproductive organs first appear in the developing embryo during the earliest weeks of pregnancy. Initially they are identical in both male and female embryos, but as the weeks pass, the reproductive organs follow separate developmental routes for each sex.

By the time a child is born the reproductive system is in place. Those parts of it that can be seen on the outside of the body are known, in both sexes, as the external genitalia, genital organs, or genitals. Those parts contained within the body are referred to as the internal reproductive organs. A baby's sex can be determined by his or her external genitalia: he has a penis, and she has a vulva. But the internal parts of their reproductive systems remain inactive until their early teenage years and the onset of puberty (see Chapter 3).

During puberty, a boy's testes produce male sex cells called sperm. The testes also then release sex hormones that stimulate the growth of other parts of the reproductive system and the appearance of secondary sex characteristics such as facial hair. At the same time, a girl's ovaries start to release sex cells called eggs, or ova, and to produce sex hormones that stimulate the development of the reproductive system and the appearance of secondary sex characteristics such as breasts.

By the time they reach adulthood, males and females are capable of reproduction. The male reproductive system delivers sperm, through the penis, into the female's vagina. If one of these sperm meets a newly released egg, it will fertilize it, and conception—the beginning of a new life—occurs. Nurtured in the "incubation chamber" of the woman's uterus, the fertilized egg develops over the next nine months into a fully formed human being.

As well as enabling us to procreate, our reproductive systems allow us to enjoy those sexual and sensual pleasures that appear to be particular to human beings. The reproductive organs, most notably the external genitalia, are richly endowed with sensory nerve endings that produce sensual feelings when stimulated. The origin of these feelings lies not in the organs themselves but in the nervous system, primarily in its supreme organ, the brain. And it is the nervous system, together with the body's hormonal system, that controls and coordinates the reproductive system.

The female reproductive system

Between puberty and menopause a woman's reproductive system releases female sex cells (eggs, or ova), provides a location for fertilization of an egg by a male sex cell (sperm), and protects the developing baby during pregnancy. The reproductive system also contains the sensory structures that aid sexual arousal.

Within the female reproductive system, the primary sex organs are the two ovaries, which produce eggs and release them during the reproductive phase of a woman's life. The accessory sex organs are the other parts of the reproductive system—internal and external—that facilitate fertilization and protect and nurture the fetus during pregnancy. The breasts, or mammary glands, are also considered accessory reproductive organs because they produce milk to feed the newborn baby.

The female internal reproductive organs

A woman's internal reproductive organs lie protected within the bones of the pelvis. They consist of two ovaries, two fallopian tubes, the uterus (womb), the cervix, and the vagina. The vagina connects the uterus with the external reproductive organs.

The ovaries

The ovaries release eggs and produce sex hormones that control a woman's fertility. Lying

---

THE EXPANDING UTERUS

During pregnancy, the uterus, normally the size of its owner's clenched fist, expands enormously to accommodate the growing fetus. Its increase in length is a result of the "stretchiness" of the *myometrium*, the muscular layer that makes up most of the thickness of the uterine wall. Microscopic studies show that the individual muscle cells that make up this layer can elongate by up to 10 times their original length. After the baby is born the uterus shrinks considerably, although it may never return to its original size.

---

in the upper pelvic cavity, one on each side of the uterus, they resemble almonds in both size and shape. At birth, a girl's ovaries already contain 2–4 million immature eggs, or ova; these are all the eggs she will ever have. In sexually mature women, many immature eggs ripen each month, although usually only one—occasionally two or more—becomes fully mature. Eggs that fail to mature are re-absorbed into the body. Once the egg or ovum is ripe, the wall of the ovary ruptures, and the egg is released into the nearby opening of a fallopian tube. This release is called ovulation and, usually, each ovary releases one egg on alternate months, although not all women ovulate every month. The ovaries stop releasing eggs around the time of the menopause *(see p.265)*.

The fallopian tubes

These are the passageways that connect the ovaries to the uterus and along which an egg travels after ovulation. For most of its 4-inch length, the inside of the fallopian tube is narrower than a strand of spaghetti. However, at the end next to the ovary the fallopian tube expands into finger-like projections called fimbriae. These do not touch the ovary, but form a funnel that directs the egg into the fallopian tube after it is released from the ovary. Lining the fimbriae, and the rest of the fallopian tube, are microscopic, hair-like cilia, which move rhythmically, transporting the egg toward the uterus. Each tube has a trumpet-shaped end that opens into the hollow interior of the uterus.

The fallopian tubes are the site of fertilization, which may occur if the egg meets a sperm within 24 hours of ovulation. Occasionally, following fertilization, the fertilized egg implants in the fallopian tube instead of in the uterus. This is called an ectopic pregnancy and requires termination to prevent harm to the mother.

The uterus

The uterus, or womb, is a hollow, pear-shaped and pear-sized organ that houses, protects, and nourishes the developing fetus during pregnancy. Its thick muscular walls stretch

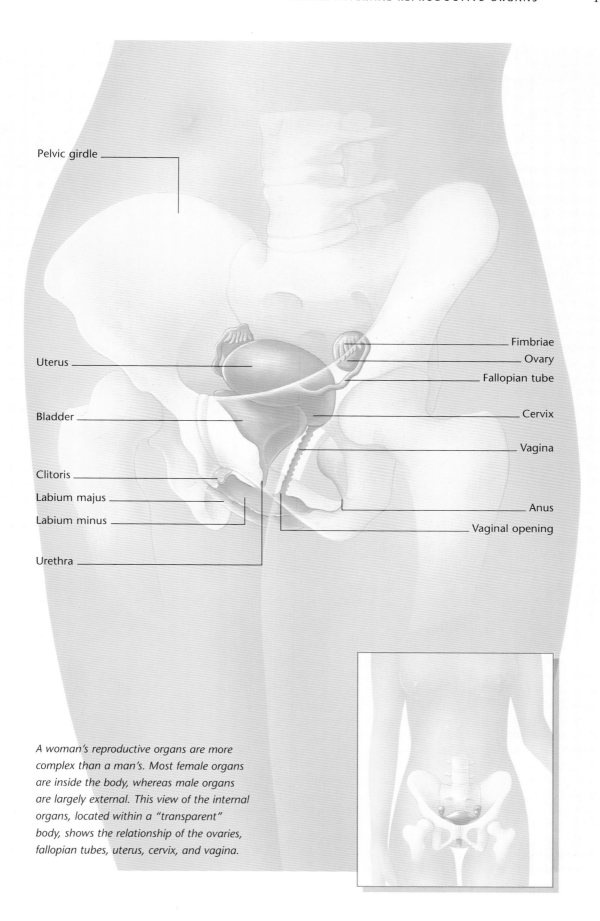

Pelvic girdle

Uterus

Bladder

Clitoris

Labium majus

Labium minus

Urethra

Fimbriae

Ovary

Fallopian tube

Cervix

Vagina

Anus

Vaginal opening

A woman's reproductive organs are more complex than a man's. Most female organs are inside the body, whereas male organs are largely external. This view of the internal organs, located within a "transparent" body, shows the relationship of the ovaries, fallopian tubes, uterus, cervix, and vagina.

considerably during pregnancy to accommodate the fetus, and contract during birth to expel the baby. The womb's inner lining is deep and velvety in texture and thickens each month as the womb prepares to receive an egg, should it be fertilized in the fallopian tube. If fertilization does not occur, the inner lining is shed during the woman's menstrual period, and grows again the following month.

THE DISPLACED UTERUS

In 90 percent of women, the uterus is tilted toward the front of the body, over the bladder—this is known as an anteversion. Some women may have a backward displacement, or retroversion, with the uterus inclining backward so that the cervix faces forward. Usually this position is simply a variation of the norm, and does not cause any problems. Contrary to what was once believed, having a retroverted uterus does not make it more difficult for a woman to have a baby.

The cervix

The lower part of the uterus is called the cervix. Its narrow cavity, the cervical canal, runs between the thick cervical walls to connect the main body of the uterus with the vagina. These cervical walls secrete a sticky mucus that usually prevents the entry of sperm into the uterus following intercourse; just after ovulation, however, the mucus becomes thinner so that sperm can travel easily from the vagina into the uterus. When a woman gives birth, her cervix widens considerably to allow the baby's head and body to emerge into the vagina.

The vagina

This muscular tube, which connects the cervix to the outside of the body, receives the penis during sexual intercourse, carries the menstrual flow during a period, and provides the passageway through which a baby passes during birth. In its "resting" state the vagina is between 3¼ and 4 inches long, and its front and back walls touch. During sexual arousal, however, the folded nature of its walls enables the vagina to expand considerably in length and width, to accommodate the erect penis. At the same time, the vaginal wall releases a type of "sweat" that assists with lubrication. The vagina, like many other parts of the body, naturally contains a healthy "flora" of bacterial and fungal microorganisms. Occasionally the natural balance of this flora is disrupted and an overgrowth of one or more microorganisms occurs, resulting in a vaginal infection, such as a yeast infection *(see p.116)*. The vagina may also be affected by diseases that are transmitted during sexual intercourse *(see pp.121–6)*.

The female external reproductive organs

A woman's external reproductive organs comprise the breasts and the genitalia between her legs. The latter, known collectively as the vulva, include the mons pubis, the vaginal lips (the labia majora and labia minora), the clitoris, and the vaginal vestibule—the area enclosed by the labia minora that surrounds the openings to the urethra and the vagina. Because of its rich supply of sensory nerve endings, the vulva is highly sensitive to touch, and so plays an important part in a woman's sexual arousal.

The mons pubis

This pubic mound (also known as the mons veneris or mount of Venus) is the only part of the vulva clearly visible from the front. Under the skin of the mons, a fatty pad covers the pubic bone at the front of the pelvic girdle, which can be felt by pressing gently in this area. At puberty, the mons usually becomes covered by a triangle of coarse pubic hair. During sexual intercourse, the mons and its covering of pubic hair cushion the pubic bones of the partners to prevent them from grinding painfully against each other. Running backward from the base of the mons pubis are two folds of skin, the labia majora.

The labia majora

The labia majora (literally the "larger lips") form the outer part of the vulva, enclosing and protecting the rest of the external genitalia. The two labia majora (labium majus in the singular) are composed of soft fatty tissue,

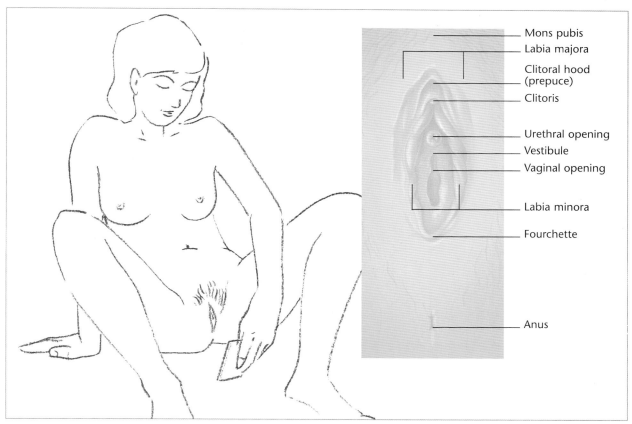

Mons pubis
Labia majora
Clitoral hood (prepuce)
Clitoris
Urethral opening
Vestibule
Vaginal opening
Labia minora
Fourchette
Anus

like the mons. Externally, each labium majus has a covering of pubic hair, although its inner surface is smooth and hairless, and contains glands that release secretions. Numerous oil and sweat glands produce an oily secretion that lubricates and softens the vulva. Apocrine (scent) glands, which are more active during sexual arousal, discharge a thickish liquid with a musky smell that can act as an attractant and stimulant for sexual partners. Like other parts of the vulva, the labia majora have many sensory receptors that make them very sensitive to touch during sexual foreplay. Just inside, and often hidden by the labia majora, are the labia minora, or "smaller lips."

The labia minora

The inner lips of the vulva (labium minus in the singular) are hairless folds of skin that are thinner and more delicate than the labia majora. They extend on each side of the vulva from the clitoris at the front to the fourchette (from the French for "little fork"), the fold of skin just behind the vaginal opening, at the

To see your vulva, sit with your legs apart and use a mirror. You should not be surprised if the labia majora and labia minora do not look exactly like these. They vary considerably in size and shape from one woman to the next.

SELF-EXAMINATION

Because of its position, the vulva is not easily visible, in contrast to a male's penis and scrotum, which hang out from the front of his body. Some women familiarize themselves with their vulva by using a mirror. Self-examination will not only increase your understanding of your genitals, it also enables you—as with the other parts of the body—to check for any incipient problems that may require medical attention. In some cases, examining her vulva can help a woman overcome any inhibitions she may have about that area, particularly if she was told as a child that she should not touch herself "down there." Familiarization may help her develop a positive attitude toward her sex organs, and thereby enhance her enjoyment of sex.

back. Depending on the individual woman, the labia minora may be concealed within the labia majora, or may protrude between these outer lips; the two labia often differ in size and shape as well. The inner lips have more oil glands than the outer lips, and the secretions they produce keep the vestibule that lies between them moist. These secretions also mix with sweat from sweat glands and secretions from the vagina, to produce a waterproof covering that protects the vulva from both urine and menstrual blood, as well as from bacteria. The labia minora have more sensory endings than the outer lips, and during sexual excitement they change color and increase considerably in size as they become engorged with blood. At the front of the vulva, the two labia minora meet to form a fold of skin, called the clitoral hood. This covers the clitoris, the most sensitive part of the vulva.

The clitoris

The clitoris (the name comes from the Greek for "key") is a small, sensitive organ that has the same component parts as the penis, albeit much smaller. Unlike the penis, however, its sole function is to provide sexual pleasure. In total, the clitoris is between ¾ and 1½ inches long, depending on the individual; however, the visible part that can be seen if the labia minora are pulled back is about ⅓ inch because the organ is bent back on itself. The clitoris consists of a tip (the glans)—packed with sensory nerve endings that make it the most sensitive part of the entire genital area—and a shaft, which can be felt as a rubbery cord leading to the glans. Internally, the shaft extends outward and backward to form the crura (crus in the singular), two columns of tissue that attach the clitoris to the pelvic bones.

The clitoris, like the penis, contains erectile tissue; when the woman is sexually aroused this tissue becomes filled with blood and engorged, causing the clitoris to become erect, almost double in size, and emerge from the prepuce or clitoral hood (equivalent to the foreskin in uncircumcised males) that is formed around it by the labia minora. Just behind the clitoris, and between the labia minora, lies the vestibule.

The vestibule

The vestibule (literally, "entrance hall") is the area that lies inside and between the labia minora. Toward the front of the vestibule is the small urethral opening, through which urine from the bladder leaves the body. Behind the urethral opening is a thin membrane called the hymen, which surrounds, and partially covers, the opening to the vagina. The size of this opening depends on the extent of the hymen. Physical activities such as climbing and cycling, or sexual intercourse, as well as the use of tampons, may all cause the hymen to be torn, so that in most adult women the hymen remains as just a few pieces of loose skin. However, in a very small number of women, the skin of the hymen is too thick to break naturally; in these cases it may be necessary to cut it surgically, under a local anesthetic.

Opening onto the vestibule on either side of the vagina are the vestibular glands, also known as Bartholin's glands. During sexual arousal, these glands release mucus around

FEMALE CIRCUMCISION

Probably 90 million women, mostly young girls, suffer circumcision each year, mainly in Africa and the Middle East, but also in ethnic communities in Western countries. Female circumcision is far more radical than its male counterpart, with varying degrees of genital mutilation. The mildest form, known as *sunna*, or traditional circumcision, involves removing the clitoral hood. Clitoridectomy, or excision, involves removing the clitoris and all or part of the labia minora. In the most extreme form, known as infibulation or Pharaonic circumcision, the clitoris and labia are removed and the sides of the vulva are stitched together, with a small opening left for the flow of urine and menstrual blood. Female circumcision was a religious rite among some peoples in prehistoric times, but today there is no religious basis for the practice (except in certain tribes, particularly in Africa). In many communities, however, it is regarded as a normal part of growing up, which protects a girl morally—by stopping her from becoming promiscuous—and so enables her to find a husband. The medical profession denounces this practice, believing it goes against all ethical codes for this operation to be performed.

the entrance to the vagina that, along with secretions from the labia minora, cervix, and vaginal walls, provides lubrication during sexual intercourse.

Breasts

Female breasts start to develop during puberty *(see pp.54–6)*, when modified sweat glands called mammary glands develop under the skin. In males, these glands remain rudimentary, and any breast development during puberty is temporary and the result of hormonal imbalance.

Each breast extends from the outer edge of the breastbone to the armpit, and overlies the major chest muscles, the pectoralis major and pectoralis minor. Externally, each breast has a cylindrical projection, the nipple, which is darker than the normal skin color. The nipple contains erectile tissue, and commonly becomes erect during sexual arousal, or in response to touch or cold temperatures. Surrounding the nipple is a circular area of skin, the same color as the nipple, called the areola (plural areolae). The size of the areola varies considerably from woman to woman, as does its color, although this is normally related to the individual woman's skin color. The areolae become permanently darker and larger during pregnancy. The sebaceous (oil) glands of the areolae—which produce a secretion that protects the nipple during breast-feeding—are larger than those in other parts of the body, and give the areolae a bumpy appearance.

Internally, each breast consists of between 15 and 20 lobes, each lobe being subdivided into lobules of milk-producing alveolar glands that resemble bunches of grapes. During pregnancy, the hormones prolactin, estrogen, and progesterone stimulate these glands to make, and eventually release, milk. The milk is carried in a tube called the lactiferous duct, which runs from each lobe; together these ducts open through the nipple. Just before they reach the opening in the nipple, each duct expands to form a reservoir called the lactiferous sinus where, in a mother who is breastfeeding, milk is stored before being released when the baby sucks on the nipple.

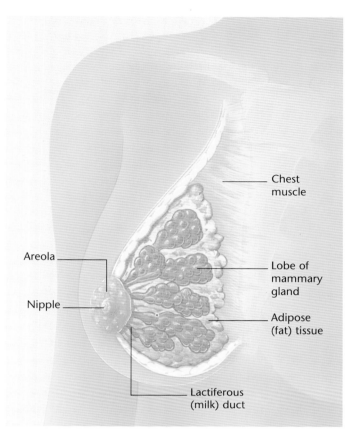

This section of a breast reveals its internal structure. The size of the breast is determined by the amount of fat tissue surrounding the milk-producing glands. These glands, shown here in a non-pregnant woman, increase in size during pregnancy.

BREAST SIZE AND BREASTFEEDING

Breast size varies considerably from one woman to the next, but size does not determine how well a woman can breastfeed her baby. Women with smaller breasts are just as capable of feeding their baby as women with larger breasts. What determines the size and shape of the breast is the amount of fat deposited inside it. This, in turn, is determined by the genes a woman inherits from her parents, her age, and whether she is overweight, underweight, or in the normal weight range for her size *(see p.88)*. Breast size and shape are independent of the network of lobes that form each mammary gland and actually produce milk. During pregnancy, all breasts increase in size as these milk-producing glands enlarge and start producing milk.

The lobes are separated by ligaments and fat (or adipose) tissue; these ligaments function like an "internal bra" that supports the breasts. Contrary to popular belief, the underlying chest muscles play no part at all in supporting the breasts.

The breasts are a common site for the development of tumors, which can be cancerous, as well as benign cysts. Breast cancer is the most common form of cancer in women: in the United States it affects as many as one in nine women, while in Britain about one in twenty suffer from the disease. After puberty, and certainly by their early twenties, it is recommended that all women examine their breasts once a month—generally, to ensure regularity, just after their period has finished —to feel for any lumps and to look for external changes that might indicate a possible problem *(for more on breast examination, see pp.100–1).* The vast majority of growths will turn out to be benign, but if a growth is malignant, the earlier it is detected and the woman begins treatment, the greater chance she has of being cured.

HORMONES AND REPRODUCTIVE CYCLES

The release of an egg and the thickening of the uterus lining that occur each month are coordinated by hormones. Those released by the pituitary gland cause the ovaries to release mature eggs. They also stimulate the ovaries to release female sex hormones, which encourage the lining of the uterus to thicken in readiness to receive an egg, should it be fertilized.

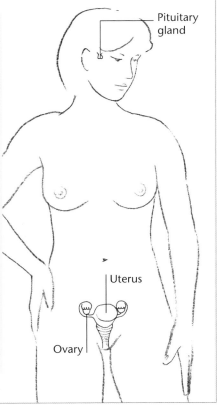

Pituitary gland

Uterus

Ovary

Female reproductive cycles

Women and men differ fundamentally in the way their reproductive systems produce sex cells. Between puberty and old age, a man's testes manufacture millions of sperm daily. During a woman's reproductive years— usually between her early teens and late forties—one egg is released each month from one of her ovaries. At the same time, her uterus prepares to receive that egg should it be fertilized by a sperm. Instead of the sex cell production line found in men, the release of an egg and changes in the uterus are synchronized processes that are repeated on a regular basis. These events are controlled by a woman's reproductive cycles.

A cycle is a sequence of events that occurs in a fixed order, and repeats itself constantly. Each month not one but two closely linked reproductive cycles take place inside a woman's body: the ovarian cycle and the menstrual cycle. During the ovarian cycle, an egg matures inside one of the ovaries and is released into the fallopian tube, where it may be fertilized if sperm are present. During the menstrual cycle, the endometrium (the inner lining of the uterus) thickens, converting the uterus into an incubation chamber where the fertilized egg can develop into a new human being. If fertilization fails to occur, the lining of the uterus is shed through the vagina. This is called menstruation, or the menstrual period, and it marks the end of one set of cycles, and the beginning of the next.

A woman's reproductive cycles are controlled by the hypothalamus (an area of the brain), the pituitary gland (a pea-sized gland situated at the base of the brain), and the ovaries; between them, these three sources release the hormones that control the reproductive cycles. During the reproductive cycles, levels of the hormones fluctuate as a result of a subtle interaction between them. Not only do these fluctuations control the length and events of the reproductive cycles, they also cause the physical and emotional changes that most women experience.

Both the ovarian cycle and the menstrual cycle are treated here as having a typical length of 28 days. However, the length of reproductive cycles may vary considerably, both between one woman and another and, in the case of each individual woman, from month to month.

The ovarian cycle

When a girl is born, her ovaries contain a stockpile of around 2–4 million immature eggs, called primary oocytes. Each primary oocyte is surrounded by a layer of cells forming a "container," the primary follicle. The aim of the ovarian cycle is to liberate one of these oocytes as a mature ovum each month.

The ovarian cycle is controlled by two hormones released by the front portion of the pituitary gland—follicle-stimulating hormone (FSH) and luteinizing hormone (LH)—and by gonadotropin-releasing hormone (GnRH) from the hypothalamus.

In this description a cycle length of 28 days is assumed, but cycles vary widely—they may be longer than 40 days or shorter than 21 days. The cycle can be described in terms of three phases. Although the first two of these can vary considerably in length, the third, the luteal phase, is usually close to 14 days long, generally ranging between 12 and 16 days.

Follicular phase—days 1 to 10
Rising levels of GnRH from the hypothalamus stimulate the release of FSH and LH from the pituitary. These hormones travel in the bloodstream to the ovaries, where they stimulate around 25 primary follicles to mature into secondary follicles (although eventually only one follicle will mature fully each month). As the follicles enlarge, the ovaries release the hormone estrogen.

Ovulatory phase—days 10 to14
By this phase, only one oocyte has continued to mature. The mature follicle bulges out from the side of the ovary. The increasing level of estrogen in the bloodstream feeds back to the pituitary gland, causing it to release a large amount of LH. This in turn causes the mature

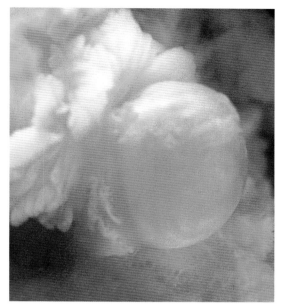

Impending ovulation: a mature follicle, about to burst and release its egg, bulges from the side of the ovary.

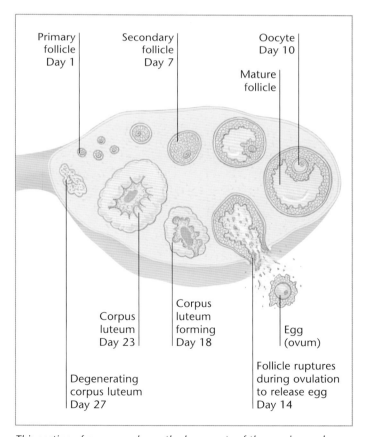

Primary follicle Day 1 | Secondary follicle Day 7 | Oocyte Day 10 | Mature follicle | Corpus luteum Day 23 | Corpus luteum forming Day 18 | Egg (ovum) | Degenerating corpus luteum Day 27 | Follicle ruptures during ovulation to release egg Day 14

This section of an ovary shows the key events of the ovarian cycle. To give a clear indication of what happens during the cycle, all the stages are shown happening together here. However, during a real cycle the stages occur sequentially, as indicated by the time scale.

follicle to rupture, releasing the mature egg into the fallopian tube. This is ovulation. When it occurs, some women feel a twinge of pain in their back or lower abdomen, which is known as *Mittelschmerz* (meaning "middle pain").

Luteal phase—days 14 to 28

Once ovulation has taken place, the ruptured mature follicle seals itself up and becomes what is known as a corpus luteum ("yellow body"). This secretes the second female sex hormone, progesterone, as well as some estrogen. Both of these hormones now suppress the release of FSH and LH by the pituitary gland. If pregnancy does not occur, the corpus

luteum degenerates, levels of estrogen and progesterone decrease rapidly, the block on FSH and LH production is removed, and the next ovarian cycle begins.

The menstrual cycle

The menstrual cycle is the series of changes that the endometrium of the uterus goes through as it prepares to provide a protective environment in which a fertilized egg can settle and develop into a baby. If a woman does not become pregnant during her menstrual cycle, the thickened lining of the uterus breaks down and its remains trickle out of the vagina during menstruation (the menstrual

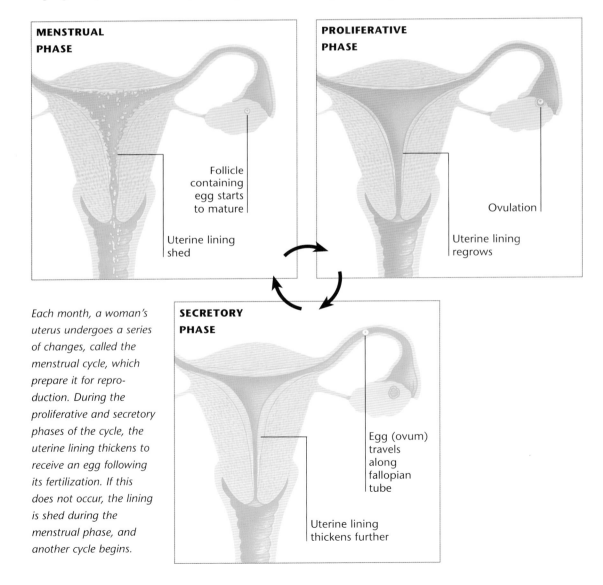

MENSTRUAL PHASE

Follicle containing egg starts to mature

Uterine lining shed

PROLIFERATIVE PHASE

Ovulation

Uterine lining regrows

SECRETORY PHASE

Egg (ovum) travels along fallopian tube

Uterine lining thickens further

Each month, a woman's uterus undergoes a series of changes, called the menstrual cycle, which prepare it for reproduction. During the proliferative and secretory phases of the cycle, the uterine lining thickens to receive an egg following its fertilization. If this does not occur, the lining is shed during the menstrual phase, and another cycle begins.

period). This monthly bleeding is one of the few signs that a menstrual cycle is taking place. The menstrual cycle is controlled by changing levels of estrogen and progesterone released during the ovarian cycle. Estrogen and progesterone are known as the sex hormones because, in addition to playing a part in the menstrual cycle, they cause the development and maintenance of a woman's secondary sex characteristics, such as breasts. The menstrual cycle can be divided into three phases. Once again, a "typical" cycle length of 28 days is used.

Menstrual phase—days 1 to 5

The beginning of the cycle is marked by menstruation or the menstrual period. With low levels of progesterone being produced by the ovaries, the blood vessels supplying the thickened wall of the endometrium constrict; deprived of its blood supply, the wall starts to fragment. The menstrual flow that passes out of the vagina from the uterus consists of tissue fragments and blood.

Proliferative phase—days 5 to 14

Estrogen released by the ovaries stimulates the repair and growth of the endometrium, so that it proliferates and becomes thicker and more spongy.

Secretory phase—days 14 to 28

After ovulation on day 14, release of progesterone and estrogen from the ovary's corpus luteum stimulates the endometrium to develop even further. The lining thickens still more, and its blood supply increases considerably. This provides a fertilized egg with a receptive, nutrient-rich environment in which to grow and develop. If fertilization does not occur, the corpus luteum breaks down, the endometrium starts to disintegrate, and the cycle comes to an end. However, if fertilization does occur, the corpus luteum receives a hormonal message from the newly implanted embryo which, by preventing its regression, enables it to continue production of the hormones that will keep the endometrium in place, prevent menstruation, and thereby maintain the pregnancy.

The male reproductive system

The basic roles of a man's reproductive system are to produce male sex cells, called sperm, and to deliver them into the vagina of his sexual partner. Within the male reproductive system, the primary sex organs are the two testes, which manufacture sperm throughout a man's life once he has reached puberty. The accessory sex organs are the other parts of the reproductive system—both internal and external organs—that nurture the sperm by producing the other ingredients of semen (the liquid that contains sperm), transport sperm from the testes to the outside of the body, and enable sperm to be deposited in the female's vagina. The external parts of the male reproductive system also contain sensory structures that aid sexual arousal in the adult male.

The male internal reproductive organs

The male internal reproductive organs comprise the ducts—the epididymis, vas deferens, and urethra—that store sperm and carry it toward their exit point from the tip of the penis, and the glands—the seminal vesicles, prostate gland, and bulbourethral gland—that produce semen. Semen contains nutrients and chemicals that activate and fuel the sperm and protect them from the hostile environment found in the vagina.

The epididymis

This is a highly coiled tube that lies around part of each testis (see p.27). Immature sperm pass from the testis, where they are manufactured, into the epididymis, where they are stored for about 20 days, during which time they reach maturity and start moving. Once they are mature, sperm pass from the epididymis into the next part of the duct system, called the vas (or ductus) deferens. Together each testis and its epididymis comprise what is referred to as a testicle.

The vas deferens

Also known as the ductus deferens, this tube, which is about 18 inches long, runs from the epididymis of each testis, over the front of the pubic bone, and around the side of the bladder, where it joins the urethra. The job of the vas deferens is to carry sperm from the testis to the urethra and to store sperm prior to ejaculation. During that journey sperm become mixed with secretions from the seminal vesicles that together form semen.

Male sterilization, or vasectomy *(see pp.165–7)*, involves a doctor making an incision in the scrotum, and cutting and tying the vasa deferentia to block transport of sperm.

The urethra

The urethra forms the final part of the duct system that links the vas deferens to the outside. It runs from the bladder to the end of the penis, serving both the reproductive and urinary systems. When the urethra leaves the bladder, where it is surrounded by the prostate gland, it is joined by the two vasa deferentia that carry sperm from the testes. It then travels along the penis, opening at the tip of the glans (the end of the penis). During ejaculation, semen is forced along the penis by the contraction of muscles near its base.

The urethra may become infected and inflamed as a result of the man contracting a sexually transmitted disease such as gonorrhea or non-gonococcal urethritis during sexual intercourse *(see pp.121–6)*. These infections require treatment with antibiotics.

The seminal vesicles

The finger-length seminal vesicles lie behind the bladder. They produce a secretion which forms about 60 percent of the semen. This secretion not only activates sperm but also contains fructose, a type of sugar that provides fuel for sperm. These secretions and sperm mix together in the vas deferens in preparation for future ejaculation.

The prostate gland

This single, chestnut-sized gland surrounds the urethra just below the bladder. Its secretions, which make up over 30 percent of semen, are squeezed through tiny, trapdoor-like openings into the urethra during ejaculation. Prostate secretions activate sperm and, following ejaculation, make the vagina less acidic and more "sperm-friendly."

The bulbourethral glands

Also known as Cowper's glands, these pea-sized glands are found just below the prostate gland. During sexual arousal they produce a clear fluid that makes the urethra less acidic —the acidity comes from traces of urine—and more amenable to sperm survival. Droplets of secretion may appear on the tip of the glans as a lubricant prior to ejaculation.

The male external reproductive organs

A man's external genitalia comprise the penis and the scrotum that contains the testes. All the external genitalia, but especially the glans penis, or tip of the penis, are well supplied with sensory nerve endings, which can produce a sensation of sexual arousal when touched or stroked.

The penis

This tube-shaped organ consists of a root, which anchors it inside the body, and a shaft, which hangs outside the body and which ends in an expanded tip called the glans or glans penis. The glans, the corona (the rim of the glans), and the frenulum (the cord of tissue that links the underside of the glans to the shaft) are all richly endowed with sensory nerve endings and contribute greatly to sexual pleasure when stimulated.

Running inside the penis, along its length, is the urethra, the tube that carries urine from the bladder to the outside of the body; it also carries semen (the liquid that contains sperm) when a man ejaculates, but it cannot carry both semen and urine at the same time. The urethra is surrounded by a cylinder of tissue, the corpus spongiosum, which also forms the glans. Two other parallel tissue cylinders, the corpora cavernosa, run along the upper side

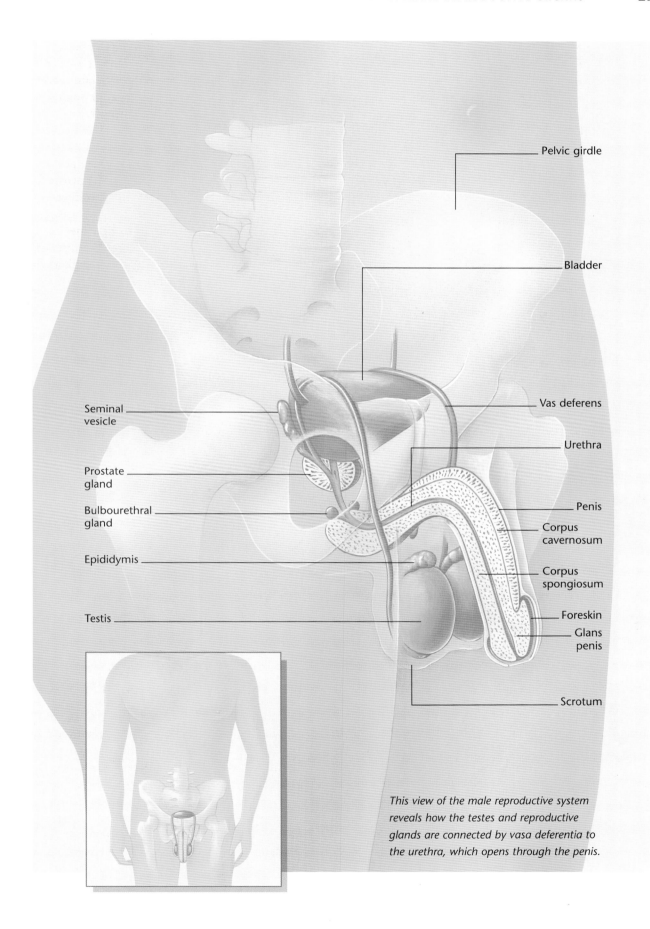

Pelvic girdle

Bladder

Seminal vesicle

Vas deferens

Urethra

Prostate gland

Bulbourethral gland

Penis

Corpus cavernosum

Epididymis

Corpus spongiosum

Foreskin

Testis

Glans penis

Scrotum

This view of the male reproductive system reveals how the testes and reproductive glands are connected by vasa deferentia to the urethra, which opens through the penis.

of the shaft above the corpus spongiosum. All three of these parallel cylinders contain tiny vascular spaces. When the man is sexually aroused these spaces fill with blood, and the penis becomes erect and projects from the body. During erection, the corpus spongiosum stands out, and can be felt as a ridge running along the underside of the shaft of the penis. The underside of the penis is particularly sensitive to touch.

There are occasions, experienced by most men, when erection is difficult or impossible to achieve. Erectile problems are most commonly short-term inconveniences caused by excessive alcohol, by medications, or by stress. More rarely, erectile failure has a physical basis and requires medical intervention to provide a possible cure *(see also pp.194–5)*.

The skin that covers the penis is fairly loose, and is folded over the glans to form the foreskin. This can be pulled back to expose the glans. In some men, the foreskin is removed in a minor operation called circumcision *(see below)*, usually carried out during infancy or childhood. Below the penis, at its base, hangs the scrotum, containing the testes.

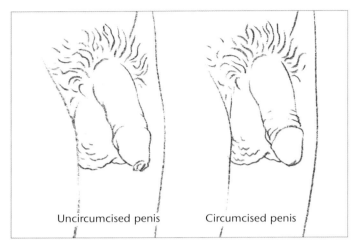

Uncircumcised penis   Circumcised penis

The glans, or head, of an uncircumcised penis is covered by a loose-fitting foreskin, which can be pulled back. Circumcision, the surgical removal of the foreskin, leaves the glans permanently exposed.

The testes and scrotum

The testes are two oval-shaped glands, measuring about 1½ inches in length and 1 inch in diameter. Every day, between puberty and old age, the testes manufacture

MALE CIRCUMCISION

Circumcision is the surgical removal of the foreskin. The glans of a circumcised penis is permanently exposed, while the glans of the intact, uncircumcised penis is covered by the foreskin, which on most men can be easily pulled back to expose the glans. In a sexual context, the glans of a circumcised penis may be less sensitive to the touch than that of an uncircumcised penis, because its protective foreskin has been removed and it is constantly rubbing against underwear (this reduced sensitivity can, however, help a man to prolong his erection).

Circumcision may be performed on newborn boys, for religious or cultural reasons, or on older children or adults for medical reasons. As a religious practice, the circumcision of male babies has been performed by Jews and Muslims for thousands of years.

The main medical reason for circumcision is where the foreskin is too tight—a condition called phimosis—causing pain when it is pulled back over the glans. This makes it difficult to wash away secretions, known as smegma, that build up under the foreskin and may cause infections. A tight foreskin can also make erection painful and sexual intercourse impossible.

In the United States, circumcision—on health grounds—became a widespread practice across all religious groups in the 20th century. Around 70 percent of newborn boys are still routinely circumcised in the United States, although this percentage has decreased over recent years.

Recent research indicates that, contrary to earlier beliefs, circumcision does not decrease the risk of penile cancer or other infections, provided standards of personal hygiene are adhered to and the penis is washed regularly. Many physicians now feel that circumcision should only be carried out for specific religious or medical reasons.

Some men and women prefer uncircumcised penises for aesthetic or sexual reasons; for similar reasons, others prefer circumcised penises. However, when a penis is erect, it can be difficult to tell whether it is circumcised or not.

millions of sperm. They also secrete the male sex hormones that produce secondary sex characteristics, such as facial hair, and that maintain male sex drive. *(Sperm and hormone production by the testes is described below.)*

The two testes are carried outside the body, supported in a pouch of skin called the scrotum. Given their reproductive importance, it may seem strange that the testes hang in a somewhat vulnerable position. The reason for this is that sperm are unviable if they are manufactured at the normal core body temperature of 98.6°F. Because the testes hang outside the body, their temperature is typically some 5°F below core temperature, ideal for the production of active sperm. In cold surroundings (and during sexual arousal), scrotal muscles contract to pull the testes closer to the body; in warm temperatures, the scrotum hangs loosely, away from the body. In this way, testicular temperature is kept constant. In addition, one testis, usually the left one, hangs lower than the other. This prevents painful collisions of the testes during walking and running.

Sperm and hormone production

Sperm, or spermatozoa, are perfectly adapted to their function of transporting, as rapidly as possible, a package of genetic information from the male and combining it with a similar package located in the egg inside a female. A mature sperm is lightweight and streamlined. It consists of a head, which contains the man's package of genetic information and, at its tip, an acrosome, which will help the sperm penetrate the outer wall of the egg; a midpiece, which supplies the energy needed for movement; and the tail, or flagellum, which propels the sperm forward.

Sperm are manufactured inside the testes. Each testis consists of around 300 compartments called lobules, each of which contains between one and four tightly coiled tiny tubes called seminiferous tubules, inside which sperm are made. A healthy man produces

INFERTILITY AND SCROTAL TEMPERATURE

Male infertility—the inability to father a child— may be the result of an abnormally low sperm count. A man's sperm count is tested by comparing the number of sperm in a unit volume of his ejaculate with that found in semen from an "average" man. With some men, tight-fitting underpants and jeans may be responsible for a low sperm count because they both pull the testes upward toward the body so that they are constantly at a temperature higher than that needed for optimal sperm production. For this reason, men with fertility problems are often advised to wear boxer shorts and looser-fitting pants in order to reduce their scrotal temperature.

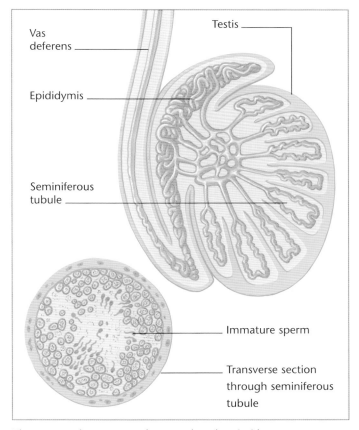

The process of sperm manufacture takes place inside the testis in a mass of narrow, tightly coiled seminiferous tubules. A section through one of these tubules (bottom) *reveals the germinal cells (pink), which divide constantly to produce thousands of tadpole-like sperm each second.*

around 1000 sperm per second (100 million per day); between 300 and 500 million sperm are released in each ejaculation. The seminiferous tubules merge and extend upward out of the testis to form the epididymis, running crescent-like down the back of the testis. This is where maturing sperm are stored.

Release of male hormones

In the tissue surrounding the seminiferous tubules of the testis are interstitial or Leydig cells. These cells release androgens, or male sex hormones, the most important of which is testosterone. Testosterone controls the growth of the body and the growth and development of male sex organs; stimulates sperm production; and maintains secondary sex characteristics, such as facial hair. It also controls a man's libido (sex drive).

Control of sperm production and hormone release

Ultimately, the brain controls both sperm production and the release of male hormones. The part of the brain called the hypothalamus

releases a hormone that stimulates the man's pituitary gland (a pea-sized gland located at the base of the brain) so that it releases both luteinizing hormone (LH) and follicle-stimulating hormone (FSH). LH stimulates the interstitial cells of the testis to release testosterone. FSH, together with testosterone, stimulates sperm production from the seminiferous tubules.

Erection

Erection—the hardening and swelling of the normally soft penis—is an obvious outward indication that a man is sexually aroused. In purely functional terms, erection serves to make a man's penis sufficiently stiff to enable its insertion into his partner's vagina so that sexual intercourse can take place. It also makes other types of sexual activity possible, such as masturbation and oral sex. A flaccid penis, which averages 3–4 inches in length, grows when erect to about 6 inches long, on average, and also increases in diameter. Smaller penises tend to grow proportionately more when erect than larger penises do, so that variation in the size of erect penises is less than the variation in flaccid ones. Although the standard "textbook" erect penis is straight and at a 45° angle to the body, the shape and angle of erections show considerable variations. Some erect penises have an upward curve, like a banana, and/or may bend to the left or right. These variations are perfectly normal and are nothing to worry about. The angle of erection can vary from horizontal to approaching vertical, depending on the individual, although the angle does tend to decrease with age.

Erection is controlled by the nervous system, specifically a part of the lower spinal cord called the erection center. Like blinking and swallowing, erection is a reflex response. It can be initiated by erotic thoughts, or by pleasurable sights, smells, or sounds. The brain sends nerve impulses (messages) to the erection center, which in turn sends out the impulses that cause erection. Additionally or alternatively, erection can be initiated by the penis being touched or rubbed. Messages

PRODUCING MALE SEX HORMONES
Released by the testes, male sex hormones stimulate sperm production and produce the sex characteristics found in mature males. Production of male sex hormones by the testes is stimulated by hormones released by the pituitary gland. Unlike a woman's pituitary and sex hormones, whose levels fluctuate during a monthly cycle, male hormone levels remain steady.

Pituitary gland

Testis

from sensory receptors on the glans and other parts travel to the erection center with the same result. Erection may also be caused by non-sexual stimuli, especially in adolescents. It occurs, too, during REM (dreaming) sleep and can be the reason why men commonly wake up with an erection. However, early-morning erections may also be caused by the man having a full bladder.

The actual mechanism of erection works like this. Nerve messages from the spinal cord's erection center stimulate the arteries that supply the tissues of the penis with blood, causing them to dilate. The blood flow into the penis increases, and the vascular spaces fill with blood. As these tissues swell, they compress the veins that carry blood away from the penis, so that more blood enters the penis than leaves it. As a result the penis becomes erect. Loss of erection occurs if sexual interest is lost or ejaculation takes place. Both result in a narrowing of the penis's arteries and a reversal of the erection process.

Ejaculation

Ejaculation is the propulsion of semen out of the penis following sexual activity. Like erection, ejaculation is a reflex action, and it is also controlled by part of the lower spinal cord called the ejaculatory center. The ejaculatory reflex is initiated when sexual stimulation reaches a certain level. It has two phases. During the first phase, known as emission, muscular contractions squeeze secretions out of the seminal vesicles and prostate gland, mix them with sperm to produce semen, and force them into that part of the urethra at the base of the penis. The bladder sphincter muscle clamps shut, preventing any flow of urine. During the second or so that the emission phase lasts, the man experiences the feeling of ejaculatory inevitability—the point of no return—and he cannot stop the second phase, ejaculation itself. So, a fraction of a second after emission, the second phase begins. Contractions of muscles at the base of the penis, at intervals of 0.8 seconds, force semen up and out of the urethra in, usually, between one and five spurts. The average

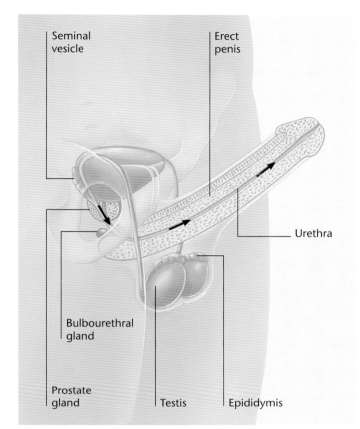

During ejaculation, which lasts only a few seconds, sperm are mixed with secretions from the seminal vesicles and prostate gland to form semen, which is forced along the urethra by muscular contractions and spurts from the urethral opening at the tip of the erect penis.

volume of ejaculate is around 5 milliliters or one teaspoonful. Following ejaculation there is a latent period during which a man is unable to achieve an erection. This period varies from minutes in young men to hours or days in older men. Although ejaculation is a reflex action, many men consciously delay their ejaculation to prolong sexual pleasure *(see also pp.195–6)*.

Ejaculation generally occurs at the same time as orgasm, although they are not the same thing. Ejaculation is the discharge of semen, whereas orgasm is the sudden pleasurable feeling and release of tension that sweeps through the genitals and other parts of the body. If ejaculation does not occur over a period of time, sperm do not accumulate inside the epididymis or vas deferens. Instead, they are broken down, reabsorbed by the body, and recycled.

Conception

Conception is the process that marks the beginning of a new life. It is the starting point of a nine-month period during which a single cell, the fertilized egg, develops inside its mother's uterus into a complex human being consisting of thousands of billions of cells. Conception covers the period from the moment of fertilization to the implantation of the conceptus—the name given to the developing offspring during its first days of existence—within the welcoming lining of the uterus, some five or six days after the egg is fertilized by the sperm.

Conception depends on the male and female sex cells—the sperm and egg—meeting and uniting in a woman's fallopian tube. Sperm are introduced into the female reproductive system during sexual intercourse. Ejaculation by the male deposits hundreds of millions of sperm in the vagina, although probably 99 percent of these do not enter the uterus and are lost. Those sperm that survive to this stage now undertake the two-to-seven-hour journey through the uterus to the fallopian tubes. By then the hundreds of millions of sperm have been reduced to several hundred. The surviving sperm remain viable, and capable of fertilizing an egg, for between 48 and 72 hours, or occasionally even longer.

Unfertilized, the woman's egg survives for only about 24 hours after its release from the ovary. If it meets viable sperm during this time, fertilization—the fusion of egg and sperm—takes place. Before fertilization many sperm mass around the egg. Their combined efforts clear a pathway through the outer covering, the *zona pellucida*, enabling a single sperm to penetrate the egg completely. Once this has occurred, other sperm cannot penetrate; those remaining outside are left to die.

Inside the egg, the nucleus of the sperm joins with the nucleus of the egg. Each nucleus contains a packet of genetic information in the form of chromosomes *(see pp.34–7)* from the parent that produced the sex cell. The combination of these two packets provides the blueprint that will determine the characteristics of the new human being, and its sex.

In the week following fertilization, the process of conception is completed. The fertilized egg travels along the fallopian tube until eventually it arrives in the uterus, settles into the uterine lining, and begins its development into a baby.

The stages of conception from ovulation, through fertilization to implantation

• Ordinarily, a woman releases a single egg from one of the ovaries into the fallopian tube each month. The egg travels slowly along the fallopian tube.

• If the egg meets a sperm within 24 hours of ovulation, fertilization takes place. As the sperm penetrates the outer membrane of the egg, its tail detaches. The sperm nucleus and egg nucleus fuse, the union resulting in the formation of a fertilized egg or zygote containing a complete set of genetic information.

• By 36 hours after fertilization, the zygote has undergone its first cell division. It is now a conceptus, or pre-embryo, consisting of two identical cells. This is the first of a series of cell divisions that will eventually give rise to billions of cells.

• Two days after fertilization, the two cells have divided again, producing a four-celled conceptus. As the journey along the fallopian tube continues, the cells of the pre-embryo divide about every 12 hours.

• By 72 hours after fertilization, the conceptus consists of a berry-shaped, solid mass of cells that is known as a morula (from the Latin for "mulberry").

• Five days after fertilization, the conceptus has arrived in the uterus. Now called a blastocyst, it consists of a hollow sphere of cells, with a small inner cluster of cells on one side.

• Seven days after fertilization, the blastocyst burrows into the inner lining of the uterus, a process called implantation. The outer cells of the blastocyst go on to form part of the placenta, the link that will supply food and oxygen from the mother to the developing baby; the inner cells become the embryo, which within another seven weeks will begin to be recognizably human. *(For gender determination see Chapter 2; for the development of the embryo see Chapter 7.)*

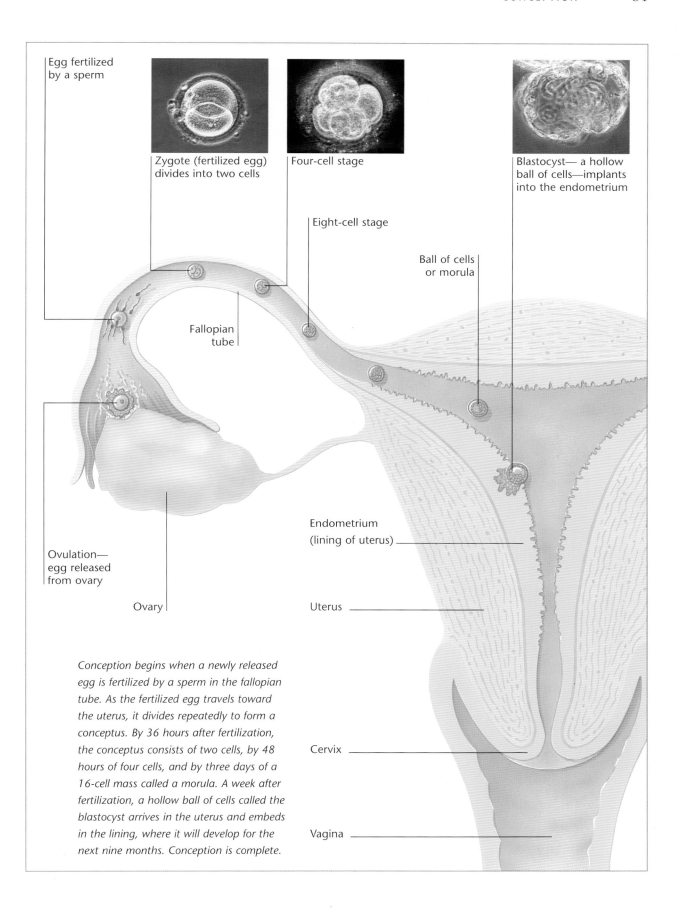

Egg fertilized
by a sperm

Zygote (fertilized egg)
divides into two cells

Four-cell stage

Blastocyst— a hollow
ball of cells—implants
into the endometrium

Eight-cell stage

Ball of cells
or morula

Fallopian
tube

Ovulation—
egg released
from ovary

Ovary

Endometrium
(lining of uterus)

Uterus

Cervix

Vagina

Conception begins when a newly released egg is fertilized by a sperm in the fallopian tube. As the fertilized egg travels toward the uterus, it divides repeatedly to form a conceptus. By 36 hours after fertilization, the conceptus consists of two cells, by 48 hours of four cells, and by three days of a 16-cell mass called a morula. A week after fertilization, a hollow ball of cells called the blastocyst arrives in the uterus and embeds in the lining, where it will develop for the next nine months. Conception is complete.

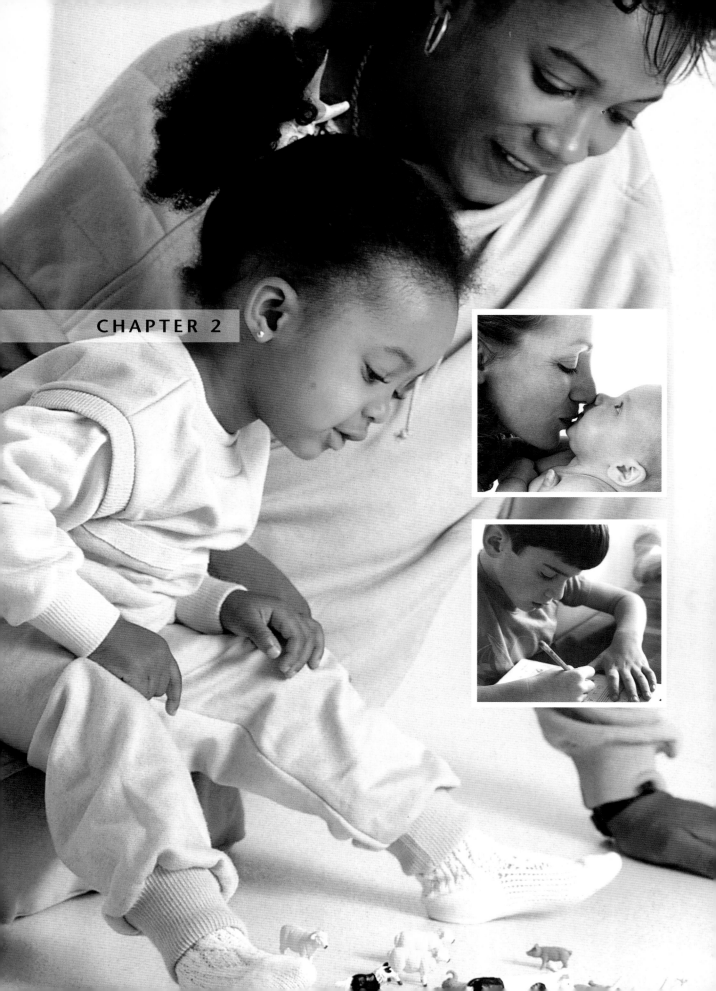

CHAPTER 2

From Baby to Child

A child's anatomical, physiological, and sexual development begins in the uterus and continues until the end of puberty. The sex of a child is determined the moment that a sperm and an egg fuse during fertilization. Chromosomes inside each cell of the developing embryo contain not only the blueprint for the child's sexual development but also the information to push development in a male or female direction. Male–female differences take shape in the fetus as the genes direct the development of the sex organs. First responses of the sex organs, such as periodic erection of a male fetus's penis, also begin before birth.

From birth onward, children gradually develop their gender identity—their awareness of themselves as female or male. Exactly how early in life children start to become aware of their own gender and sexuality is a complicated question that has been the subject of much discussion and research. Although we do not know exactly what babies are thinking and feeling, there is clearly a stage—usually between 18 months and 3 years old—when children become conscious of their own body parts, including their external sex organs. However, as time passes, their gender and sexual awareness is also determined by their cultural environment—the influence of parents, relatives, friends, other children, teachers, and the media.

As they get older, children first become aware of their own gender, and then of the fact that some other children do not belong to the same gender. Whether gender-based differences in behavior are genetically determined or the result of a child's environment, including family behavior and attitudes, has provoked considerable debate over the years. However, it now appears that, although we may not be able to determine the exact extent to which each factor is responsible, boys behave like boys and girls like girls due to the combined influence of genes and environment.

From about the age of two, children take an active interest in the differences between themselves and members of the opposite sex, both children and adults. They begin asking questions about these differences, and this can provide an opportunity for parents to begin a subtle program of sex education.

At the same time parents should realize the important position they hold as sexual role models for young children. It helps if a parent has a positive attitude toward sex. For example, children may derive pleasure from touching their genitals, and a rebuke from a parent for doing so may cause a child to have a negative attitude toward sex. Parents should always try to make their child aware of what is appropriate sexual behavior without implying that natural curiosity about sex is wrong.

Sex determination and chromosomes

During fertilization, a sperm and an egg unite to begin a new cycle of life. But what is it within that newly fertilized egg that determines whether the baby born some nine months later will be a boy or a girl? The answer lies in the chromosomes, the tiny structures within a cell that control all its activities, and more specifically, within the sex chromosomes.

Cells, chromosomes, and sex chromosomes

A human body consists of billions of microscopic living units called cells. Each one of those cells has something in common: inside its control center—the nucleus—are 46 microscopic structures called chromosomes. Chromosomes contain the information necessary to build, maintain, and run a cell. And because the body's cells work together to form the tissues, organs, and systems that make up a functioning human being, the chromosomes ultimately control all processes in the body.

A chromosome is divided into units called genes. Each of the many genes on a chromosome—there are over 100,000 genes in each nucleus—contains an instruction for a specific part of the body's structure and function, such as eye color or blood type. Together, this genetic material—the sum total of all the information contained in the genes—forms an instruction manual for life.

The 46 chromosomes of each cell are arranged into 23 pairs. One half of each pair is provided by the baby's mother, the other half by the father. In 22 of these pairs, called autosomes, the two halves match each other in size and shape, and contain the same sequence of genes. Each pair of genes controls one characteristic, although they may produce conflicting versions of that characteristic.

Consider, for example, two chromosomes carrying the paired genes that control eye color. If the gene from the baby's mother produces brown eyes, while the gene from the baby's father produces blue eyes, the baby will have brown eyes. This happens because the brown gene dominates the blue; this dominant gene is "expressed," while the other, the recessive gene, has no effect. However, if the baby inherits two recessive "blue" genes, he or she will have blue eyes, because no dominant genes are present. Collectively, the interaction of all the dominant and recessive genes inherited from both parents produces the individual characteristics shown by each baby.

In addition to the 22 matched pairs of autosomes, there is another pair of chromosomes. This pair determines whether a child is male or female, and the two are therefore called the sex chromosomes. Female cells contain a matching pair of sex chromosomes known as X chromosomes, while male cells contain one X chromosome paired with a much smaller Y chromosome. Accordingly, the pair of female chromosomes is identified as XX, while the male chromosomes are identified as XY.

Sex-cell formation

Sperm are produced in the testes continuously after puberty; eggs are produced before birth in the female fetus's ovaries, and remain in the woman's ovaries in immature form unless "called upon" to ripen and be released. Formation of both eggs and sperm, however, involves a common process. Both are produced by cell division. This process is found in most body cells—it enables us to grow and to

DNA—THE GENETIC BLUEPRINT

DNA—deoxyribonucleic acid—is a remarkable molecule that makes up each chromosome. Each DNA molecule consists of two linked spiraling chains that resemble twisted ladders. The DNA contained within the chromosomes of every cell is remarkable because its chemical structure contains the coded blueprint for the construction of a complete human body. It is also unique in being able to duplicate itself, splitting down the middle to produce two identical copies of itself so that its vital information can be passed on uncorrupted when cells divide repeatedly during the development of a new human being. The genes that control the production of the body's characteristics each consist of a short piece of a DNA molecule—a few rungs of the genetic ladder.

replace the millions of our body cells that wear out every day. But the cell division that produces sex cells is slightly different. Each sperm or egg cell that results from this special type of division contains just 23 chromosomes instead of the normal 46, including just one sex chromosome instead of the normal two.

Fertilization and sex determination

When the sex cells—the male sperm and the female egg—fuse during fertilization, each carries its own cargo of chromosomes. Although the egg (or ovum) is enormous compared to the sperm, they both contribute the same amount of genetic material to the new individual: 23 chromosomes each. After fertilization, the zygote—the name given to the complete cell formed by the combined egg and sperm—contains the standard 46 chromosomes (23 pairs), including one pair of sex chromosomes.

The sex of the resulting child is determined by the sex chromosome carried by the sperm. The paternal cell from which a sperm is produced contains both an X and a Y chromosome, so there is a fifty-fifty chance that an individual sperm will carry the X or the Y. An egg, on the other hand, always has an X chromosome, because the maternal cell from which the egg is produced contains two X chromosomes. If an egg is fertilized by a Y-carrying sperm, the child will be a boy; if it is fertilized by an X-carrying sperm, it will be a girl. So any one conception has a 50-percent chance of producing a boy and a 50-percent chance of producing a girl.

When a child is born, his or her sex should be apparent from the external genital organs. A boy has a penis and scrotum, while a girl has labia (genital lips) and a clitoris. The girl will also have, internally, a vagina, uterus, fallopian tubes, and ovaries, while the boy has two testes (inside the scrotum) and an internal system of reproductive ducts and glands. These are the primary sex characteristics, present at birth, that distinguish a female from a male.

Yet despite the obvious sex differences between boys and girls at birth, the male and female sex organs have identical origins in the embryo (the name given to the developing human being between the second and eighth week after fertilization; thereafter, until birth, the unborn child is known as a fetus). Whether the embryo goes on to develop male or female sex organs depends on the sex chromosomes that are contained in every one of its cells; specifically, it depends on whether there are two X chromosomes or one X and one Y chromosome.

Genital development in the embryo and fetus

Six weeks after fertilization, the human embryo is no bigger than a large grape. Internally, its reproductive system is developing, but at this stage it is identical in both sexes. The same is true of the external

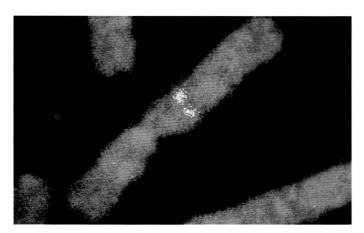

This rodlike structure, seen here using a powerful microscope, is one of the 46 chromosomes found inside the nucleus of each one of the body's billions of cells. The yellow-green areas on this chromosome indicate the locations of specific genes.

genitalia. But it is around this time that sexual separation begins: if the embryo is genetically female (with XX chromosomes) she develops a female reproductive system; if the embryo is genetically male (with XY chromosomes) he develops a male reproductive system.

The first move toward sexual separation is made by the Y chromosome; without the influence of the Y chromosome, the embryo will go on to develop naturally into a female. The Y chromosome sends out a signal that says, "Make testes!" In fact, it is just one gene on the Y chromosome that sends this message, triggering the development of testes in the so-far uncommitted reproductive system. This is the SRY (sex-determining region of the Y chromosome) gene (sometimes called the TDF—testis-determining factor). A female fetus has no Y chromosome, hence no SRY gene, so ovaries develop rather than testes.

As the testes develop they begin to release hormones into the fetal bloodstream. Hormones are chemical messengers released by glands (in this case the testes) that instruct certain parts of the body to alter their activities in some way. The hormones released by the testes are sex hormones called androgens, the most important of which is testosterone. The androgens "instruct" the external genitals to develop into a penis and scrotum. That this message has been acted upon is evident in the male fetus just 12 weeks after fertilization (*see panel, below*). In the

DEVELOPMENT OF EXTERNAL GENITALIA

At six weeks the external genitalia are identical in both sexes. At this indifferent stage, the embryo has a projection called the genital tubercle and an opening called the urethral groove surrounded by urethral folds, which are in turn surrounded by labioscrotal swellings.

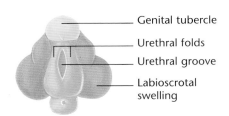

Genital tubercle
Urethral folds
Urethral groove
Labioscrotal swelling

UNDIFFERENTIATED STAGE—SIX-WEEK EMBRYO

By 12 weeks, the external genitals are beginning to look different. In the male the genital tubercle expands to form the glans of the penis and the urethral folds are fusing to form the penile urethra. In the female fetus, the urethral folds and labioscrotal swellings remain separate to form the labia minora and majora, and the genital tubercle forms the clitoris.

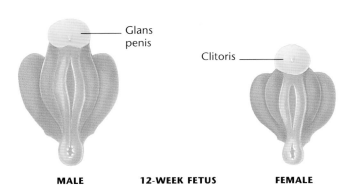

Glans penis

Clitoris

MALE   **12-WEEK FETUS**   **FEMALE**

At 38 weeks, male and female genitals are recognizably different. Two months before birth, a boy's testes descend from his abdomen into his scrotum, formed by the fused labioscrotal folds. A girl's ovaries also descend, but only as far as the upper part of her pelvis.

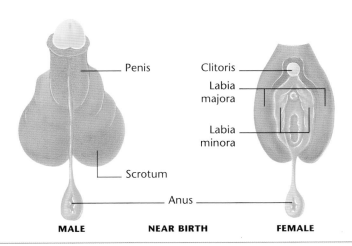

Penis

Clitoris
Labia majora

Labia minora

Scrotum

Anus

MALE   **NEAR BIRTH**   **FEMALE**

female fetus, uninfluenced by testosterone, the external genitalia develop labia and a clitoris. By the time the baby is born, the external genitals are readily distinguishable as male or female.

The contribution of androgens to sexual differentiation raises an interesting point. Without the presence of androgens, particularly testosterone, the growing embryo will naturally develop into a female. For male development to take place, the input of androgens is required.

There is also evidence that prenatal (before birth) hormones not only determine genital differences between boys and girls but also affect the pattern of brain development, thereby influencing differences in male and female behavior—the gender differences—that become apparent during childhood.

ABNORMAL SEXUAL DEVELOPMENT

If the sex hormones called androgens fail to act normally inside the male fetus, or if they are produced by some genetic error in the female fetus, genital abnormalities can result. These may be evident to parents and doctors when a child is born, or may become evident as a child gets older. In the case of testicular feminization, the fetus is genetically male (XY chromosomes) and the testes develop normally. The developing reproductive system does not respond to androgens released by the testes, however, and the male baby's sex organs are indistinguishable from a female's. Alternatively, in the case of adrenogenital syndrome, a genetically female (XX chromosomes) fetus develops ovaries, but is exposed to androgens, either from her mother or from her own adrenal glands. As a result, she may be born with an enlarged clitoris or, in more severe cases, she can develop a penis and an empty scrotum (the ovaries are inside the body), and look like a male externally. Individuals whose primary sex organs (testes or ovaries) do not match their external genitals are known as pseudo-hermaphrodites. Some may seek gender-reassignment (sex-change) operations in later life in order to match their external genitalia to their sexual identity (see p.188).

Sex and gender

So far, we have seen how genetic information passed on from a mother and father determines their baby's biological sex. Girl babies have female sex organs, while boy babies have male ones. As babies grow into children, however, other differences become evident: boys and girls also behave differently. So what is it that makes girls behave like girls, and boys behave like boys? Is it innate? Do their genes "instruct" them to behave as males or females? For example, research has indicated that male babies are often more active and irritable than girl babies, while girls often mature and talk sooner than boys. Or do infants and children learn to behave in a way "appropriate" to their biological sex because of the way they are influenced by their environment—their families, peers, and society in general? Certainly all of us are perceived as sexual beings from birth, as indicated by the most basic question asked by new parents: "Is it a boy or a girl?" Or are genetic influences and learned behavior both significant factors in determining our identity as males and females, and as sexual beings? These are the questions raised by the "nature versus nurture" debate.

Nature versus nurture

"Nature" refers to the contribution made by our genes to the way we look and function. There is no doubt that the genes contained inside all of our body cells hold the blueprint needed to construct a functional human being. However, some of our characteristics are certainly influenced by "nurture," or our surroundings. For example, a healthy human infant is born with the capacity to learn a language, because of their gene endowment, but whether or not any of us actually goes on to learn a language depends on a number of factors, including whether, when, where, and how we are spoken to.

Basically, the two sides in the nature versus nurture debate have been:
• For nature—the argument that the differences in behavior between boys and girls are

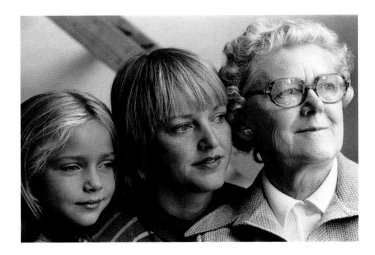

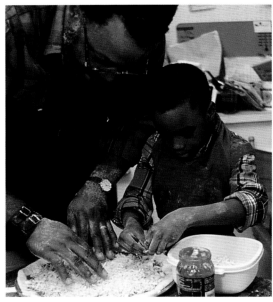

The sex and physical features of the three generations of females (top) *are determined purely by their genes. But is this boy's gender role determined by his genes or by his father's and other influences, or by both?*

determined by their genes, and in particular by the influence of prenatal hormones on the brain.

• For nurture—the argument that differences between boys and girls are acquired by learning as a result of environmental influences.

Factors that may cause the differences in behavior between boys and girls are explained briefly below. Before looking at these factors, it is probably useful to distinguish between two words—sex and gender—that are often used synonymously.

The difference between sex and gender

Sex is a word used to define whether a person is biologically male or female. A child belonging to the male sex has male sex chromosomes and can be identified by his male sex organs. Similarly, a child belonging to the female sex has female sex chromosomes and can be identified by her female sex organs. In a very few cases, however, the external genitals may not "match" the sex chromosomes *(see p.37).* Biological sex is determined by the influence of prenatal hormones on the developing fetus. The production and release of these hormones is, in turn, controlled by the fetus's genes. So, biological sex is fundamentally the result of "nature."

(The word "sex" is, of course, also used in another context to describe the whole area concerned with erotic or sensual experiences, and used, for example, in a question such as "Did you have sex [that is, sexual intercourse] with him?" or in calling a book about sexual matters a "sex manual.")

Gender involves a person's femaleness or maleness and is commonly used in phrases such as "gender identity" and "gender role."

The term gender identity refers to a person's self-awareness and inner perception of his or her identity as male or female. Thus gender identity is an individual experience, but it can be expressed through interaction with other people as gender role.

Gender role is defined by everything a person does in his or her behavior that socially conveys a gender identity as male or female. A gender-role stereotype is a set of behaviors, attitudes, opportunities, risks, or burdens that a given culture imposes on males or females. For example, in many cultures, the traditional stereotypical gender role has been for boys to be aggressive and assertive and play with guns, and for girls to be passive and reactive and play with dolls.

Acquiring gender identity and gender roles during childhood

Research has shown that by the time a baby is between the ages of 9 and 12 months it responds differently to female and male faces. By the age of two, a child can usually pick out a photograph of a child of the same sex as itself and knows its own body parts. By two and a half, a child can identify the sex of other children and has established a gender stability—that boys become men and girls become women. By the age of three, children have developed gender constancy, which becomes an irrevocable part of their personality. This involves the recognition that they will stay male or female throughout their life—and that a person stays the same sex regardless of the clothes they are wearing or the length of their hair. Gender-role stereotyping becomes evident between the ages of two and three. By this age, children begin to identify that certain possessions or tasks are associated with either women or men.

So to what extent are gender identity and gender role innate, the product of a child's genetic makeup (nature); and to what extent are they environmental, a result of influences encountered during childhood (nurture)?

Nature—the biological determination of gender identity and gender role

Some psychologists and biologists suggest that gender-role behavior can be explained by our genetic inheritance. Humans, they say, like other species, have evolved sexual traits that maximize the chances of successful reproduction in order to ensure continuation of the species. Boys and girls have different levels of hormones in their bodies, and it is thought that these condition their brains, both before and after birth, to produce behavior appropriate to their particular gender role. But although boys certainly have higher levels of the hormone testosterone than girls do, from before birth, and this appears to affect their behavior, the evidence for biological determination is not clearcut.

As babies, boys are on average bigger, sleep less, and are more active and more irritable than girls. Girls are usually healthier than boys, and tend to mature faster and talk sooner. The argument is that these differences depend on differences in hormone levels, and are therefore genetically determined. The same argument is put forward to explain why boys expend more energy in play, and why

NONSEXIST OR TRUE TO NATURE?

Should parents treat their children in exactly the same way regardless of gender, or should boys be treated as boys and girls as girls? This dilemma brings the nature versus nurture debate into sharp focus. Are parents going "against nature" if they treat their children identically? Or are they behaving in a sexist way if they bring up boys as "typically male" and girls as "typically female"? The answer, in the end, may be out of their hands. The influence of society, as expressed through peers, relatives, and television, will probably be more important in persuading children to conform to their particular gender role. Where parents can be influential, however, is in helping to provide their child with a strong sense of self-esteem, whether they are male or female. While accepting that boys may differ from girls in some ways, parents can still strive to ensure that their children have equality of opportunity and support, regardless of gender.

attention to personal appearance between the sexes differs, as do patterns that rehearse parenthood, such as playing with dolls.

There seems little doubt that such behavior differences become clear soon after birth. Some people consider this to be evidence of their genetic origins. Others argue that later behavior is clearly affected by differences in the ways parents and other adults treat and respond to male or female children (see box above) and that the only "genetically induced" behavioral difference is that boys are more likely to be aggressive than girls.

Further evidence that the influence of "nature" is not clear-cut has come from studies of girls with adrenogenital syndrome (AGS), who are genetically female (XX) but, at birth, have genitals that may appear more "masculine," because they have been exposed to high levels of androgens (male sex hormones) in the uterus. As a group, these girls show greater energy in play and less interest in dolls; they often become unusually tomboyish, preferring the company of boys. All of these are factors that suggest genetic determination of behavior. However, girls with AGS whose external genitals were less masculine, and who had been "assigned" as girls at birth and been brought up as girls, typically had relationships with boys, got married, and had children. Those whose genitals were more masculine, and who were brought up as boys, later reported their gender identity as male, and behaved in ways more in keeping with male gender-role stereotypes. These examples suggest that gender assignment and rearing are more important in establishing gender identity than are genetic factors.

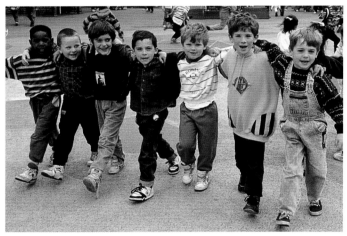

Boys will be boys? Nurture, in the form of social factors, plays a major role in determining that boys behave in a "gender-appropriate" way. But how social determination of gender role actually happens is still debatable. Several theories (right) have been advanced to explain it.

SEXUAL IMAGES IN MOVIES AND ON TV

To what extent television, videos, and movies influence children has for many years been the subject of fierce debate. It is true that children may benefit from seeing programs that show them how people live in different countries or in other parts of their own country. On the other hand, children who are allowed limitless access to the visual media, especially television and videos, may receive negative or confusing messages that may not be acceptable to their parents. Sexual stereotypes and sexual violence are an integral part of popular entertainment and, without any other information to counteract it, may influence the way children feel about sex and relationships. This possibility underlines the importance of parents giving truthful, thoughtful, and developmentally appropriate answers to their children's questions about sex. Parents also need to supervise what children actually watch.

Nurture—the social determination of gender identity and gender role

There are several theories that put forward the idea that social factors are very important, or are the only factors, in determining behavioral differences between the sexes.

Social learning theory

This suggests that children learn to behave in a way "appropriate" to their gender by modeling themselves on adults of the same sex; by being punished by parents and peers alike for gender-inappropriate behavior, and rewarded for gender-appropriate behavior; by exposure to gender stereotypes in movies, in books, and on television; and by observation of social customs.

Cognitive development theory

This suggests that children are not the passive recipients portrayed by the social learning theory. Instead, children acquire their gender role by stages in the same way that they acquire other cognitive skills, such as thinking and reasoning, by being active agents in the learning process. Once children establish their gender identity, between the ages of two and three, and recognize that they will always remain male or female, they become highly motivated to learn to behave in a manner appropriate to their gender.

Gender schema theory

This argues that gender is a major focus around which society chooses to organize its view of reality. Most cultures construct a network of practices and beliefs based on the distinctions between females and males. As children develop, they are brought into this network by learning that gender is crucial, and that all aspects of society are seen in the context of the differences between males and females. In this way, they learn to pose the question, "Am I enough like a boy?" or "Am I enough like a girl?"

There appears to be no clear answer to whether genetic or social factors are the main cause of behavior differences between boys and girls, and later between men and women. But these differences are now seen as determined by the combined influences of nature (genetically determined development) and nurture (social reinforcement).

A child's sexuality from birth to puberty

How old are children when they first become aware of their own sexuality, and when do they come to recognize the differences between their own body and those of the opposite sex? At the end of the 19th century, it was widely believed that sexual awareness first appeared at the same time as the reproductive system matured during puberty. Childhood was perceived as an age of innocence, untainted by any sexual thoughts or actions. Now, at the end of the 20th century, current thinking is that although children become full-fledged sexual beings during adolescence, they experience pleasurable feelings associated with genital and other physical contact from their earliest years. Children develop sexually, and take an interest in sexual matters—albeit not with anything like the intensity apparent during adolescence—throughout childhood. They begin to identify their own gender, and to differentiate between themselves and members of the opposite sex, from around the age of two. The development of sexual awareness in a growing child is described here by dividing childhood into several stages.

Infancy—the first 12 months

In the first months of its life, a baby responds to skin contact, either through being held close to its mother's (especially while being breast-fed) or father's body, or by touching and stroking. All these stimulations produce a pleasurable response, as indicated by smiles and gurgling sounds, and although this may not appear sexual in the adult sense, the nature of the response it produces suggests sensual satisfaction.

As the baby grows, and motor coordination improves, he or she will start touching and exploring his or her own genitals. Seeing this may cause parents to worry if they think that genital touching at this age is a sign of sexual precocity. In fact, it is perfectly normal and natural for young children to be interested in the different parts of their bodies.

Another issue in a boy's developing sexuality is the observation that he has erections. These can occur during breastfeeding, and it may be that oral stimulation is pleasurable at this age.

From one to two years

As children develop greater control over their hands, they will touch their genitals in a more purposeful way and may start to masturbate. Children in this age group may also stimulate themselves through rocking movements or thrusting with their pelvis. These types of sexual activity can be profoundly worrying to some parents who may feel they should take measures to stop their child's actions. However, most masturbatory behavior is perfectly natural. In any case it is likely that at the toddler age children will ignore attempts to stop them from touching their genitals. Rarely, children may indulge in explicit sexual behavior, such as simulated intercourse. This is most likely learned by

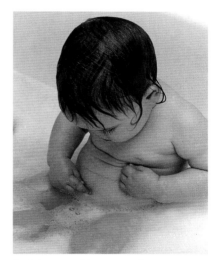

Bathtime provides an excellent opportunity to explore interesting parts of the body, including the genitals.

direct observation of older children or adults. In these situations parents should try to figure out when and where the child might have been exposed to such behavior, and take steps to remove those influences.

From two to four years

By this age, children are becoming more fully aware of their gender identity and taking a much greater interest in their genitals, as well as those of siblings and other children. They will soon realize that girls and boys look different. Toilet training leads to an intensified focus on the genitals, and it is important for parents at this time not to imply that there is something "dirty" about the genitals because of their proximity to the anus.

In this age group, "sex" play between children is normal and common. It may involve affectionate interest in each other, rough-and-tumble play, hugging and kissing, lying down together, or exploring each other's genitals—for example, if they bathe together. Slightly older children of about six or seven may seek privacy to play "doctors and nurses," play that can involve showing and touching each other's genitals. If parents discover children doing this they should avoid an angry response, and should certainly not punish the children. Attitudes in Western society to childhood sexuality lead some parents to worry about this kind of play, but such exploratory behavior should be accepted as normal.

The acquisition of language gives children another means of exploring sexual matters. This is the age of the "why" question, and children will want to know why they are different from their brother or sister or friend, why (if parents appear naked in front of their children) mother and father look different from each other, where do babies come from, or how do babies get out of mother's stomach? It is usually best that such questions are not dismissed with a trivial answer, and that children are given a clear, straightforward reply appropriate for their developmental stage, even if they don't fully understand conceptually what they are being told. For example, to be told in reply to the question "Where do babies (where did I) come from?" that a baby grows inside its mother's womb may be puzzling to a three-year-old. But as the child gets older—and, perhaps, sees the arrival of new brothers or sisters—they will realize they can trust their parents to give honest answers. It is far better to be truthful about where babies come from than to tell tales of storks or leave to a child's imagination possible ways a baby could emerge from a stomach (they usually believe it is through the navel).

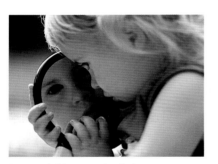
Young children gradually become aware of their own gender identity, and also realize that girls and boys look different.

From four to eight years

At four and five, children become more familiar with differences between the sexes, and may become more self-conscious or aware of their nakedness, and more modest when they get undressed. As children begin to understand more, they become aware of certain sexual taboos in society. A child will begin to appreciate that walking around naked is not generally acceptable and that asking certain questions can be intrusive—such as demanding of an elderly aunt whether she has a penis! Children will also respond to a kind but firm statement that masturbation in public is not something that people do. If parents take this approach, rather than punishing a child for touching themselves, the child should understand that masturbation is not a bad thing, but something that should be done in private.

Similarly, parents should not be surprised if children in this age group form special friendships that can involve "erotic" play such as cuddling, kissing, and embracing.

As children get older, their questions about sexual matters can become more demanding. Although they may still ask where babies come from, they may want to know what breasts are for, why dad doesn't have breasts, why mom doesn't have a penis, or what the man and woman were doing to each other on television. Once again, the best approach is to

QUESTIONS AND ANSWERS: HOW TO RESPOND?

Q. My three-year-old keeps asking me where she came from. What should I say to her, and how much detail should I go into?
A. Tell her quite plainly that she grew inside you and that she came out through your vagina. Keep it accurate but simple—let her questions and comments guide you as to how much detail she is ready to hear and understand.

Q. I have always picked up and cuddled my young niece and nephew without thinking about it, but now they are getting older I am concerned that other people might feel that this behavior is not appropriate. What should I do?
A. Providing you use touching and hugging to show genuine nonsexual affection and care, and the children enjoy your attention, you should continue to give them this affection.

be straightforward and explain in simple, straightforward language what they want to know. A clear answer will satisfy a child; avoiding the issue will make children more curious and may lead them to become confused over their parents' attitude toward sex.

Late childhood

With the approach of puberty *(see pp.47–68)*, children often take more interest in how their own body and those of their friends are beginning to change. They may appear less openly curious about sex, but their interest will undoubtedly still be present. It may be helpful at this age for parents to use simple books written for children to explain to them what sorts of physical changes to their body they can expect as they near their teenage years.

Sexual development and parental influence

Parental attitudes and influence play a vital part in all aspects of a child's development, including sexual development. Of course, sexual development does not occur in isolation, but is an integral part of the development of gender role and personality. It is important that parents take an open, informed, and positive attitude toward sexual matters to ensure that their child reaches adulthood with well-balanced and healthy perceptions about sex and relationships.

If children sense that a sexual subject is taboo, they will feel inhibited and unable to talk freely about that or related subjects later in childhood. Children also sense if their parents have hang-ups about sex and are unwilling to talk about or answer questions about certain topics. This can affect the child's normal gender development. If a parent's attitude toward their child's developing sexuality is repressive, or if it reflects their own sexual anxieties, the child may be affected for life. On the other hand, parents need not feel compelled to be more open than they are comfortable with—whatever the level, a relaxed attitude is the key.

As children get older, parents may find it helpful to anticipate children's questions and to talk to them about the changes that will happen to their bodies as they grow up, as well as about sexual relationships. This is especially helpful if school provides little or no sex education (often the case). If parents feel relaxed enough to talk about sex, then sexual matters can be brought casually into conversations from time to time, rather than making a special time for "sex education." There are books on sex and growing up, often with clear illustrations, that can be read by

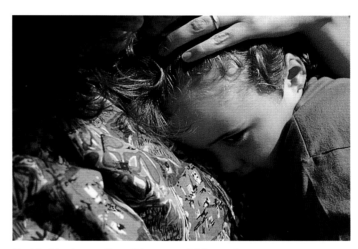

Cuddled by her mother, this young child experiences not only the physical warmth of her embrace but also the emotional feelings of love, comfort, and security.

children, either with their parents or on their own. Children will also be influenced by the hidden elements of parental sex education— what their parents don't or won't say about sexual matters.

Attitudes toward nudity

Being open and relaxed about nudity within the family can prevent a child from perceiving the body as strange or shameful. Some parents allow their children to see them naked from an early age, not only when walking around the house but also by sharing a bath with the child. Parents who do this should not be surprised when children ask questions about pubic hair, their mother's breasts, or the size of their father's penis because these are all the result of a child's natural curiosity.

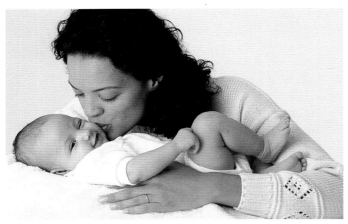

Parental influence on a child's development starts from birth. By holding, touching, talking to, and caring for her baby, this mother gives him a secure start in life.

TALKING ABOUT SEX TO CHILDREN

How and when should parents educate their children about sex? The best answer is that parents should, to a certain extent, let the flow of everyday family life and a child's curiosity lead the process of sex education. Very young children often become aware of the difference between males and females when they see their siblings, friends, or parents naked, however briefly and innocently. Straight answers to questions raised by nudity will ensure that the child knows that differences between males and females are normal. Naming of genital parts is an individual matter, but parents may feel it is a good idea to encourage children to use correct terminology rather than nursery names for their genitals. If a child calls his finger a finger, why give his penis a special name? Similarly, the arrival of brothers or sisters may prompt questions about how babies are "made." Again, clear answers (with detail appropriate to the child's developmental level) are usually best.

CHILDREN WITH SPECIAL NEEDS

Children with special needs, or with learning difficulties, have as much need for sex education as other children. If parents find it difficult to talk to their children about sexual matters, it may be that the child's school can provide some help, or suggest other sources of help.

Other parents find that nudity embarrasses them and the child; for those who are not prepared to field frank questions, it is probably better not to encourage nudity at home. Our society today also takes a dim view of parental nudity. Some experts view the practice as a form of child abuse, forcing children to confront adult visual information before they are ready to process it.

Which approach to take is a matter of personal choice for each family. For parents who worry about whether and when to appear nude in front of their children, the best advice is never to behave in any way that makes either parents or children feel uncomfortable.

Touching and hugging

A positive attitude toward sexuality does not come from words alone. It's important to hug and touch children, to give them a sense of comfort and being loved, and the knowledge that being close to someone else is not wrong. Similarly, seeing their parents hug and kiss each other, or behave with affection, sends a positive message to children. For many parents, hugging and touching children is a natural progression from the loving care given to them as babies. But if the parents themselves were not hugged or kissed when they were children, they may feel inhibited about touching their children. In these circumstances it may help to try and overcome inhibitions by realizing that natural, affectionate contact reduces a child's anxieties and generally makes him or her a happier person.

Talking to children—sex education

Traditionally, sex education is taught in a series of classes that take place in middle or junior high school. They are designed to inform children about the reproductive system, what sexual intercourse involves in a physical way, and how to avoid having an unplanned pregnancy or contracting a sexual disease, but there is seldom any mention of sexual feelings and relationships. Sex education varies from school to school and from state to state; some children may receive little or none. But whether children attend sex education classes at school or not, parents must appreciate their own role as sex educators. The most important lesson for parents to teach is that sex is not wrong, shameful, or dirty but a natural—private—part of a healthy life. Communicating this message and its conditions can be extremely challenging.

As children get older they may ask parents difficult questions about sexual matters. Some families are very open about sex, while others are more inhibited. In either case it is vital that the child's assumptions and ideas be voiced and heard, and that clear answers to questions be provided, if necessary at a more appropriate time and place. The child should not be made to feel that the topic of sex is forbidden territory in family conversations.

In later childhood, as a child approaches puberty, parents who talk to their children about sex should clearly and explicitly discuss, but not overemphasize, issues like sexually transmitted diseases and contraception, in order to ensure that their children develop a responsible attitude toward sex without fearing that the expression of sexual feelings will be threatening or dangerous. Parents can emphasize the positive aspects of sex, and that it is a way to express love and pleasure in relationships between mature adults. Above all, children should be aware that their developing sexuality, and the changes that happen to their bodies, are simply part of growing up, and nothing to be frightened of or ashamed about. If a parent is worried about how to tell their child about sex, it may help if they reflect on their own childhood. How much did they understand about sexual matters at different ages? What concerns and worries did they feel? What do they wish they had known while growing up?

Protecting children from sexual abuse
Telling a young child that all strangers pose a threat will probably frighten a child; not telling them that a stranger may pose a threat is irresponsible. So, what is the right thing to say to a child about contact with strangers and at what age should it be said? Once children have a reasonable grasp of language, between the ages of two and four, they can be told that some people are bad, and that they

PROTECTING CHILDREN

Parents can advise children about possible dangers in the outside world, but what action can a parent take to help their child avoid the various dangers? Parents should:
• make sure that they leave a child only with someone they know and trust
• make sure that a baby-sitter can contact them in case of emergency
• make sure that a child understands the arrangements if they are being left with someone else
• tell children that they should tell their mother or father immediately if anyone touches them in a way that they feel is wrong, too friendly, or too personal
• tell children that if they feel threatened by a stranger it is perfectly all right if they shout or run away
• tell children to report to parents or teachers any strangers whom they see hanging around near their house or school, in the park, or on a beach.
Children who are aware that there may be dangers around them are much less likely to be abused, physically or sexually (see also Chapter 12, Sexual Offenses).

should not talk to people they do not know in case they belong to this "bad" group. It may be helpful to refer to books or cartoons that feature "good guys" and "bad guys." As the child gets older, the message can be repeated more subtly, perhaps being brought up in everyday conversations. At bathtime, parents can casually mention to children that their bodies belong to them, and that they should not let anyone touch or look at the private areas of their body if they don't want them to, even if the person is known to the child. Repeated often in the context of everyday life, messages about not talking to strangers and keeping bodies private should become part of a child's knowledge. If children are encouraged to talk about their day, this can give valuable clues as to how much they understand about sexual matters, and gaps in information or a sudden change in communication can alert parents to shifts and dangers in the child's life. At school, it is helpful if teachers can tell children—in a calm way—about not talking to, accepting candy from, or getting in the cars of strangers, because this reinforces the message received at home.

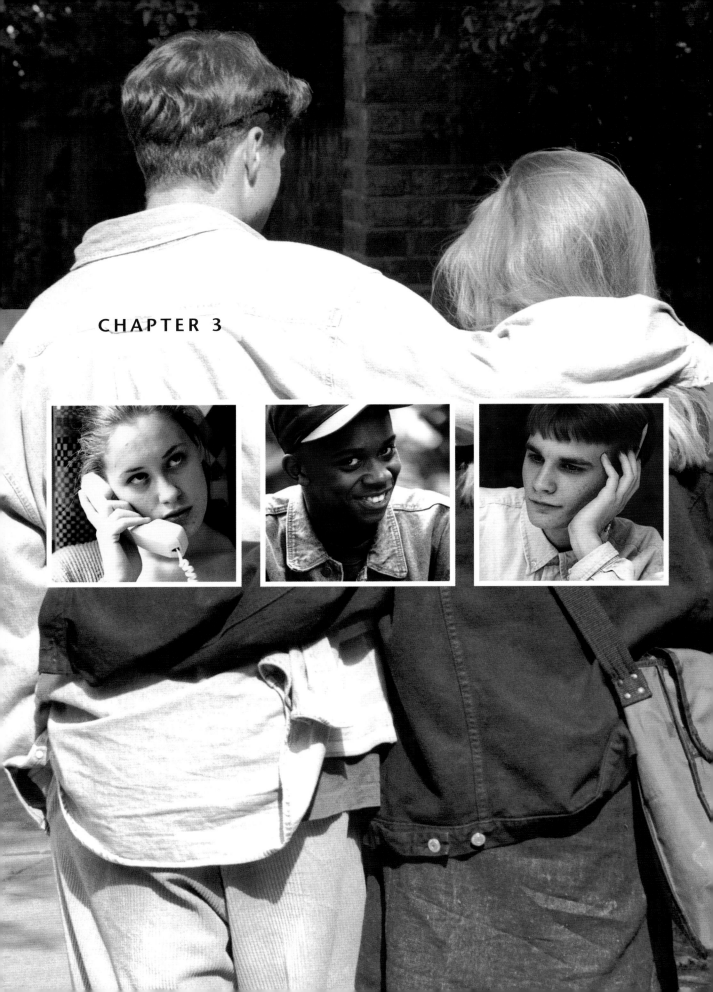

CHAPTER 3

Adolescence

Between the ages of 9 and 18, young people go through a phase of rapid growth, development, and maturation. At the beginning of this process they are children. At the end of it they are physically, sexually, and psychologically young adults. Two terms—puberty and adolescence—are often used interchangeably, and confusingly, to describe this time of change. In fact, the word "puberty" describes the physiological and physical changes that take place during adolescence, while the term "adolescence" refers to the complete period of a person's physical and psychological transition between childhood and adulthood.

Adolescence can be a difficult time, especially if neither the young person nor their parents are prepared for what is going to happen. However, contrary to popular belief, adolescence is not necessarily a time of endless arguments, upsets, and turmoil. Indeed, for many adolescents—the descriptive name given to young people as they pass through this phase of their life—it is an exciting and positive time when they can revel in newfound freedoms, discover new interests, and make new friends. Equally, parents should not see adolescence as a time when they may lose a child but as one where the parent–child relationship enters a more adult stage.

As the body changes shape and develops sexually, so the emotions change and adoles-

cents mature mentally. Although the general patterns of adolescence are the same, no two individuals share the same experiences. Some pass through adolescence quite smoothly; others experience emotional upheaval that can make them feel happy one day and miserable the next. Some—regardless of when their bodies began to change—may race through adolescence; others mature more slowly.

During adolescence and puberty, young people begin to understand themselves and one another. They tend to become less focused on their families and more focused on their friends. Friendships often become more intense than they were in childhood. Parents should not feel anxious about such friendships because they help teenagers learn important skills, such as how to get along with other people—both individually and in groups. In their early teens, boys and girls tend to form close friendships with members of their own sex, but as they get older they begin to "hang out" in mixed groups.

Many of the changes in adolescence and puberty are sexual. Teenagers start to have sexual thoughts and feelings and will probably have their first intense relationships, which may become sexual. As their bodies change, they may worry about their looks and feel confused about their self-image and identity. As they seek greater independence and parents question their attitudes, friendships, or behavior, their relationship with their parents will certainly change. In their search for their own personal identity, some young people may appear to be in rebellion against their parents and teachers. Adults should remember that behind the seemingly confident or stubborn facade presented by most "difficult" teenagers often lie serious doubts about their future role in life or worries about their attractiveness and/or sexual identity. Although such worries are a natural part of growing up, they may cause a young person to seem tense and uncommunicative.

Adolescents have so many changes to get used to—physical, emotional, social, and sexual—that it is sometimes easy to forget that parents have some adjusting to do, too. It can be difficult for parents to watch their children growing up, maturing sexually, and breaking away from the family. Despite the almost inevitable clashes, adolescence is generally least painful if parents and their children can be relatively open with each other about day-to-day subjects, including sex and relationships. Misunderstandings and major conflicts are also less likely to occur if each makes an effort to understand the other's point of view. A contributing factor to the problem may be that many parents tend to respond to their teenage children's behavior rather than taking the initiative in dealing with them. They may feel that their children's increased desire for freedom is a threat to their family structure, and may tend to react in a negative way, for instance, by telling their son or daughter that they cannot stay out late, or shouldn't wear

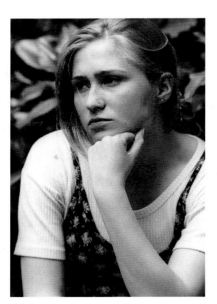

Adolescence is a time of great changes, but knowing what to expect during the teenage years can help both children and their parents weather the storm.

certain clothes or see certain friends. Instead of *reacting* like this—and probably causing a fight—parents should try to recall the feelings they had in their own teenage years and the conflicts they may have had with their parents. While adults often need to set firm guidelines for teenagers, young people equally must be allowed to develop their independence—and this should all take place within a framework that is acceptable to the whole family. For their part, adolescents must remember that if parents appear to criticize or nag it is probably only out of love and a sense of responsibility.

What is puberty?

Puberty consists in both sexes of a period of rapid growth; a change in body shape; the "switching on" of the maturation process of the reproductive system, which ends in the capacity for sexual reproduction; and the development of secondary sex characteristics such as breasts and pubic hair. All these changes do not appear overnight, however. Puberty typically takes between two and five years, and proceeds in a series of stages that vary in length from one individual to the next. On average girls start, and complete, puberty before boys. However, for both sexes one sign of puberty is the sudden increase in height, the growth spurt, that typically occurs between the ages of $10\frac{1}{2}$ and $12\frac{1}{2}$ in girls, and between $12\frac{1}{2}$ and $14\frac{1}{2}$ in boys.

These are the main changes that occur in both sexes during puberty.
• The body undergoes a period of rapid growth—the growth spurt—that brings it close to its adult size.
• The primary sex organs, or gonads—the testes in boys and ovaries in girls—are "switched on," so that they become more active and start releasing more sex hormones.
• The secondary sex characteristics appear. These are adult body features that indicate that the sexual maturation process is under way. In girls, the secondary sex characteristics that develop during puberty include the breasts, pubic and armpit hair, and changes to

the vulva. In boys, the secondary sex characteristics also include pubic, facial, and armpit hair, as well as the increase in the size of the penis and testes, the darkening of skin on the scrotum, and the deepening of the voice. In both boys and girls, adultlike body odors and acne may develop.

The sequence in which the changes of puberty take place varies very little from one person to another (see box, right). However, the changes do not begin at the same age in everyone, nor do they take the same amount of time. Some children or parents may be concerned by the apparently early or late onset of puberty; changes to the body, such as the appearance of breasts or pubic hair, may cause delight to one adolescent and distress to another, and be a matter of indifference to a third. Worried children or parents might try to take comfort in the thought that puberty is something which happens to everyone, and that it doesn't last forever.

In girls, the sign that the body is attaining sexual maturity is menarche, the first menstrual bleeding. In boys, approaching maturity is evidenced by the increased size of the testes and the ejaculation of semen, often in nocturnal emissions or "wet dreams." But in neither case do these signs mean that the young person is completely sexually mature. The release of an egg from the ovary (ovulation) may not occur until the first few periods have occurred; and, similarly, the first ejaculations do not contain any sperm.

The puberty timeline (right) features the average age at which the various changes of puberty begin. Although the events of puberty typically occur in the same sequence in all girls and boys, the age at which they occur varies enormously. Only if the signs of puberty start very early or have failed to start by the middle teenage years should children be referred to a doctor to see if their precocity, or lack of development, is a cause for worry.

Why puberty happens

Puberty is initiated and regulated by chemicals called hormones, which are produced by the body. These stimulate physical growth and the development of the sex organs and secondary

PUBERTY TIMELINE

GIRLS

9½–14½ YEARS
- The breasts start to develop; as they begin to enlarge, they are known as breast buds (see p.55). Consult a doctor if breast buds have not appeared by the age of 13.
- The growth spurt—a time of rapid growth—begins. Consult a doctor if it has not begun by the age of 14.
- The first pubic hairs appear.
- Armpit sweat glands start working—girls start to produce adult body odor.
- Internally, the vagina, ovaries, and uterus grow.
- Many girls experience a discharge of clear or whitish fluid from the vagina.

11–14 YEARS
- Periods begin (see pp.59–62), usually two years after the start of breast development. Consult a doctor if periods start before the age of 10 or have not begun by 16.
- Changes occur to the vulva—the external part of the reproductive system (see p.58): the clitoris becomes larger; the inner and outer labia (lips) become fleshier; and pubic hair becomes coarser and spreads over the mons pubis.
- Armpit hair darkens and coarsens.
- Sebaceous (oil) glands become more active; acne may develop.
- Pelvis increases in size. Fat deposits change a girl's body shape to that of a woman. Total body-fat content rises from about 8 percent to 25

BOYS

11–12 YEARS
- The testes grow, and the skin of the scrotum—the "bag" that holds the testes—gets darker. Consult a doctor if the testes have not enlarged by the age of 14.

12–13 YEARS
- Pubic hair starts to grow.
- The penis gets longer, initially, and then thicker.
- Boys may notice a tender lump of tissue behind the nipple (gynecomastia—see p.67) on one or both sides. This is a normal phase that may last up to 18 months.
- Armpit sweat glands become active—boys start to produce adult body odor
- The growth spurt—a time of rapid growth—begins. Consult a doctor if the growth spurt starts before the age of 11 or has not begun by 15.

13–15 YEARS
- Boys start to ejaculate semen, either during masturbation or during "wet dreams" while asleep. Initially it does not contain any sperm.
- Pubic hair becomes coarser and spreads farther over the pubic area.
- Armpit and other body hair starts to grow.
- Hair starts growing on the face, starting at the corner of the upper lip, and spreads toward the center.
- Sebaceous (oil) glands become more active; acne may develop.

14–15 YEARS
- The voice "breaks" and becomes deeper as the larynx (voice box) enlarges.

sex characteristics, and may be related to some of the behavioral changes that teenagers tend to go through during the period of adolescence.

Hormones are chemicals that are released into the bloodstream by organs called endocrine (hormonal) glands, which are scattered around the body. Carried by the blood, a hormone acts like a messenger: when it reaches a target organ in the body it "delivers a message" which causes the activity of that organ to change. For example, growth hormone—which plays a part in the pubertal growth spurt—targets bones and "instructs" them to grow. The collective action of many hormones plays a vital role in controlling specific body activities. Typically, the effects of hormones are slow and long-acting, unlike those of the body's other control and coordination system, the brain and nervous system, where effects are rapid and short-lived. For example, the development of a girl's breasts during puberty—a process controlled by hormones—takes years; moving your hand to pick up a cup—an action controlled by the nervous system—takes only seconds. Although hormones regulate many aspects of life, it is only those that affect growth and sexual development that are considered in this chapter. The involvement of hormones in the process explains why the changes of puberty do not occur suddenly overnight, but unfold over a long period of time.

Overseeing the hormonal process is part of the brain called the hypothalamus. In late childhood, the hypothalamus begins secreting substances known as releasing hormones, which are carried by blood vessels to the nearby pituitary gland, a pea-sized endocrine gland that hangs from the base of the brain. One of these releasing hormones (gonadotropin-releasing hormone—GnRH) triggers the release of gonadotropic hormones by the pituitary gland. These in turn stimulate the testes in boys to produce a hormone called testosterone and the ovaries in girls to produce the female sex hormone estrogen. Testosterone encourages growth, triggers the development of male secondary sexual characteristics, and eventually causes the testes to produce sperm. Estrogen stimulates the development of girls' breasts and initiates the menstrual and ovarian cycles, during which a female's body is prepared for potential pregnancy and an egg is released from one of her ovaries.

At the same time, other hormones cause the release in both sexes of the growth hormone, which encourages the growth of bones and muscles. Pituitary hormones also encourage the adrenal glands (located on top of the kidneys) to release hormones called adrenal androgens, which are similar to testosterone. In girls, these adrenal androgens influence the growth spurt, as well as stimulating the growth of pubic hair.

TALKING TO CHILDREN ABOUT PUBERTY

Change disturbs most people, and if the change concerns their own body and happens at an age when they have little experience of life, it can cause great confusion and distress. Yet this is what can happen to children in their early teens if they are not aware that puberty is a normal part of growing up. Despite improvements in sex education and the more open approach to sex in the media, some girls are still taken by surprise by their first menstrual period, and some boys by their first ejaculation. Misinformation from peers does not help either. Parents can help by talking to their children about growing up and developing sexuality, a task that is made easier if they have already discussed the subject when the child was younger. Books can help as well, either read by the child and parent together or left for the child to read on their own. Even the best-informed adolescents may have doubts about what is happening to them, and may need parental reassurance.

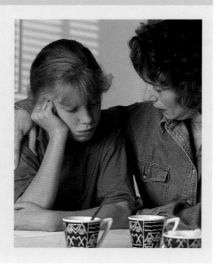

Changes common to girls and boys

Many of the physical changes of puberty are similar in boys and girls. Changes specific to either sex are described in later sections.

The growth spurt

This is the rapid period of growth in height and increase in body weight caused by the growth of bones and muscles to their adult size and, in the case of girls, the deposition of fat under the skin to produce the adult female body shape. In addition, the hipbones grow wider in girls and the shoulders grow wider in boys.

The growth spurt begins in girls, on average, between the ages of 10 and 11. Growth is fastest between the ages of 12 and 13, and has slowed by the time a girl reaches 14. The growth spurt in girls is one of the most obvious signs that puberty has started. Most boys begin their growth spurt between the ages of 11 and 12, grow fastest at 13 or 14, and have started to slow down by the age of 15. In boys, the growth spurt usually begins after early changes to the sex organs have occurred. During the growth spurt, girls can grow by as much as 3 inches in one year, and boys by up to 4 inches. The earlier start made by girls explains why 12-year-old girls are frequently taller than the boys in their class at school. But although boys start later, their overall growth period is longer and their peak rate of growth is higher compared to girls, so that by the end of puberty they are typically taller than girls of the same age. By adulthood, on average, men have one and a half times the muscle mass and bone mass of women, while women have twice as much body fat as men.

Like the other changes of puberty, when the growth spurt starts depends on a number of factors, including the characteristics inherited from parents and current and past general health and nutrition. These factors will also determine how tall and heavy a person becomes, and what body shape they have as

an adult. Children may or may not resemble one or the other of their parents in adulthood; their final shape and size will depend on their own individual genetic makeup. There is no connection between the age at which the growth spurt begins and the final height of a person: someone who starts growing early

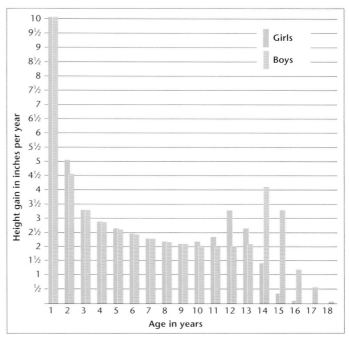

This graph illustrates yearly height gain in boys and girls from birth to the age of 18. Two things are immediately obvious. First, the rapid phase of growth during the adolescent years is second only to that occurring in the first two years of life. Second, the adolescent growth spurt occurs earlier in girls than in boys.

GROWING PAINS

Growing pains are aches and pains that may occur in the legs, and sometimes the back, of adolescents and sometimes younger children. The cause of growing pains is unknown, although it does not appear to be linked to the rapid growth that occurs during puberty. Attacks of growing pains are usually felt at night, lasting usually for a few minutes, but occasionally for up to an hour. Although growing pains are not medically significant and require no professional attention, a child who experiences them may be sufficiently disturbed or frightened to require calming and reassurance, especially if she or he is kept awake at night. However, if a child experiences persistent and repetitive joint or muscle pain, he or she should be referred to a doctor because these symptoms may indicate a more serious condition.

could complete their growth spurt quickly and not be particularly tall as an adult.

Sudden growth can produce problems for teenagers, especially boys, if they feel gawky or awkward. Such awkwardness is usually caused by the order in which bones grow, with the bones of the hands and feet lengthening first, followed by the lower leg and forearm, followed by the thigh and upper arm, followed by the hip and shoulder girdles. The lengthening of the trunk and an increase in the front-to-back diameter of the chest are the final stages of the growth spurt. If young people feel uncomfortable while their bones are undergoing this period of growth, it may help to reassure them that they will soon "catch up" with their rapid expansion in size and feel confident and coordinated again.

Stretch marks

Growth during the growth spurt may be so rapid that the skin loses its elasticity. If this happens, pale lines called stretch marks (or striae) can develop on the skin's surface. They may also appear if an individual is overweight or if there is an abnormal hormone function. In most cases, stretch marks fade with time, although they rarely go away entirely.

Body hair

Before puberty, most of the body of both boys and girls has a fine covering of vellus hair, the short, fine hair that covers the bodies of children and adult women. Only on the eyebrows and scalp are longer, thicker hairs to be found. At puberty, sex hormones called androgens are released inside the bodies of both sexes, although a higher level is released in males than females. The most important of these androgens is testosterone. During puberty, the androgens stimulate growth of hairs around the genitals (pubic hair) and in the armpits. In both sexes, the hair on the arms and legs becomes longer and darker, although this change is more pronounced in boys. Many girls decide to remove their underarm and sometimes leg hair, using a razor or, in the case of legs, creams or waxing. However, some girls prefer to retain their body hair. In boys, hair typically appears on the face (see p.67) and, eventually, on the chest and perhaps the back.

Perspiration—new hygiene problems

Skin—in both children and adults—contains sweat glands that release sweat in hot conditions to cool us down. But during puberty, another type of sweat gland becomes active. These glands, known as apocrine sweat glands, are confined mostly to the armpits, the area around the genitals, and the anus. Apocrine glands produce sweat not only when an individual is hot but also when he or she is excited or anxious. The sweat they produce is thicker than "ordinary" sweat, as it contains proteins and fatty substances. Freshly released apocrine sweat is odorless, but as it is decomposed by skin bacteria it takes on the unpleasant, musky smell known as body odor. Fortunately there are effective ways to keep body odor to a minimum (see box, left).

AVOIDING BODY ODOR

Avoiding body odor is relatively simple. A daily bath or shower removes old sweat, and application of an antiperspirant to the armpits reduces sweat release from the glands there. As far as the area around the genitals is concerned, however, washing is enough. The skin around the vulva is particularly sensitive to chemicals, and products marketed as vaginal deodorants should not be used.

BOYS' AWKWARDNESS WHEN GROWING

As all boys' bodies change radically in shape and size during their teenage years—more suddenly than girls' bodies do—it is natural that many boys feel for a while as though they're living in the wrong body. This is hardly surprising when you consider that their body is halfway between their childhood body and their adult body. The feeling of awkwardness is caused by the different bones in the body growing at different times during the growth spurt—for example, feet may reach their adult size long before the rest of the body. If during this period boys feel awkward or gangly, the best thing to do is try to think positively about their body, and remember that this stage doesn't last for long.

Acne

Acne is a common problem for both sexes during adolescence, affecting 60 to 80 percent of teenagers between the ages of 14 and 17. What causes acne? The androgen hormones that produce the changes visible during puberty in boys, and some of the changes, such as growth of pubic hair, in girls, also cause changes in the skin. In the skin there are glands, called sebaceous glands, which produce an oily secretion called sebum that lubricates both skin and hairs and keeps them soft and waterproof. At puberty, sex hormones increase the number, size, and activity of these sebaceous glands and the thickness of the sebum. If the duct leading from a sebaceous gland to the surface of the skin becomes blocked by dead cells or hardened sebum, small white or black pinpoints—called whiteheads or blackheads, respectively—form. But if the sebaceous gland behind a blackhead becomes infected, it swells, becomes reddened and sometimes sore, and often produces a pus-filled cyst on the skin's surface. These cysts are called acne, and are most commonly found on the face, neck, and shoulders, although they may extend down the back.

Acne causes great distress to young people because this is a time when they are very sensitive about their looks and want to appear attractive to their peers. Acne can be treated initially by washing with antibacterial soap, lotions, and face washes; these remove excess oil from the skin's surface and stop the acne from spreading. Alcohol-based cleansing lotions are less effective than water-based cleansing lotions because they cause excessive drying of the skin, which can make the situation worse. Nonprescription skin creams containing benzoyl peroxide or other agents, obtainable at drugstores, can help to unblock pores by removing sebum and destroying bacteria. Mild exposure to sunlight may also help, although excessive exposure will cause burning, which will aggravate the acne and, more importantly, may increase the risk of developing skin cancer later in life. Avoid picking or squeezing pimples, as this can spread the infection and thereby make the

acne worse. If acne persists, a doctor may prescribe a course of oral antibacterial drugs. In most cases, acne does not continue to be a problem beyond the late teens, although a few people still suffer from it as adults. Occasionally in the past, people with severe acne that persisted into adulthood became scarred, but nowadays, with modern treatments, scarring is extremely rare.

There is no conclusive evidence that diet affects acne. Contrary to the commonly held view, it appears that fatty and fried foods, chocolate, and soda do not increase the chances of developing pimples. However, some people—both children and adults—are sensitive to certain types of food, and this sensitivity may affect their skin.

How can adults help a younger person who has acne? It is probably not helpful to

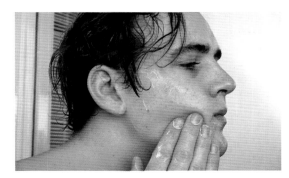

Keeping the skin clean and free from excess oil and dirt by regular washing with an antibacterial soap can help to reduce the incidence of skin problems that are very common among adolescents.

say to him or her that acne is common among people of their age or that their pimples will disappear in a year or so. It may help to explain what is causing it, tell her or him about simple remedies (such as cleansing lotions), and advise them not to pick or squeeze their pimples. If necessary, parents can buy lotions or soaps for their teenager if he or she is too embarrassed to buy them. If the acne is very bad, a parent should arrange an appointment, or encourage the teenager to make an appointment, to see the doctor. Above all, the best thing that parents can do is to provide support and help their teenager to maintain their self-confidence.

Puberty in girls

During the years of puberty a girl's body grows rapidly, her ovaries develop and become active, her internal and external reproductive organs mature, her secondary sex characteristics appear and, in the later stages of puberty, she has her first period. The main changes she will notice include:

• development of the breasts
• growth of pubic hair
• changes in the vulva (the external genitals)
• widening of the hips
• menstruation begins.

Breast development

Breast development is one of the first signs that puberty has started *(the internal anatomy of breasts is described on p.19)*. Throughout childhood, girls' breasts, like those of boys, are flat except for the raised nipple and the colored area around it, the areola. Somewhere between the ages of 8 and 16—on average between the tenth and twelfth birthdays—small mounds called breast buds *(see stage 2, opposite)* gradually appear around a girl's nipples, which during the years of puberty grow into fully developed breasts. The age at which breasts start growing bears no relation to how quickly they will develop or how large they will be.

Breasts generally reach their full size by the time a girl is 18. They may feel tender and a bit sore as they develop. If a girl has started her menstrual periods, her breasts may feel tender in the week or two before menstruation, as a result of the hormonal changes happening in her body at that time.

How breasts develop

Breast development is described here in five stages. In practice these stages merge into each other, but they are useful for girls who want to monitor their breast development. How long it takes to get from one stage to the next depends on the individual. From stage 2 to stage 5 could take six months or six years,

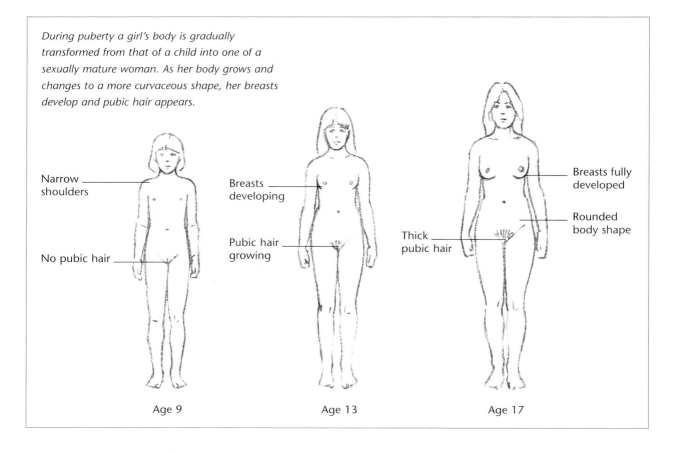

During puberty a girl's body is gradually transformed from that of a child into one of a sexually mature woman. As her body grows and changes to a more curvaceous shape, her breasts develop and pubic hair appears.

Narrow shoulders

No pubic hair

Breasts developing

Pubic hair growing

Thick pubic hair

Breasts fully developed

Rounded body shape

Age 9

Age 13

Age 17

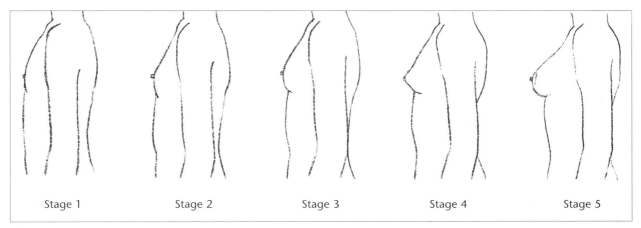

| Stage 1 | Stage 2 | Stage 3 | Stage 4 | Stage 5 |

although typically it takes around four years for the breasts to develop fully.

Stage 1

During this stage, which lasts from birth to the start of puberty, the breasts are flat.

Stage 2

This is the breast bud stage, which starts, on average, between 10 and 12. The area around the nipple starts to swell as fat tissue is laid down under the skin and the first milk glands develop. Usually the nipples get larger and the areola becomes wider at this stage.

Stage 3

Now the breasts are almost cone-shaped; the nipple and areola have usually darkened.

Stage 4

The areola and nipple form a separate, secondary mound or bump on the breast. However, not all girls experience this stage; some go straight from stage 3 to stage 5.

Stage 5

During this final stage, a girl's breasts become fully developed. The areola, which is now at its full size, no longer forms a separate mound but is part of the main, rounded breast shape; generally, the nipple projects outward. Inside the breast the milk glands and ducts are in place, and are surrounded by fat tissue (although milk will not be produced unless a woman has recently had a baby).

Breast shape and size

Many girls worry about the size of their breasts and their appearance. Girls may be concerned by how quickly or slowly their breasts are developing, or by how large or

This sequence shows a girl's breasts developing during puberty. Because everyone differs, however, a girl may find that her breasts do not grow exactly like this; and that by stage 5 her breasts, or her nipples or areolae, may be larger or smaller than those shown here.

small their breasts will be when they are fully grown. Such fears are compounded by images in magazines and films of "perfect" breasts, supposedly of a size and shape that women prefer and men find sexually attractive. In reality, breasts come in all shapes and sizes. What a girl's breasts look like depends on the genes she has inherited from her parents. However, although they may resemble her mother's breasts, or the breasts of women in her father's family, they may be unlike either in terms of shape and size. Some girls may also worry because one or both of their nipples sink into the areola (are inverted) instead of sticking out. They should be reassured that their nipple or nipples may not start sticking out until they get older, and that even if their nipples never protrude outward, there is nothing wrong with their breasts; many women have inverted nipples.

Breast self-examination

Breast self-examination *(see also pp.100–1)* is something that adult women are encouraged to do on a monthly basis—usually just after their period has finished—in order to check for any unusual lumps that might indicate the presence of a disease of the breast such as breast cancer. It is suggested that younger women get into the regular habit of examining their breasts in their early twenties.

QUESTIONS AND ANSWERS: BREASTS

Q. My breasts are so large and heavy that my bra straps cut into my shoulders. The weight of my breasts also makes me easily tired. Is there anything that can be done to help me?

A. Girls who wish they had bigger breasts often don't realize how much stress and physical pain very heavy breasts can cause, not only from bras but sometimes from backaches as well. If you are overweight, losing weight should help. In some cases, there is also the possibility, when you are adult, of having breast-reduction surgery, although you need to discuss the pros and cons of this operation very carefully with your doctor and the plastic surgeon, who will advise you whether such intervention is suitable in your case.

Q. I measured the diameter of the dark skin around my nipples. It was 3¼ inches wide! Is anybody else like me?

A. The dark skin around the nipple (the areola) varies in size in just the same way that the breasts and nipples themselves do. Some women have very small areolae, some very wide ones, and others are somewhere in between. All of these are perfectly normal.

Q. When I look in the mirror I can see very clearly that my breasts are different sizes. All the models I see in magazines seem to have equal-sized breasts. How is it that I am such a freak?

A. It is very common for breasts to develop at different rates during puberty. Generally, in time, the smaller breast develops to approximately the same size as the larger one. But most adult women do not have two breasts of equal size. Like most of our other external features, breasts tend to be lopsided—even on famous models or actresses. (Padding is often used to make these women appear perfectly symmetrical.)

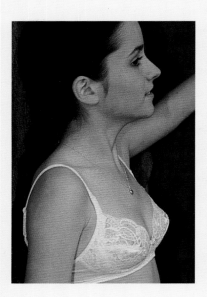

Bras come in many different sizes, shapes, and styles, and it's all too easy to buy one that is uncomfortable, too tight, or too loose, or gives too much or too little support. Some women's clothing and lingerie stores have charts to help you calculate your bra size, as well as salespeople trained to measure customers and advise on size and style.

However, even though breast cancer is very rare in teenagers, it might be wise for girls to begin examining their breasts on a routine basis as soon as they start to have their menstrual periods, hopefully thereby establishing the habit for life.

Bras

A bra covers and supports the breasts. Exactly when a girl should start wearing a bra, or whether she needs to wear one at all, varies from individual to individual. Certainly if her breasts are small a girl may not feel the need to wear a bra; on the other hand, if she has larger breasts, she may feel uncomfortable if she doesn't wear one. Many girls either feel embarrassed about going out without a bra on or want to support their breasts and keep them from moving around when they are dancing or exercising; some girls prefer the rounded breast shape a bra produces. Breasts will not sag and droop immediately if a girl chooses to go without a bra. But over time, if the breasts do not have any external support, they may start to become elongated and flatter—especially in the case of larger, heavier breasts—because the ligaments that support the breast from the inside will eventually become stretched.

Although many parents, especially mothers, will notice when their daughter needs her first bra, others may not, and their child may have to broach the subject herself. Even if a girl doesn't really need a bra, it's better for her to wear one of the smaller training bras than to be told she is too young or doesn't need one.

Pubic hair

Coarser, curlier, and often a different, darker color than the hair growing on the person's head, pubic hair is found around the genitals in both sexes. In girls it commonly first appears between the ages of 11 and 12, although it may start growing as early as 8 or as late as 16. By the end of puberty, pubic hair covers the mons pubis and the outer lips (labia majora) of the vulva, the external part of the reproductive system.

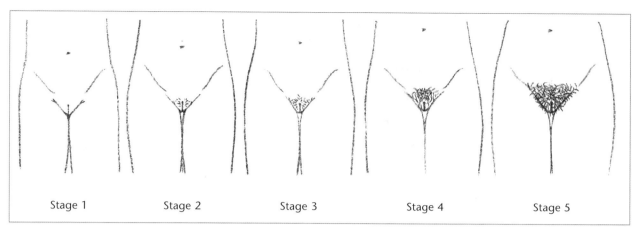

| Stage 1 | Stage 2 | Stage 3 | Stage 4 | Stage 5 |

Growth of pubic hair

Like breast development, the appearance of pubic hair during puberty can be divided into stages (see above and below). In reality, of course, these stages merge into each other. However, it is often reassuring for a girl to know both that the appearance of pubic hair is not unusual and that she is following the same path of development as her friends. The age at which each stage is completed will vary considerably between individuals.

Stage 1

During this stage, which lasts from birth to the start of puberty, no pubic hairs are present.

Stage 2

Pubic hairs appear, usually between the ages of 11 and 12. Identifiable by being longer and probably darker than other body hairs, the first pubic hairs may appear along the edges of the outer lips of the vulva, or on the mons itself.

Stage 3

This stage is generally reached between the ages of 11 and 13. More hairs appear, and these are curlier and darker than those in stage 2.

Stage 4

Between the ages of 13 and 15, pubic hair becomes coarser, providing a more extensive and denser covering than before.

Stage 5

This is the adult stage. The pubic hair is typically coarse and often tightly curled, and covers a triangular area extending over the edge of the thighs.

The first wisps of pubic hair appear on a girl's genitals between the ages of 9 and 13, gradually spreading over the mons pubis. Adult pubic hair varies greatly in thickness and extent from person to person.

QUESTION AND ANSWER: PUBIC HAIR

Q. How much pubic hair should a woman have when puberty is finished?
A. Like all other body characteristics, this depends on the individual. Generally, pubic hair extends out into a triangular shape over the mons pubis, although it may form a narrower vertical band in some women. Pubic hair may grow outward onto the inside of the thighs. It may also appear to grow upward toward the belly button, although this extension is actually formed by softer body hair.

Removing pubic hair

Pubic hair protruding from the sides of a bathing suit is a frequent cause of embarrassment and annoyance to young women. Some people resort to plucking out these hairs from the "bikini line," which is a painful and not particularly effective solution. Others shave the area, but this can leave the skin red and irritated, and it may feel rough when the hairs start to grow back. If a girl wants to remove the hair from this area, the best procedure is to do so with a commercial depilatory (hair-removing) cream intended for that part of the body (follow the instructions carefully), or by hot or cold waxing, which can be done easily at home but is probably best done at a beauty salon.

Changes to the vulva

The vulva is a girl's external genitalia—those parts of her reproductive system that lie on the outside of the body (see pp.16–20). These are the mons pubis (or mons veneris)—the fatty pad that covers the pubic bone, the outer lips (or labia majora), and the inner lips (or labia minora), the clitoris, and the openings of the urethra and vagina, which all lie between the outer and inner lips.

During puberty, the vulva changes as the external sexual organs mature and develop.
• Before puberty, the inner lips of the vulva are scarcely visible, and the outer lips are relatively small.
• During puberty, the outer lips become plumper, while the inner lips appear fleshier and moister. The mons pubis becomes thicker and more prominent. Pubic hair begins to grow on the outer lips and the mons pubis. Both the vaginal opening and the clitoris become larger.
• After puberty, when a young woman is sexually mature, both the inner and outer lips of the vulva are more fleshy. Pubic hair typically covers the mons pubis and the outer lips. However, the shape and color of the lips and the extent of pubic hair vary greatly between one individual and the next.

If a girl examines her vulva with a mirror she may feel she is "abnormal" because it does not resemble the standard textbook picture of a vulva. In fact, vulvas differ considerably from one person to the next, most obviously in the shape and size of the outer and inner lips. The inner lips may project beyond the outer lips, or be contained within them; and they may be of equal or unequal length. During puberty the outer and inner lips start to produce secretions from tiny glands which change the way the vulva smells. Again, every woman's personal scent is different—practice good hygiene, but never use vaginal deodorants.

The clitoris, a small budlike organ, is a highly sensitive part of the vulva that plays an important part in a woman's sexual arousal and her enjoyment of sex. During puberty the clitoris becomes larger. The tip of the clitoris can be felt where the inner lips join just below the mons, and it can be seen—using a mirror—by gently pulling the inner lips apart.

Changes inside the body

The female internal reproductive organs consist of the ovaries, fallopian tubes, uterus, and vagina (see also pp.14–16). During puberty, all of these organs change as a girl becomes sexually mature.

The ovaries
The ovaries become larger during puberty and, in the later stages, start to release eggs. When a girl is born her ovaries contain around 2–4 million primary oocytes ("unripe" eggs). Some of these remain in "suspended animation" from birth until puberty, while others are broken down and reabsorbed into the body; by a girl's first menstrual period about 400,000 unripe eggs remain. In late childhood, the ovaries start to respond to hormones from the pituitary gland (see also pp.20–3), which stimulate them to release the hormone estrogen. This produces some of the external changes visible during puberty. It also causes some of the oocytes inside the ovaries to ripen. Eventually, toward the end of puberty and usually after a girl's menstrual periods have started, a ripe oocyte—now called an egg or ovum—is released from the ovary. This marks the beginning of a regular process of egg release, or ovulation, that will occur every month until a woman reaches menopause, usually in her late forties or early fifties.

The uterus
During puberty, a girl's uterus grows to about the size of her clenched fist, and it generally becomes tilted forward over the bladder. The inner lining of the uterus, the endometrium, becomes thicker, with a more extensive blood supply, in response to hormones released by the ovaries. By the time the first ripe egg is released from the ovary, the endometrium is ready to receive it, should it be fertilized. If, as is usual, it remains unfertilized, the uterus sheds its thickened lining and the girl experiences her first period.

The vagina and cervix

During the growth spurt that occurs at the beginning of puberty, the vagina becomes longer and wider. By carefully inserting a finger inside the vagina it is possible to feel, at its upper end, the cervix. This is the neck of the uterus that projects into the vagina. In the early part of puberty, some two years before a girl has her first period, the vagina produces a clear or milky discharge. This is perfectly normal and natural, and is the result of the cervix and vagina producing fluid that cleans the walls of the vagina. If the discharge has an offensive smell, changes color, or causes irritation, a girl or woman should see her doctor, as these can indicate a vaginal infection. After her periods start, a girl will find that normal vaginal discharge changes on a regular basis during the month. This is because the cervix produces mucus of varying consistency on different days of the menstrual cycle *(see pp.59–60)*.

Menstruation

No event shows more clearly that a girl is becoming sexually mature than the occurrence of her first menstrual period. The menstrual period, also known as menstruation, marks the end of a monthly cycle. In the early part of the cycle, the lining of the uterus thickens in preparation to receive an egg should it be fertilized on its journey from the ovary. Then, if fertilization has not taken place, the spongy tissue of the uterine lining breaks down and menstrual bleeding (menses) begins. For three to seven days the lining of the uterus, along with some blood, flows from the uterus and through the vagina out of the body.

A girl's first period (menarche) marks a rite of passage from childhood to womanhood. This section deals with the beginning of menstruation. *(The menstrual cycle is described in Chapter 1; menstrual problems and pads and tampons are covered on pp.93–5)*

Menarche

Menarche is the time when a girl has her first menstrual period. It usually occurs sometime between the ages of 11 and 14, although it is

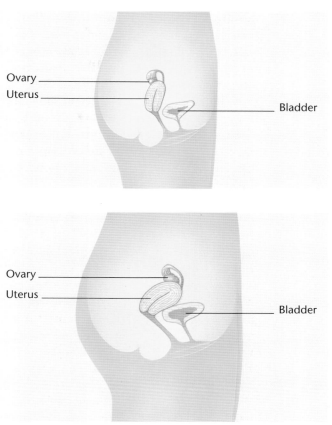

These illustrations of the female body show how the reproductive organs change during puberty. In a young girl (top) the uterus, ovaries, and other reproductive structures are much smaller than in the body of an adult woman (bottom). A girl's uterus is also upright, whereas in an older woman it is normally tilted over the bladder.

THE HYMEN

Just behind the opening of the urethra, through which urine passes, is the opening to the vagina. This opening is partially covered by a membrane called the hymen. The hymen may be torn when a girl first has sexual intercourse, causing a little pain and a small amount of bleeding. However, in many girls, the hymen is already sufficiently stretched that there is no pain, tearing, or bleeding during her first intercourse. The hymen is of little functional value and has only a cultural significance. In some societies, women who are deemed not to have intact hymens are assumed not to be virgins (a virgin is a person who has never experienced sexual intercourse) and are banished or even killed. In other societies, the bed sheets are displayed after the wedding night to show off the bloodstains that indicate the bride was a virgin. Yet to elevate the hymen to such importance is unfair and may cause suffering. Nobody can tell for sure by looking at a woman's hymen whether or not she has ever had sexual intercourse.

quite normal for it to occur earlier or later. Starting her periods is commonly one of the later events of a girl's puberty, generally occurring during stage 4 of development, well after the appearance of breasts and the growth of pubic hair. Occasionally, however, one or two periods may occur in the earliest stages of puberty, and there may then be no more periods for a year or more. Some girls menstruate at intervals of several months all through their pubertal years.

When menarche occurs depends on the individual, although it may be related to the

THE TIME OF MENARCHE

A hundred years ago, the average age for menarche—the first menstrual period—in the United States and Western Europe was 15 years. Today the average is just under 13 years. The reason for this decrease is believed to be improved standards of nutrition. Today, girls at 13 are heavier than their predecessors were at the same age a hundred years ago and carry more body fat. However, the decrease in the average age for menarche has now leveled off and is unlikely to drop much farther.

PREPARING FOR MENSTRUATION

Even if girls have been told what to expect, they can still be confused and uncomfortable about their first periods. Far better than sex education at school, or information from a book, is a personal explanation by a girl's mother (or older female relation, female family friend, or teacher). This personal touch is more effective because an older woman can draw on her own experience of periods, reassure the girl about what will happen, and give her advice about sanitary protection. She can help her understand that periods are a natural part of life and not something to be hidden away. Ideally, an older women should talk to a girl about periods before puberty begins. Obviously, this is easier if parents (or a teacher) have talked about sexual matters to a girl during her childhood. It is also a great help if, when a girl's periods do start, her "coach" is on hand to help with any problems.

time at which a girl's mother started her periods—"early" and "late" starters tend to run in families. But whatever the family pattern, a primary requirement for menarche seems to be a girl's body weight and proportion of body fat. Periods are unlikely to start before the body weighs about 100 pounds and is at least 17 percent fat by weight. This is why young dancers and athletes, who typically have low body weight and body fat, often begin their periods late, or have irregular periods during their teenage years. If a girl has not started her periods by the age of 16, it would be wise to consult a doctor.

The first period may start anywhere—at home, at school, during the day or night. Its arrival may be heralded by small spots of blood in a girl's underpants, so that she has time to use some sort of sanitary protection. More often, it remains unnoticed until a girl detects a slight feeling of wetness. However, some girls only find out their periods have started when friends point out that some blood has soaked through their clothes. Being prepared, by carrying a spare pair of underpants and some sanitary protection, can be a big help if this happens away from home.

First menstrual periods
Once periods have started, they may be irregular with long intervals in between for the first year or so. The reason for this is that the ovary is not yet releasing eggs on a regular basis, nor is it releasing the levels of hormones that produce a regular, monthly menstrual cycle. Like all other aspects of puberty, the regularity of the first periods depends very much on the individual. By the age of 16 or 17, however, many teenagers have regular periods. When she first starts menstruating, a girl shouldn't worry if she misses or has irregular periods, unless she is very underweight (sudden weight loss can cause periods to stop) or unless she has sexual intercourse, in which case she may be pregnant. Other girls may find that the length of each menstrual cycle—the time between one period and the next—varies from month to month. During the first months they have periods, many girls find it helpful to mark the days of their

periods on a calendar so that they can keep track of this new part of their life, a habit that may continue to be useful in adult life.

Just before her periods start, a girl may find she has headaches or feels irritable. At the start of each period, some girls experience menstrual "cramps" *(see pp.95–7)*. These may range from mild aches to acute muscular pain, and some girls also suffer from sweating, nausea, and backache. Relaxation techniques, a hot-water bottle on the abdomen, or pain medication such as ibuprofen may help. Girls tend to outgrow this type of period pain.

For the first few months the menstrual flow may be brown in color, and not the bright red found when periods become more regular. Very often the amount of blood loss is very little during the first few periods. In fact, blood loss during periods is much less than most people imagine. On average, a woman loses about three tablespoonfuls, although anything between 1 teaspoon and ½ cup is normal. In any case, a woman is not losing that volume of pure blood; it is diluted by mucus, and also contains small fragments of the lining of the uterus. And blood loss does not happen suddenly, but over a number of days. Menstrual flow may be light initially and then heavier in the middle of the period, or may be heavy to start with but decrease toward the end of the period.

Pads and tampons

When her periods start, a girl will need to use some sort of sanitary protection to absorb the menstrual blood, and will probably ask her mother what to use. Most girls can use tampons, although they may find insertion a little difficult at first until they get used to it. Mothers may advise their daughters to use pads at first, or to use pads during the night and tampons by day. Girls should be told about the need to change tampons at least every four to six hours, and how to dispose of

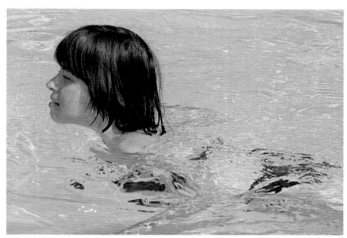

So long as you feel OK, there's no need to change your lifestyle when you have a period. Swimming may even help relieve menstrual cramps if you have them—but if you do go swimming, use a tampon rather than a pad.

QUESTIONS AND ANSWERS: PERIODS

Q. I had my first period six months ago and I haven't had another since then. What should I do about this?
A. When periods first start, the levels of sex hormones—the chemical messengers in the bloodstream that control the events of the menstrual cycle—may still be fluctuating considerably. This means that it is not uncommon for girls to miss periods for months on end, although there is nothing wrong. However, if you have missed your periods for six months you should consult your doctor to see if there is a medical problem. If you have had sexual intercourse since your last period, you should use a home pregnancy test immediately, or ask your doctor to give you a pregnancy test.

Q. I am fourteen and my periods started last year. Can I use tampons instead of pads?
A. Yes, you can use tampons. There is a myth that girls cannot use tampons if they have never had sexual intercourse, but this is not true. The vagina and its opening are quite stretchy, although it might be better to use a small, thin size of tampon at first (some brands offer "junior" sizes). However, if you find that tampons are uncomfortable, use some other type of sanitary protection—such as a pad—and try tampons another time. Tampons should be changed regularly: at least every four to six hours, and usually more frequently at the heaviest time of the period. Be sure to remember to remove the last tampon when your period comes to an end.

pads (and tampon applicators) hygienically, wrapping them in paper or plastic and putting them in a trash can, rather than flushing them down the toilet and risking blocking it.

In a few very rare cases, tampons can cause toxic shock syndrome *(see p.95)*. Anyone who experiences sudden unexplained symptoms when using tampons should stop using them immediately and see a doctor.

Preparing girls for periods

It is best to explain about periods to girls (and boys) as part of a general discussion about

DEVELOPING FASTER THAN OTHERS

Although the changes to your body during puberty take place in a fairly set order, you will find that exactly when they begin and how long they take to complete varies a great deal from one girl to another. You may also find that friends and other girls at school react differently to these changes. As their bodies change shape (or because they haven't yet changed shape), some girls may feel embarrassed or shy about undressing at school, while other girls may feel more confident and adult because they now have a more "grown-up" figure. The thing to remember is that the bodies of adult women come in all shapes and sizes—thin, plump, "boyish," curvy, tall, and short. And while we are all dissatisfied with our bodies and their shape at some time or other, you should try to appreciate your "best" points—and learn to like your body as a whole.

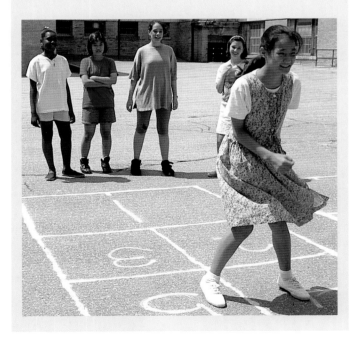

sex. Certainly a girl should have any questions about periods answered by the time she is nine years old. It may be a good idea to explain the following points to her.

• Although accurate prediction of when her periods will start is not really practical, if her body weight is around 100 pounds, she is 11 years of age or over, and her breasts are quite well developed, a girl should be prepared for the start of her periods.

• In theory a girl can get pregnant when she has her first periods, even though ovulation (the release of eggs from the uterus) might not occur during the first menstrual cycles. For this reason contraception should be used if a girl has sexual intercourse at this age. Of course, it is also valid to ask whether a girl is mentally and emotionally mature enough to consent to or embark upon a sexual relationship involving intercourse at this age.

• Periods should not stop a girl from doing anything she wants. For example, if she uses tampons *(see pp.93–4)*, she can go swimming at any time, provided she feels well enough and her periods are not excessively heavy—swimming may ease cramps, but can also make menstrual flow heavier. If she uses pads, she will not be able to go swimming when she has a period, unless it is very light.

• Although girls may experience menstrual cramps either just before or during their periods, they are not an inevitable accompaniment to menstruation. Menstrual cramps can range widely in intensity and duration, depending on the individual. (*Methods for pain relief are described on pp.96-7.*)

• On average, a period lasts from three to seven days, with the heaviest flow on days two and three. But every woman is different and a period may last for one day or eight days, and may vary in length from month to month. The first periods are usually shorter, with little blood flow, but they become longer as the menstrual cycle settles down.

• In theory, the menstrual cycle is 28 days long. In actual fact, some women do have 28-day cycles, but others' cycles are longer or shorter and may vary from month to month. The first menstrual cycles tend to be irregular and then settle into a more regular pattern.

Puberty in boys

For most boys, the first changes that occur during puberty involve the growth of the penis, testes, and pubic hair. As these develop and the body grows and becomes more muscular, body hair appears and the voice becomes deeper. In later puberty a boy experiences his first ejaculation as his internal reproductive organs produce seminal fluid and his testes begin to manufacture sperm. By the end of puberty, boys are typically larger and more muscular than girls of the same age.

Development of the penis, testes, and pubic hair

In much the same way as the development in girls of pubic hair and breasts can be divided into stages (see pp.54–7), so the changes to a boy's penis and testes, and the growth of his pubic hair, can also be divided into five stages. It should be remembered, however, that these stages give only an indication of the order in which changes occur during puberty and that in reality the stages merge into each other. When each stage begins, and how long it lasts, depends on the individual. Some boys may start changing at the age of 9; others may not show any changes until they are 16. The stages of development are illustrated below and on the next page. Note that the penis shown here is uncircumcised (circumcision is described on p.26).

Stage 1

This is the childhood stage of development, between birth and puberty. The penis and testes grow gradually, as the rest of the body grows, but there is none of the pubic hair that can be seen in adults. During the later part of this stage, when a boy is about 10 years old, hormones that will initiate the external changes to his body are released from his testes.

Stage 2

The changes that occur during this stage, which generally starts between the ages of 11 and 12, mark the beginning of puberty. The

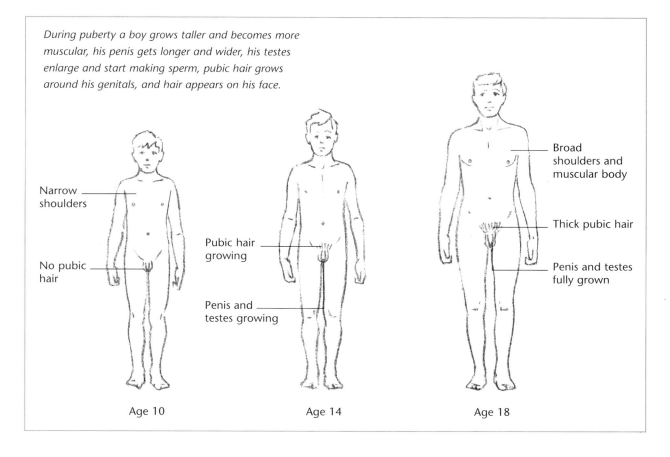

During puberty a boy grows taller and becomes more muscular, his penis gets longer and wider, his testes enlarge and start making sperm, pubic hair grows around his genitals, and hair appears on his face.

Narrow shoulders

No pubic hair

Pubic hair growing

Penis and testes growing

Broad shoulders and muscular body

Thick pubic hair

Penis and testes fully grown

Age 10   Age 14   Age 18

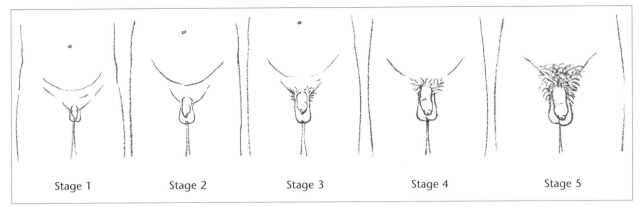

| Stage 1 | Stage 2 | Stage 3 | Stage 4 | Stage 5 |

Between the ages of 10 and 18 a boy's genitals take on an adult appearance. Shown here are the typical changes that occur, although these vary, as do the shape and size of penis, the amount of pubic hair, and whether the penis is circumcised or, as here, not.

two testes, which lie behind the penis and between the legs, grow at a much faster rate than they did during childhood, as they prepare for their role of sperm production. The testes also release the male sex hormone testosterone, which will control the production of the secondary sex characteristics that appear in this and the following stages. The skin of the scrotum, the "bag" of skin that holds the testes, thins out, becomes looser and more wrinkly, darkens or becomes redder, and hangs lower between the legs. The "baggy" scrotum enables the testes to hang away from the body's core, thereby keeping them at a lower temperature than the rest of the body, one which is optimal for sperm production.

During this stage, many boys also find their first pubic hairs growing at the base of the penis, where it joins the body. At first, these hairs are often straight and fairly similar to the hair on the head, but over time, as they spread around the base of the penis, they become curly, coarse pubic hair. Although his testes increase in size, the boy's penis remains much the same length. On average, stage 2 lasts about 13 months.

Stage 3
Sometime between the ages of 12 and 13, on average, the penis starts to grow, although at first it gets longer rather than wider. During this stage, the testes continue to grow and the scrotum becomes even darker in color. Most boys will notice at this stage, especially if they look in the mirror, that one testis—usually the left—begins to hang lower than the other. This is perfectly normal and is an

adaptation to stop the testes from pressing on each other during walking or running; squashed testes, as all men are aware, are extremely painful. Another change visible on both the scrotum and parts of the penis are small dots or bumps on the skin's surface. These are either the points from which pubic hairs are growing, or are about to grow, or they are skin glands that start to release an oily type of sweat—which gives the genital area a different type of smell—during puberty. In either case they are completely normal. Finally, pubic hair, now more coarse and curly, spreads across the base of the penis to reach the legs. Some hair may also sprout around the anus at this time. On average, stage 3 lasts about 10 months.

Stage 4
This stage generally starts between the ages of 13 and 15. The testes and scrotum continue to enlarge, while the penis gets both wider and longer. The glans or tip of the penis also becomes larger. During this stage, the testes and the internal glands that produce semen become fully functional, and many boys experience their first ejaculation, through masturbation *(see pp.72–4)* or during a "wet dream" *(see p.66).* The covering of pubic hair extends to form an upside-down triangle, with its apex at the base of the penis. It may also extend upward toward the navel, although, strictly speaking,

this growth consists of ordinary body hair rather than pubic hair. By this stage the pubic hair also looks and feels more like adult pubic hair in texture; it is usually coarser-textured and noticeably darker in color than the hair on its owner's head. On average, stage 4 lasts about two years.

Stage 5

By the time a boy reaches the age of 15 or 16, on average, he will have started to resemble a young adult in terms of his physique. His penis, testes, and scrotum are reaching full adult size. However, it must be remembered that these stages of development are not always the same. Some boys may reach this final stage earlier than 15; others may not reach full physical maturity until they are 17 or 18.

Penis shape and size

Of all the worries most males have about their body, penis size reigns supreme, whether the individual is 15 or 50. During puberty, penis size is probably more of an issue than it is during adult life for two reasons. First, because boys mature at different rates, boys of the same age will naturally show variation in penis size. And second, they have plenty of chances to compare penis size when changing or showering at school before or after gym or sports practice.

It is true that, when soft, not all penises are the same length, although they are generally between 3¼ and 4¼ inches. But when erect, most penises are between 5 and 7 inches long from base to tip. During erection *(see pp.28–9)*, smaller penises increase proportionately more in size than larger penises. Another factor is that boys and men usually view their own organ by looking down at it—a process that makes it seem shorter—while inspecting other boys' penises from the front or side—which makes others' penises look longer in comparison. Boys who are overweight may think that they have a small penis, although it is probably the normal length, "buried" in the mound of fat at its base. The greatest damage, however, is probably done by the locker-room discussions that perpetuate the myth, as they probably have done for thousands of years, that penis size is an indicator of sexual prowess. In reality, penis size has nothing to do with how many erections or orgasms you can have, and little or nothing to do with whether you can satisfy your partner during sexual intercourse.

QUESTIONS AND ANSWERS: EMBARRASSMENTS OF PUBERTY

Q. I am 14 and my penis is really tiny. I feel so depressed because I wouldn't dare take my clothes off in front of anyone in case they laughed at me. I have to cover myself up in the showers at school. What can I do?

A. The sizes of penises when soft are very variable. But the sizes of erect penises are very similar, usually between 5 and 7 inches in length. You will probably find that, when erect, your penis is much the same size as those of your friends at school. It may also be that, because you are still only 14, your penis has not yet grown to its full length and width. However, if your testes have enlarged, and your pubic hair is widespread, and you are worried that your penis is too small, you should consider consulting your doctor to check there is no problem.

Q. After a football game we were in the showers and I got an erection. Everybody laughed at me and said I must be gay. But I'm not interested in other boys in a sexual way. Is there something wrong with me?

A. During puberty, erections seem to happen with annoying frequency at the wrong time. A boy is just as likely to get an unexpected erection while sitting in a boring class as he is by looking at a sexually exciting picture. The sexual turmoil of puberty tends to give the penis a "mind of its own"; erections can happen at any time, so having an erection in a shower full of boys is perfectly normal.

Q. I am 15 and I keep having wet dreams. I get so embarrassed because I know my mother must see the stains on the sheets. How can I stop having them?

A. Having wet dreams is a perfectly normal part of puberty. It just means that the sperm-producing part of your reproductive system is in full working order. The marks on the sheets can be embarrassing, although most parents will understand. Try wearing underpants in bed, and keep some tissues by the bed to wipe away the semen. That will help reduce the staining.

Erections

Erections do not start happening at puberty. Boys experience erections from before birth, when they are still in their mother's womb. However, it is during puberty that erections become more frequent and are noticed more, as sexual feelings and thoughts develop as a natural part of growing up. During an erection, the penis becomes stiffer and harder because blood floods into its spongy tissues. The biological reason for this is to facilitate its insertion into the vagina during sexual intercourse. The penis becomes erect in response to messages from the brain. And the reasons why the brain sends out these messages are varied. It could be because the boy is having thoughts about sex or looking at sexual images, or is touching himself or being touched sexually. Or it could be because he is feeling excited about something, or for no particular reason. Many boys and men wake up in the morning

DEALING WITH UNEXPECTED ERECTIONS

Unexpected erections are one of the more unwelcome aspects of developing sexuality in boys. They can happen at any time: on the bus; reading a magazine; in a gym class; talking to a girl; or walking down the street. A boy will probably not be thinking about anything sexual at the time, but his body will still send messages along the relevant nerves so that he has an erection. Remember two things. First, that it happens to most boys. And second, that if you think of something dull (like homework) the erection should go away.

TALKING TO BOYS ABOUT WET DREAMS

Ejaculation is a sign that a boy is becoming sexually mature and reaching the end of puberty. For many boys, their first experience of ejaculation is a wet dream. If this is the case, but they are not prepared for it, a wet dream may be confusing or frightening. The feeling of waking up with a cold, damp patch on the sheets can be unpleasant: a boy may think that he has wet the bed with urine, or that he has some strange disease. It is a great help to a boy if his father or mother can talk to him about ejaculation and wet dreams in a matter-of-fact way early in puberty so that he regards them as perfectly normal. Fathers can be especially helpful because they can refer to their own experiences when talking to their sons.

with an erection. This is because erections occur naturally during dreaming (whether or not the dream is about something sexual), or because they may be stimulated by having a full bladder. Frequent and unexpected erections during the teenage years causes many boys some embarrassment *(see box, below)*, however, these are perfectly normal and their frequency decreases considerably as a boy gets older.

Ejaculation and wet dreams

During puberty many boys find pleasure in touching and rubbing their penis during masturbation. Initially they may find that although they reach orgasm—a peak of pleasure *(see p.177)*—they do not ejaculate *(see p.29)* because sperm and semen production are not yet in full operation. But eventually most boys discover that as they reach orgasm during masturbation, they also ejaculate, the muscles at the base of the penis contracting to squirt out sperm-containing semen. This is normal and an important sign that the body is growing up, just as the first period is an indicator of impending biological sexual maturity for a female during puberty.

Many boys also experience wet dreams (or nocturnal emissions, to give them a fancier name). These happen automatically when a boy is asleep and dreaming, although not necessarily dreaming about anything sexual. It can be a confusing shock to experience a wet dream for the first time, waking up in a sticky puddle of semen, especially for a boy who does not know what is happening or has not ejaculated before. But, once again, wet dreams are perfectly normal. They become less frequent with age and increasing sexual activity, but may still occur during adult life.

Body hair

Testosterone, the male sex hormone that causes the growth of pubic hair during puberty, also encourages growth of coarser, longer hair in the armpits, and on the chest, face, arms, and legs. A similar hormone encourages growth of pubic and armpit hair in females. The first hairs generally appear in the center of the chest and around the nipples. How hairy a man's body becomes depends, like his other features, on what characteristics he has inherited from his parents. Some men have a thick covering of body hair on their chest and back, while others have completely bare chests and backs. However, hairiness generally increases with age.

Facial hair and shaving

Sometime between the ages of 13 and 15, hair that is longer than the normal fine vellus hair (which covers the body in childhood) starts to grow on a boy's face, and the first signs of a mustache and beard appear. The amount and extent of this facial hair vary enormously from one individual to the next, depending on the characteristics a boy inherits from his parents, and on his ethnic origin: males from some ethnic backgrounds tend to have more facial hair than others. The first facial hairs, often looking like peach fuzz, appear on the upper lip. Over time, they spread outward to the cheeks and chin, although many men cannot grow a full beard until some years after puberty has ended.

Once the first facial hairs arrive, many boys feel the need to get rid of them by shaving. Shaving is a sign of growing up that some boys deal with very easily but others feel embarrassed about. Many fathers, or other adult males, are willing to recommend a type of razor for shaving, although the disposable razors available in supermarkets and drugstores are easy to use. Initially, shaving is only necessary once or twice a week, but by the early twenties it is usually a daily or even twice-daily requirement.

Voice breaking

As the body grows during puberty, so does the larynx or voice box, the expanded upper region of the windpipe that produces sounds. This larger larynx produces the "Adam's apple" that protrudes from the front of the throat. When the larynx grows, the vocal cords—membranes that stretch across the inside of the larynx and vibrate when air passes between them, so producing sounds—get thicker and longer, making a boy's voice sound deeper. This generally occurs between the ages of 14 or 15, but may be earlier or later. Some boys experience a gradual transition from the high-pitched voice of childhood to the deeper adult voice, while others appear to switch overnight, an experience which is described as the voice "breaking." In either case, boys may find, much to their embarrassment, that their voice suddenly switches back from sounding deep to sounding high-pitched and squeaky. This phase does not last long.

What is normal?
Developing at different rates

As has been described already, boys start puberty at different ages, and go through the stages of puberty at different rates. A boy who starts maturing early may feel more confident

---

QUESTION AND ANSWER: A MANLY BUILD

Q. Some of my friends at school have become more powerful with bigger muscles during the past year. I still look like a skinny kid. Will I ever look like them without doing daily weight training?
A. You may feel as though you are lagging a bit behind your friends in terms of your development, but you will soon catch up. Everybody reaches the stages of puberty at different times and the increase in muscle bulk occurs during the later stages. But you have to remember as well that all boys (and adults) have different body shapes.

BREAST DEVELOPMENT

Some boys experience a small degree of breast development during puberty. This comes as a shock to many boys because they think of breast development as a female characteristic. Sometimes a small bump appears under one or both nipples and occasionally a larger growth appears. Such breast development, which can cause the type of soreness or aching that girls feel as their breasts grow, is called gynecomastia. It can be upsetting for boys, especially if they are teased by their friends, but these growths are perfectly normal, a temporary product of the hormones that appear during puberty. Breast swellings generally last for between 2 and 18 months.

than his peers and see his early maturity as an advantage, but these feelings will probably disappear as his contemporaries catch up with him. A boy who starts puberty later than his contemporaries may worry that he will never catch up and that he will be mocked by his peers; however, all boys eventually reach a similar stage of maturity.

Emotions and relationships

At the same time that the physical changes of puberty are taking place in their bodies, adolescents' mental and emotional attributes are also evolving. Typically, they progress through some or all of the changes mentioned below before reaching adulthood.

A major worry for many adolescents is their appearance as they consciously seek a self-image. They can be moody and argumentative with members of their family. They need more privacy than they had in childhood and may no longer be as close to their family as they were. They often form close friendships, at first with friends of their own sex and later with members of the opposite sex; these friendships may develop into intimate, sometimes sexual relationships. Adolescents recognize their developing sexuality and sexual preferences. Overall, adolescence sees a young person becoming more independent, acquiring a greater sense of self-identity, and achieving an increasing mental capacity as he or she progresses from childhood to adulthood. By the end of adolescence they will usually have adult feelings of independence and self-reliance.

Self-image and body image

Adolescents in particular are very concerned about their self-image—their own perception of their personal attractiveness—and link this very closely to their body image, the way they see their own bodies. This concern is evident from the way many teenagers constantly check their appearance in the mirror and

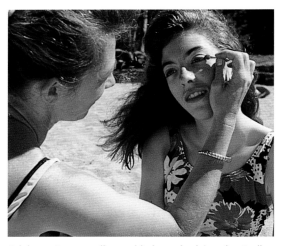

Adolescents generally need help and advice about all kinds of matters from parents, as shown here by a mother helping her daughter with her makeup.

worry about their body shape and their weight and height. Such obsession with self-image is encouraged by the prevalent idea in some societies that personal worth is to be measured by the way people look, and is heightened by the fact that during adolescence the body is undergoing rapid change. Secondary sex characteristics cause particular concern, because of the differences in the degree and timing of their development. Girls are especially aware of their breast development because the size of their breasts can be seen when they are fully clothed and easily appraised by other teenage girls, who may have larger, smaller, or more "desirable" breasts themselves. Boys will also take notice of girls' breast development for many reasons, both sexual and social.

A boy's physical features are less visible, until he removes his clothes in the locker room. Here boys who are making slower progress with the changes of puberty may be mocked for their small penis, lack of pubic hair, or undeveloped body muscles. There seems to be no doubt that there is a strong relationship between personal attractiveness and social acceptance during adolescence. Adolescents' deep concern with body image appears to underpin this relationship and explains the pain and depression that many young people experience if they have negative feelings about their self-image.

Communicating with parents

Contrary to popular belief, adolescence is not necessarily a time when teenagers and their parents have a stormy relationship, nor is it a time when a generation gap develops. True, many adolescents seek the advice of their peers about matters such as clothes, music, and relationships, but they usually still refer to their parents about important matters and, in early adolescence at least, show a high degree of dependence.

Conflicts between children and parents during adolescence commonly arise over relatively minor matters such as loud music, messy bedrooms, and general selfishness. Parents may also indicate their unhappiness with their child's—especially their daughter's —burgeoning sexuality by disapproving of any overtly sexy clothes she may want to wear when going out with her friends. There is a tendency for conflicts to take place particularly between teenagers and their mothers —regardless of the child's sex—probably because mothers are often the family member who organizes and regulates the household.

Teenagers are often characterized as being egocentric and selfish. This can happen for a number of reasons. First, many adolescents are obsessed with their own self-image and style, so what can seem like tiny matters of detail to others—such as the desire to have a particular brand of jeans—becomes all-important to the teenager. Second, they have a different concept of time from that of their parents: forgetting to do the chores may be the result of daydreaming rather than selfishness. Third, young people tend to assume that others share their own preoccupations and therefore automatically understand why they appear so obsessive in their behavior.

Parents can be as confused as their children by the arrival of adolescence. The child who has always been close suddenly demands privacy, may be short-tempered and rude, no longer wants to join in family activities, and wants to spend more time with their friends. Adolescents need to understand that, in general, although parents may irritate them by their attitudes, a parent's main concern is to safeguard their children's well-being. If both sides—parents and children—know what to expect during adolescence, then it is easier for both to adjust to the changes and reach the compromises necessary to ensure that the child is allowed to grow up, while still following the rules of the family.

It is important for both parents and adolescents to develop a working relationship in which the parents still maintain the family system. However, it is equally important that adolescents be allowed some independence and the right to have a say in family issues.

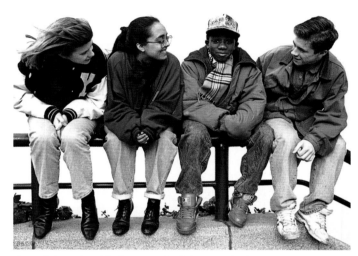

One of the enjoyable features of adolescence is the formation of strong friendships that enable boys and girls to develop a separate identity outside the family.

PEER PRESSURE

Pressure from friends of the same age can be irresistible. The urge to conform to a certain image during a time of change and uncertainty is very strong. Friends may try to convince an adolescent to skip school, take drugs, or have sex, when he or she may not want to do these things. The point to remember is that if saying no to peer pressure means that those friends drop you, they may not be very good friends. It is generally far better for you to make your own deliberate decisions, to be assertive, and to say "no" if you are being pressured into doing something you feel is wrong. Don't allow yourself to drift into unpleasant situations in response to peer pressure.

Friendships

Friendships are important because they allow the adolescent to develop a different identity outside the family context, experimenting with their self-image, developing a social life, and having new experiences without direct parental supervision. The first friendships during adolescence are often with members of the same sex. These friendships are frequently stronger than those experienced in childhood; they usually last longer and involve a greater degree of commitment and sharing. Good friends are people with whom everyday problems and the ups and downs of life can be shared, and who do not try to impose their will on anyone else.

Some children develop friendships with members of the opposite sex from an early age that continue throughout adolescence. Others may not wish to develop close friendships with the opposite sex until they reach their late teens or early twenties. Still others may have close relationships with both sexes

PARENTS AS ROLE MODELS

Adolescents may act as though their parents are aliens from another planet, but in fact they watch and are influenced by what their parents do and say. This is especially important when talking to adolescents about "boundaries" as they get older. It is easy to tell a child that he or she should not smoke or drink, but parents should bear in mind that if they smoke or drink themselves, the message they are trying to send will be devalued. Similarly, a parent who has just been through a divorce may not be perceived by their teenager as a reliable authority on the suitability of a boyfriend or girlfriend.

Parents must remember that they are also sexual role models. Even if they find it difficult to talk to their children about sex, they must be aware that children are affected by adult attitudes toward sex. If parents have negative attitudes about it that they convey to their children, adolescents may adopt similar views. Similarly, if parents are disparaging about specific aspects of sex (homosexual relationships, for example), children may develop similar prejudices or incur deep feelings of guilt if their own sexuality appears to differ from the "norm." When couples are open and positive about sex—while at the same time maintaining privacy with regard to their own sexual relationship—their children are more likely to have a positive and informed view of sexuality.

throughout adolescence but eventually find that their sexual preferences are homosexual. As mentioned elsewhere in this book, every individual is different, and there is no universally wrong or right pattern of behavior during adolescence.

Dating

Adolescence is a time when teenagers begin to get to know about themselves and about members of the opposite sex. In their early teens, boys and girls tend to form close friendships with members of their own sex. As they get older, they start going around in mixed-sex groups. Then, typically between the ages of 14 and 16, a teenage boy and girl may feel that they want to spend more time together on their own and get to know each other on a one-to-one basis, so they start to go out on dates together. Young women generally start dating from around the age of 14 or 15, while young men tend to start about a year later. Sometimes dating involves little more than a special friendship; in other cases it may become physically intense, or develop into a serious steady relationship.

Parents may be pleased to see their teenagers starting to date, taking it as a sign of their teenager's popularity, independence, and developing maturity. In some cases, however, parental intervention is wise if a teenager becomes obsessed with a boyfriend or girlfriend and does not have time for any other interests. On the other hand, parents should be careful not to belittle a son or daughter's first relationship as trivial, just when he or she is starting to learn about developing intimate relationships.

Dating can be fun, but it can also be painful. Many adolescents may find it difficult to build up the courage to ask out a boy or girl that they like. Inevitably, attraction is not always mutual, and rejection can be hard to take. And if a close relationship comes to an end, the teenager may suffer even more terrible feelings of rejection and depression. When things do go wrong, parents, brothers, sisters, and other members of the family circle should try to be supportive.

Starting a relationship

All sorts of factors may attract one person to another *(see pp.181–4)*. It could be the way they look, their sense of humor, the things they say, the way they listen to what another person is saying, or all of these things. It may be difficult at first for a teenager to communicate the feelings they have for someone else for fear of being embarrassed or rejected. However, if two teenagers are attracted to each other, this may be clear from their body language. Body language *(see box, below)* is the way in which we communicate with one another without using words. We use body language every day to "say" things like: "You are standing too close," "I find you really attractive," or "I wish you would go away."

Relationships may last for just one date, or for months or years. In long-lasting relationships the other person may become all-important in someone's life. A good relationship is one in which neither partner is dominant and both maintain their self-esteem, while being good friends to each other.

Just because a relationship has become established does not mean that it has to be sexual. Nobody should be forced into having sex against their will. Everyone should make a decision about what is the right time and who is the right partner. And remember that it is illegal for young men or women to have intercourse under a certain age, although the specific ages vary from state to state.

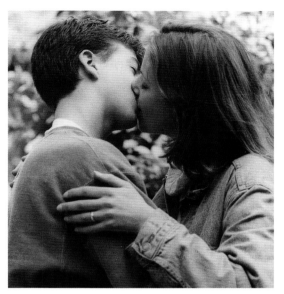

These two kissing teenagers are clearly very attracted to each other, although at this age their relationship may be short-lived.

BODY LANGUAGE

You can't expect to have instant rapport with everyone you meet, so don't feel rejected if you don't. You may find someone a complete bore...and they might feel the same about you! Try not to take it personally. This is where body language—using the body to convey a message—can be used. By reading another person's body language it is possible to avoid wasting time with someone who is not interested. Alternatively, you can improve your chances of attracting someone else if you make your body language more positive, and especially by maintaining eye contact with them *(see also pp.182–4)*.

BEING ASSERTIVE

Being assertive means saying what you feel without being aggressive, without compromising your position, and, hopefully, without hurting someone else. Being assertive will help you avoid painful and embarrassing misunderstandings. There are a number of situations where it helps to be assertive:
- **When someone you don't like asks you for a date.**
Be honest and say that you are not really interested. If you put it off by saying "maybe next week" or "give me a call," you are being cruel because you are giving the impression that you might be interested. And when they do find out that you are not interested, they will feel both rejected and patronized.
- **When your boyfriend or girlfriend wants to do something that you don't want to do.**
When you care passionately about someone, it is difficult not to feel you have to do what they want. For example, your boyfriend may try to pressure you into having sex with him. But if you don't want to, be firm and refuse. Just because you are dating, it doesn't mean that you have become someone else's possession.
- **When a close friend asks about changing your relationship to a more romantic or sexual one and you don't want to have that kind of relationship with them.**
The best strategy is probably to say that you feel that if you had a more intimate relationship with him or her it might ruin a good friendship—and you would prefer to remain friends. They may feel rejected and hurt for a while, but if you really are good friends, your friendship should recover, given time.

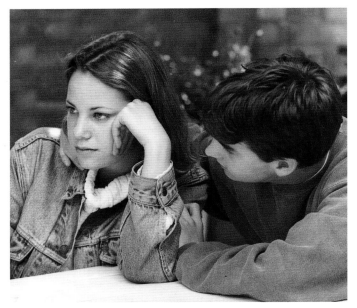

Relationships do not always work out. One of you may just lose interest. Or you may sometimes find it difficult to express, or even to know, how you feel.

When relationships end

Relationships rarely run smoothly. One moment it appears that two people care about each other very deeply, and then suddenly —be they adolescents or emotionally experienced adults—everything seems to collapse. Bear in mind that everyone, not just adolescents, sometimes misinterprets how someone else is feeling: it may be that the problem is just a question of miscommunication, and simply talking to each other may be enough to straighten things out.

But relationships do fall apart. It is in the nature of a relationship to become focused on another person, who becomes an important part of one's life in a number of ways—as friend, lover, critic, flatterer. If feelings change, and a relationship ends, suddenly all that disappears, leaving an individual with a gap in their existence. At first, the feeling of loss can be almost too much to bear, especially for the partner who has been left. With time, however, the hurt will usually become less until—older but wiser—the individual looks back and wonders why that person ever played such an important part in their life. Despite the pain, it is best to make a clean break rather than going through the motions if the feeling has gone: a final good-bye may be less hurtful in the end than continuing the relationship until it grinds to a halt.

Parents and the end of relationships

The end of a relationship—especially the first one—can be very painful, leaving an adolescent with a feeling of loss similar to bereavement. It helps greatly if parents can listen and be supportive, even if from their perspective the situation is not so serious. It probably won't help to tell a teenager they will get over it, but sympathy—and a shoulder to cry on—means a lot to most young people.

Becoming a sexual being

During adolescence, many teenagers start to have strong sexual feelings, think about sex a lot, and find themselves becoming sexually aroused. They may develop a crush on a teacher, a movie or rock star, or an older friend of their brother or sister, although they may not be ready to have an actual sexual relationship. Other teenagers do not experience such strong sexual feelings, but that does not mean that they will not do so in the future. By the time they reach their late teens, a majority of adolescents, both boys and girls, will have had some kind of sexual experience, and many will have had sexual intercourse.

Parents may feel unsettled as they recognize their children's developing sexuality. It is probably best to try to talk about sexual matters, to ensure that teenagers understand the need for sexual partners to respect each other and the importance of contraception and safe sex—and to help them have the confidence to make decisions responsibly.

Masturbation

One of the main ways that teenagers learn about their sexual body is by self-exploration. As they change and develop, adolescents inspect their bodies to check on what is happening to them. Boys will look at, and even

QUESTIONS AND ANSWERS: SEXUAL EXPLORATION

Q. I often masturbate at least once a day. Is this wrong? Will I run out of sperm by the time I get older?

A. There is nothing wrong with masturbation. It allows individuals to explore their own sexuality and discover what gives them sexual pleasure. And there is no danger of sperm running out when you're older. The testes manufacture sperm by the millions each and every day. Nor do sperm build up if you don't masturbate. They are eventually broken down inside the testes and their raw materials recycled.

Q. My friend and I are both 16 and we have just started going out with boys. Our boyfriends have both asked us if we would like to try oral sex. What does it mean?

A. Oral sex means arousing your partner by kissing or licking his penis, or for him to stimulate your clitoris and vaginal lips in the same way. While many people enjoy this as a part of sex, some people do not. Neither attitude is wrong. But however you feel about the idea of oral sex, don't be persuaded by your boyfriend into having any kind of sex until you are ready.

measure, the size of their penis, at the same time discovering the pleasurable sensations experienced when it is rubbed and stroked. Similarly, girls may examine and perhaps measure their breasts, and start exploring and stroking their clitoris and vulva, often when they are lying in bed, or bathing or showering.

Gradually, adolescents tend to focus on their genitals and spend time masturbating—arousing themselves sexually. Besides discovering it on their own, they may also find out about masturbation from brothers, sisters, friends, books, or magazines. Masturbation is a normal part of adolescent behavior, and one that often continues on into adult life. Not all adolescents masturbate, however: not masturbating is perfectly normal as well.

Boys usually start masturbating earlier than girls because, initially at least, their sex drive is more genitally focused. Younger adolescent girls are traditionally more involved with romantic feelings at first, and they generally take longer to explore themselves sexually in this way. For young people of both sexes, however, masturbation often provides their first sexual experience. There are no fixed ways to masturbate. Each individual has their own way of giving themselves sexual pleasure, although there are certain patterns common to many people.

Boys can become aroused by thinking about something sexual, or by stroking their penis or other parts of their body that are especially sensitive. As he becomes aroused,

the boy's penis stiffens and becomes erect. A boy usually masturbates by grasping the shaft of his penis and moving his hand up and down rhythmically to stimulate the shaft and the glans (the head of the penis), its most sensitive part. Some boys may also stimulate their penis by rubbing it against a pillow. As a boy becomes more and more aroused, the muscles start to tighten around the base of his penis, anus, and buttocks; he generally increases the speed of rubbing or stroking until he reaches orgasm and ejaculates semen from the tip of the penis (although at first he may find he has an orgasm but does not ejaculate, because his semen-producing organs are not yet working fully). Boys may use a tissue or their hand to catch the semen when it comes out, to stop it from leaving stains on the bed or wherever they may be masturbating. The penis then rapidly becomes soft, and it takes some time before a boy can become aroused again.

Like boys, girls may also become sexually aroused by having sexual thoughts or by touching sensitive parts of the body, such as the breasts and vulva. Many girls masturbate by using their fingers to stroke and rub around their clitoris and vulval lips. As a girl becomes aroused, her clitoris enlarges and her vagina, and often her labia, become wet. Some girls moisten their fingers with saliva, or with vaginal liquid, before rubbing around the clitoris, so that the friction does not make the area sore. As arousal increases, and clitoral stimulation continues, muscle tension builds in the pelvis and buttocks until orgasm is reached and a feeling of intense pleasure ripples though the genitals, uterus, and the rest of the body. Masturbation can happen in other ways as well. Some girls like to rub their vulva against a pillow or to tighten and release the muscles that surround their vagina and anus, or to spray water against their clitoris when taking a shower. In contrast to boys, girls may be able to have several orgasms, one following the other, in the course of a single masturbatory session.

Guilt about masturbation is common. This may result from adolescents being admonished as children for touching their genitals (see p.41). Such guilt feelings are often reinforced by stories from peers, and perhaps parents, to the effect that masturbation can make a person go blind, insane, or sterile, or cause other harm. These stories, now fortunately proved to be completely unfounded, are a legacy of the 19th century, when many authorities regarded masturbation as not only harmful but evil as well, and did their best to scare adolescents sufficiently to stop them from practicing it. Another fear is that indulging in masturbation will stop adolescents from enjoying a normal sex life with

SEXUAL FANTASIES

Fantasies are daydreams or imaginings experienced by most people. A person might fantasize that they are a famous singer or a great tennis player. Fantasies are not real and lie purely in the realms of the imagination. Sexual fantasies are exactly the same, except that the focus is erotic and sexual. It is quite common and perfectly normal to fantasize sexually while masturbating. Often the fantasy takes the form of visualizing a sexual situation with one or more partners. What may worry adolescents is that familiar people such as brothers, sisters, teachers, or friends of the same sex may appear in their fantasies, or that the fantasies involve doing things that they would never do in real life. If adolescents are worried about this, they should be reassured by the fact that fantasies have nothing to do with real life and are just one way to enhance sexual stimulation.

any future partner. In fact, however, most people find that learning to understand how their body responds sexually through masturbation actually helps them to enjoy sex even more, and enables them to communicate to their partner what they enjoy and what arouses them (see also p.180).

Same-sex experiences

Although masturbation is usually a private experience, it is not uncommon for some boys to masturbate together, or sometimes to masturbate each other, when they are in their early teens. This is all part of learning about their body's sensuality and does not necessarily mean that they are developing homosexual feelings and will grow up as gay adults— although, of course, that may happen. Girls may also masturbate together, although it seems that this is generally less common than in the case of boys. Once again, this is simply part of the process of growing up and should not be taken as an indicator of someone's future sexual preferences.

Early sexual experiences

Most teenagers go on their first dates between the ages of 14 and 16. Their first sexual experiences are likely to start with kissing and hugging, and to progress to more intimate sexual exploration, known as petting. Initially, this can involve touching each other's clothed body, including the breasts and genitals. With more intense petting, a boy may touch a girl's breasts and stroke her vulva, especially her clitoris, while the girl may touch a boy's penis and scrotum. In both cases they may give each other an orgasm.

Some couples use their lips and tongue to stimulate each other's genitals. This is known as oral sex. It may lead to orgasm but carries no risk of pregnancy; however, there is a risk of passing on sexually transmitted diseases.

Early sexual experiences depend very much on the individual and what they enjoy. Neither partner should feel obliged to do anything they feel unhappy about. They may choose to abstain from intense sexual contact until they are in a settled relationship.

Becoming sexually active

Intercourse takes sexual intimacy a step further. During sexual intercourse, a man or boy puts his penis into a woman or girl's vagina, and they move together in a way that stimulates his penis and her vagina and clitoris. Often he, and sometimes she, will reach orgasm through such intercourse. If they do not use contraception, the risk of pregnancy is substantial. And if they fail to use a latex condom, properly and with every encounter, there is the possibility of catching or spreading a sexually transmitted disease—including the HIV virus (which causes AIDS).

Provided both partners are willing participants and both accept responsibility for their actions and take the right precautions, sexual intercourse can be pleasurable and fulfilling. At first, intercourse may be awkward because of lack of experience. But partners usually become more relaxed and proficient with time, and often their sex lives become more enjoyable as they mature.

However, having intercourse with a partner within a relationship requires trust and responsibility. There is no need for anyone to be more active sexually than they themselves feel ready for, and no one should be cajoled or forced into having intercourse against his or her wishes. Some boys may try to persuade their partner to have intercourse by threatening that they will reject them or break up with them if they do not. If he does this he should be told "no" very clearly and firmly. Boys themselves should not feel pressured by their male friends' accounts of their own sexual activities, which may well be exaggerated. Apart from the fact that all states have an "age of consent" (usually around 16) below which sexual intercourse is illegal, research has shown that many adolescents who have intercourse at a young age regret it later and wish that they had waited until they were older.

Sexual intercourse is, of course, not the only form of sexual contact. Many couples enjoy mutual masturbation and oral sex. In the end, everyone is different; there is no right or wrong way to be sexually active.

SEX THE FIRST TIME

Whatever it was like, most people never forget the first time they had sexual intercourse. How you will feel is difficult to predict—it depends on the individual. It may help if:
• you can find a quiet, comfortable place to have sex where you will not be disturbed
• you know how to arouse each other, so that the girl's vagina is lubricated and the boy's penis slips in fairly easily without causing discomfort
• you are not expecting fireworks—sexual pleasuring is something that has to be learned
• a boy is not upset if he ejaculates very quickly —this often happens the first few times.
Finally, it is important to use contraception and practice safe sex the first time—and every time.

Nor is it wrong to not have sex at all. It is worth remembering that, although adolescents are physically able to have a sex life, they are not required to be sexually active. Some adolescents may actively choose abstinence and want to delay having any sexual relationship until they have found a partner to whom they feel fully committed, or until they get married. Other adolescents may show little interest in sex. This, too, is quite normal.

Talking about sex

Many of the problems that all couples, and not just adolescents, have with their sex lives are caused by simple lack of communication. Talking—tactfully—about sex with a partner will help him or her to understand what you enjoy during sex, and teach you what stimulates your partner. Unless a person actually tells, or shows, a partner how to touch them, or lets them know whether something they do is pleasurable or unpleasant, it is difficult for the couple fully to enjoy sex with each other. It is not usually possible to read someone else's mind! But all conversations about sex, between adolescents, just as much as between adults, should be handled with great sensitivity for the other person's feelings: it is all too easy to undermine someone's self-esteem by telling them what they are doing wrong in bed. Girls especially may underestimate how vulnerable an apparently confident teenage boy may feel about his sexual performance, especially if his friends are boasting of their own (often fictional) sexual prowess.

Sexual orientation

Part of adolescence involves discovering one's sexual orientation and identity. Some teenagers become concerned that they have sexual feelings for someone of the same sex, perhaps a friend, an older pupil in their school, or even a teacher or other adult. They may even have engaged in sexual contact with a friend of the same sex, perhaps through mutual masturbation, although this tends to be more common between boys than girls.

TALKING ABOUT BEING HOMOSEXUAL

A difficult choice for homosexuals is whether to hide their feelings or admit them openly and hope that friends and family will accept the way they are. Telling parents can be the greatest barrier, although most parents, however upset they may be initially, will come to accept their son or daughter's sexual orientation because of the love they have for him or her. Friends, too, are often accepting; those with a negative attitude may be so prejudiced that losing their friendship turns out to be a benefit. But it is probably wise to be certain and happy about your sexual orientation before telling people.

ACCEPTING THAT A CHILD IS HOMOSEXUAL

Many parents are initially upset or angered when a son or daughter tells them that he or she is gay. But for an adolescent to make this move usually takes a great deal of courage, and may have involved months of anguish and soul-searching. Parents can feel pleased that their relationship with their teenager is strong enough for him or her to express their sexual orientation openly. If the young man or woman knows he or she is homosexual, nothing will change the situation. So support from their parents, rather than anger, is most helpful to the adolescent.

Same-sex sexual attraction can be quite common in early adolescence and is indicative of an individual's developing sexuality rather than their final adult orientation. However, by their mid– to late adolescence, most teenagers will have discovered the nature of the sexual preferences that will continue throughout their adult life. Most will recognize that they are heterosexual, attracted to the opposite sex. But some will find, perhaps confirming what they may have felt instinctively since childhood, that they are homosexual, attracted to people of their own sex. Others may realize they are bisexual, with an affinity for partners of both sexes, although this may not become obvious until they are older. Finding that their sexual preferences are not heterosexual—and thus not fitting in with the expected norms of society—can make adolescents feel very isolated and depressed.

Being homosexual

Young people who see their sexual orientation as homosexual—gay or lesbian—may feel uncomfortable with this identity. Society, their friends, and often families as well, can have a negative attitude to gays and lesbians, and these adolescents may feel lonely because they do not fit in with what they and others perceive as "normal," even though common sexuality and sexual activities cover a wide spectrum. Being homosexual is part of an individual's identity, just like the color of his eyes or the shape of her ears. Ignoring sexual orientation because of the intolerance and prejudice of other people only makes the problem worse. Many young people suffer intolerably because they feel trapped by their own sexuality. If you are homosexual, often the best strategy is to be proud of your sexuality, and to meet and mix with other people who feel the same way.

Contraception

Whether or not teenagers are sexually active, it is important that they understand about the importance and use of contraception and the practice of safe sex. First, they must prevent unplanned pregnancy. Second, they must not place themselves at risk of acquiring a sexually transmitted disease such as the HIV virus (which causes AIDS), herpes, gonorrhea, chlamydia, or syphilis *(see pp.117–26)*.

Unfortunately, many teenagers don't find out about contraception until after they have become sexually active. There is a great need to provide clear information about contraception by early adolescence. In this way, teenagers will be aware, by the time they start a sexual relationship, of the consequences of their actions and their responsibilities in preventing unplanned pregnancies or acquiring or transmitting STDs. In reality, however, many teenagers "learn" about contraception during sex education at school, by which time some of them are already sexually active. Such education often consists of a dull display of contraceptive methods, some of which are not appropriate for adolescents. This can reinforce a negative attitude toward contraceptives, making their use as a normal part of sex more unlikely. Many girls who are not sufficiently informed about sexuality and contraception see "being prepared" as unromantic, as well as open to the interpretation that they are "looking for sex." These unfortunate realities may explain why so many teenagers in the Western world become pregnant unintentionally—nearly one million each year in the United States, including 30,000 under the age of 15.

Which are the "best" contraceptives for teenagers? The most effective method, of course, is abstinence from sex, which reduces the risk of pregnancy and the chance of contracting an STD to zero. As is emphasized in other parts of this chapter, adolescents can be reassured that whatever images they see of sexual activity in the media, and whatever peer pressure there is to conform by having sex, they should only have sex if and when they are ready. But when they are ready, they will need to use some form of contraception (unless they share their parents' objections to the use of contraception for religious or cultural reasons). The majority of adolescents who are sexually active, and regularly use contraception, choose either condoms or the combined oral contraceptive pill—better

DOES CONTRACEPTIVE KNOWLEDGE MAKE ADOLESCENTS MORE SEXUALLY ACTIVE?

Some parents worry that giving their young teenager information about sex and contraception will make them more likely to engage in sex. In fact, research has indicated that in countries such as the Netherlands, which have a comprehensive program of sex education that begins before puberty, and where sexual matters are openly discussed, the average age of first sexual intercourse (taken as a measure of sexual activity) is older than in countries like the United States, where such programs do not exist. And the younger adolescents are when they become sexually active, the less likely they are to use contraception, or to use it properly, and the higher the risk of pregnancy. The conclusion to be drawn is that if children are equipped with knowledge about sex and contraception in their early teens, they are more likely to wait until they are older before starting their sex lives. They are also more likely to use contraception, as indicated by the lower figures for teenage pregnancies in countries that provide early, consistent, and thorough sex education.

TALKING ABOUT CONTRACEPTION TO CHILDREN

Parents can play a part in informing their children about contraception, whether or not they approve of their child having sex. Research has shown that when parents talk to young people about contraception and discuss the different options available, young people are more likely to show a responsible attitude about contraceptive use and be properly aware of the consequences of their actions. Contraceptive awareness also helps adolescents plan ahead—not a natural adolescent attribute!—ensuring that they do carry and use contraception as a matter of course if they have sex.

WITHDRAWAL AS A FORM OF CONTRACEPTION

Withdrawal, or coitus interruptus, is one of the oldest known methods of contraception. It involves a man pulling his penis out of his partner's vagina just before he ejaculates. The problem with this method is that it depends on the male's timing to ensure that he withdraws before any sperm are released. Younger men have less control over ejaculation, so are more likely to ejaculate before they can withdraw from their partner. Most authorities agree that withdrawal is better than nothing as a method of contraception, but may be less effective for inexperienced adolescents. *(Contraceptive methods are discussed fully in Chapter 5, STDs in Chapter 4.)*

known as "the pill." Each of these birth control methods has its particular advantages and disadvantages.

Condoms

The condom is a barrier method of contraception that stops sperm from getting into the uterus. It is readily obtainable from drug stores and supermarkets and does not require a doctor's prescription. Most importantly, the condom helps to stop people from acquiring the HIV virus (which causes AIDS), as well as other sexually transmitted diseases (STDs), which can have serious consequences for health and fertility if they remain untreated, especially in young women.

The main disadvantage of the condom is that if it is not used properly it will not be very effective in preventing pregnancy. If a boy's only previous experience with condoms is seeing them filled with water and thrown out of a window, he may find it difficult to use one correctly during his first sexual encounter! Common problems include putting the condom on the penis inside out; not putting the condom on as soon as the boy gets an erection, so that there is a risk of sperm leakage near the vagina; and withdrawing from the vagina after ejaculation without holding the condom to the penis *(see also p.134)*, so that the used condom remains inside the vagina and its contents spill out. It helps, therefore, if the boy has an opportunity to get some practice using the condom before actually wearing it for the purposes of sexual intercourse.

Some young men will complain that condoms are uncomfortable or reduce penile sensation. However, precisely because of this, condoms often make adolescent boys "better lovers": by decreasing the intensity of penile sensation, they reduce the likelihood of premature ejaculation (reaching orgasm more quickly than he would like to, before his partner has had time to become fully aroused, or even, in some cases, before he has had time to insert his penis into her vagina). If a boy refuses to wear a condom it is best not to have sex: the risks of pregnancy and spread of STDs are too great.

The pill

The pill contains synthetically made equivalents of hormones naturally produced at certain times in the body. These stop a girl from ovulating—that is, releasing eggs from her ovaries. If no egg is released, she cannot get pregnant. The pill is very effective, providing that it is taken as directed, usually at approximately the same time every day. To start taking the pill, a girl must see her doctor, or go to a family planning clinic, and be examined to ensure that there are no medical reasons why she should not use this form of contraception *(see also pp.143–7)*. A disadvantage of the pill is that it does not prevent the spread of sexually transmitted diseases. Therefore, if a girl uses the pill she is strongly advised to use a condom as well.

Teenage pregnancy and parenthood

Sexual maturity physically equips a young woman to have a baby. By convention in most Western countries, women tend to wait until they are in their twenties before they start a family. However, there is no physical reason why they cannot start a family in their teenage years. Usually other considerations dominate in a young woman's decision-making: the desire to be sure of a committed relationship or the need to gain an education or become financially secure precludes early pregnancy. In the early teenage years pregnancy can be harmful for a girl, both physically and psychologically, because she is not likely to be prepared for the trauma and responsibility of giving birth and having a child. Young pregnant adolescents are at higher risk of anemia, hypertension (high blood pressure), and other complications of pregnancy. These heightened risks, however, are not necessarily caused by the mother's physical immaturity. They may be bound up with social factors—a high proportion of teenage mothers are likely to come from poorer backgrounds, and therefore to have less access to information and prenatal health care, along with a greater probability

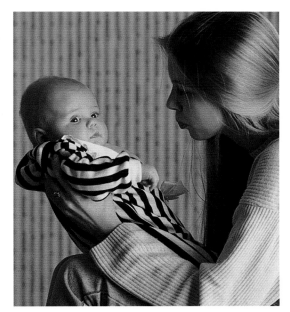

Although unplanned pregnancy may disrupt the lives of both a girl and her parents, there is no reason why a teenager should not be a good mother to her baby.

of suffering from a nutritionally inadequate diet. Not only are infants born to very young teenage mothers more likely to die during their first year of life than those born to more mature women, but they are also frequently born prematurely and at a low birthweight.

Unplanned teenage pregnancy

Many adolescent girls and boys choose to be sexually active. As measured by the age of first sexual intercourse, sexual activity among adolescents has increased over the past 20 years in most Western countries, mainly as a result of a more permissive attitude toward sex. Although some data show more frequent and regular use of contraception in certain countries, there has not been enough of a change of attitude toward preparing young people to understand and deal with their new-found sexuality, and unplanned teenage pregnancy is generally on the increase in Western countries. While television, movies, and magazines arguably show sexual images in excess— thereby probably encouraging sexual adventurousness—parents and schools may be unwilling or unable to do two things to protect teenagers: to provide them with a thorough understanding of what contracep-

tion is, how it works, the consequences of not using it, and easy access to it; and to give them a straightforward account of how their bodies work sexually.

Without this information, adolescent sexual partners are less likely to communicate with each other about sex or make preparations for safe participation in sexual activities. Unfortunately, many teenagers take a negative attitude toward contraception, at the same time as they are engaging in sex. The link between poorly informed adolescents and high pregnancy rates is revealed by comparing two countries with similar levels of teenage sexual activity but contrasting attitudes toward sex education and different levels of access to contraceptive methods. In the United States, where sex education is still a controversial issue, 95 girls (aged 15–19) out of 1,000 become pregnant annually. In Sweden, where sex education starts young and aims to give a clear understanding of all aspects of sex and to represent it as a natural part of life, the teenage pregnancy rate is 35 girls per 1,000 per year. And in the Netherlands it is lower still: just 15 girls out of 1,000 each year.

So why do teenagers get pregnant? Many girls simply believe that they cannot get pregnant and that they are in some way immune. This sense of immunity, combined with lack of planning for sexual encounters, impulsiveness, poor access to health care, a general reluctance to use contraception, and the high fertility rate of teenage girls, puts teenagers at high risk of unplanned pregnancy. Too many young couples fail to use any form of contraception when they first have sexual intercourse. Drinking alcohol, or using other drugs that lower inhibitions and decrease the ability to make deliberate choices, increases the chances that sex will take place and that it will be unprotected. In addition, some girls get pregnant deliberately because they want to have someone (a boyfriend or a baby) in their lives to love and be loved by. And some boys just do not care if their partner gets pregnant.

But, putting statistics and explanations aside, how does a teenage girl feel when it dawns on her that she may be pregnant? And what action can she take?

Signs of pregnancy

For a young woman to be pregnant she must have had sex, but the chances of being pregnant depend on the type of sexual contact and when it happened. If she has had unprotected sexual intercourse (without the use of contraception) since her last period, there is a chance of pregnancy. However, the likelihood is greatly increased if she and her partner had intercourse at the time of the month when she was most fertile *(see p.157)*, and increases even more if intercourse was frequent around the fertile time. If, on the other hand, she and her partner used contraception, the possibility of being pregnant is much reduced. Other forms of sexual contact, such as oral sex, will not cause pregnancy, although if her partner ejaculates near her vulva, without entering her, there is still a small risk of pregnancy.

So if a young woman has had unprotected intercourse in the previous few weeks and her next period has not started at the expected time, she may be pregnant. If a girl knows that she has had unprotected sex in the previous 72 hours, she can ask a family planning clinic for emergency contraception *(see pp.167–8)*. However, during adolescence, periods may be irregular until they settle down into their adult pattern. And, if she has had unprotected intercourse, the stress induced by fear of being pregnant may delay the onset of her period. Other common signs

of early pregnancy can include nausea and morning sickness, feeling the need to urinate all the time, sore or swollen breasts, fatigue, or even that clothes feel tighter than usual.

Many teenagers, especially younger ones, are terrified at confronting the fact that they may be pregnant, especially if they have not told anyone. Some simply ignore signs and symptoms, and hope that the pregnancy will just go away. But the longer an unplanned pregnancy is left to proceed, the fewer the options available to deal with it. The first step, to be taken as soon as possible, is to confirm the pregnancy.

If a period is late, or two periods have been missed, reassurance that a girl is not pregnant, or confirmation that she is, can be obtained by using a pregnancy test. Home pregnancy tests are widely available from drugstores. Using a sample of urine, they usually give a clear indication of whether a girl is pregnant. Follow directions on the pack carefully. If the home test proves positive, or uncertain, it is a good idea to visit a doctor or family planning clinic for confirmation.

Making decisions about a pregnancy

When a teenager discovers she is pregnant, and that fact has been confirmed by a reliable pregnancy test, it is time to make a major decision. Making that decision should not be left to the girl alone. Parental support, and

TELLING PARENTS ABOUT YOUR UNPLANNED PREGNANCY

If you think you may be pregnant, confiding in anyone can be difficult. But telling your parent or parents can seem like an insurmountable obstacle for two reasons. First, you may feel ashamed and guilty about what has happened. Second, you may be terrified that they will be angry or even reject you. It may help if you have an older sister or brother or close family friend you can tell first, so that they can help you break the news to your parents. Your parents will probably feel shocked and angry at first and may seem to be incapable of accepting the situation. As the dust settles, however, you may find that they are most helpful and supportive, and will talk openly about what

can or should be done. If you are pregnant and feel, for whatever reason, that you cannot tell your family or partner, you should seek advice from a family planning clinic or other counseling service.

Some boys will make a quick exit when told that their sexual partner is pregnant. Others will be upset and confused. If your partner builds up the courage to tell his parents, and if he wants to stand by you, he may find that one or both sets of parents—or even you yourself—resist the idea. The only answer is to talk about things. Try to remember that however angry or upset they may seem at first, most parents are ultimately supportive in a crisis, whatever the cause.

especially support from her mother, will provide a degree of reassurance for her. It will also lend the necessary experience, which adolescents have yet to acquire, to help her look ahead and imagine what life could be like if she had her baby. Being supportive and openly voicing opinions are probably the right strategies to adopt here; forcing a daughter to do what she is told—for instance, to have the baby and marry the father—will not be helpful to a young person who already feels confused and bewildered. If the boyfriend is accepting his responsibility toward the girl, he should be encouraged to participate in discussions. Alternately, if help is not available from home, a girl may seek counseling from an outside agency, such as a doctor or family planning clinic. (Avoid advertisements that offer to "help"; these clinics often have a political agenda.) Providing the pregnancy has been confirmed in time, a girl has two options: either to have her pregnancy terminated by abortion or to have the baby. The teenager herself should have the final word on these decisions: ultimately she is the one who must bear the responsibility for them.

Having the baby

Deciding to have the baby may be an easy decision. The family and their daughter may share strong religious or moral beliefs that preclude abortion as an option. Alternately, a girl may have planned her pregnancy, and be determined to have her baby whatever happens. Or the entire family may welcome the pregnancy. But both parents and daughter need to think carefully before deciding whether to have a baby, and whether to keep the child once he or she is born.

Once a girl has decided to have a baby, she has to make another decision: is she going to bring up the baby herself, or put it into foster care until she is in a position to look after it, or put the baby up for adoption? Bringing up a child is hard work and costly. Babies and young children are very demanding, and the pressure of caring for a child may be too much for a lone parent if she is already having to cope with such worries as money, tiredness, housing problems, and loneliness. If she is living with the baby's father, the relationship may be strained because of a feeling that it has been forced upon both of them because of the baby. On the positive side, however, the girl's parents—and those of the father—can provide a great deal of support, both emotionally and practically. They can give her the confidence, using their own experiences as parents, to be a competent and caring mother, proud of her new status as a care-giver and nurturer of a new life. They can also help her—by looking after the child themselves and being active grandparents—to continue some of the interests, education, and activities that she might have pursued if she had not become pregnant. In addition, the girl or her parents should look for any services in the community that will enable her to continue her education while she is pregnant, and by providing daycare facilities, to return to school or college after the child is born.

Abortion

Abortion means bringing a pregnancy to an end by medical means. It is legal in many countries, although the laws concerning it do vary from country to country and from state to state. Abortion itself raises many emotional and moral issues. Some may reject it because of their religious beliefs. Others may worry about the safety of the procedure, although for girls in the 15-to-19 age group, giving birth to the baby at full term is 14 times more likely to result in the death of the mother than having a legal abortion in the first 12 weeks of pregnancy.

In general, at an abortion clinic, a health-care provider offers appropriate counseling and collects a thorough medical and social history. If the woman decides to have an abortion, the earlier it is carried out, the easier and safer it is. Up to the thirteenth week of pregnancy, abortions are done surgically, on an outpatient basis. Later abortions may require an overnight stay in the hospital. Doctors worry more about abortions after 13 weeks because of the possibility of complications and the increased chance that the girl may have problems with future pregnancies (*see also pp.230–1*).

Adolescent health

Adolescence tends to be a period of good health. The colds and other infections so common during childhood are much less evident. Good health is also encouraged by a diet that is healthy and well balanced, and by plenty of exercise. However, the upheavals of adolescence can have an impact on a teenager's mental health, which can affect their development and may continue into adult life.

Healthy eating during adolescence

All adolescents need a balanced diet that supplies their bodies with the raw materials, and sufficient energy, for normal growth and development. The growth in body tissues during the adolescent years is greater than at any time except the first years of life. Because of this incredible rate of growth and high activity levels, adolescents need more energy per day than at any other time in their lives. An average adolescent boy in his mid-teens will need around 3,000 calories per day, while a girl of the same age will need to consume about 2,250 calories.

The sources of this energy are important. The main energy providers in the diet are carbohydrates and fats *(for more about diet, see pp.88–90)*. In particular, the growth spurt leaves adolescents very vulnerable to energy

HEALTHY EATING

While junk food and soda are often the staple diet of adolescents, there is no reason why healthy eating should not be compatible with youth. Parents can help their children eat more healthfully by setting an example themselves. If Mom or Dad is a frequent consumer of pizzas and burgers, their children will probably follow suit. Healthy foods do not have to be boring. There are plenty of pasta and rice dishes, baked potatoes with fillings, exciting salads, vegetarian burgers, grilled chicken and fish, and fruit dishes that can excite the taste buds while supplying vitamins and healthy ingredients in the right amounts, without piling on the calories or saturated fats.

and nutrient insufficiency. Teenagers need energy to support growth and development, muscle activity, and metabolism—the constant daily work of cells and tissues. A diet of white bread, burgers, and fries may provide adequate calories, but it will prevent a child from growing to his or her optimal height. Also, poor eating habits continue into adulthood and may over the years result in higher risk of obesity, heart disease, and diabetes.

The ideal healthy diet for an adolescent consists of the same components as one recommended for an adult—but in greater quantities. The diet should include a range of foods that supply sufficient carbohydrates for energy, proteins for growth and body repair, vitamins and minerals for general health, and fiber for an efficient digestive process, avoiding too much fatty food or protein. This is best illustrated by the food pyramid *(see p.89)*. Adolescents, and their parents, should aim to eat foods from all but the top food group every day, and to eat different foods from each group every day in order to obtain a balance in their diet. The foods should be eaten in proportion to the sections of the pyramid. This means that each day adolescents should eat plenty of carbohydrate-rich food, such as bread, pasta, and rice, as well as fresh fruit and vegetables, but smaller quantities of meat and other protein-containing foods and dairy products.

However, as many parents will recognize, adolescents tend to be grazers and snackers who do not worry too much about what they eat providing there is some food available. Uncontrolled, this sort of indiscriminate eating tends to create a diet that is high in fats and salt, and may lead to a pattern of unhealthy eating that will affect health in later life. If possible, teenagers should be encouraged to eat fresh fruit or nuts rather than candy or potato chips as snacks. If at least one meal each day is eaten as a family, this may help to encourage a healthier eating pattern, providing, of course, that the food on the table is itself healthy. And if children want to diet, because they think they are overweight (an individual's "ideal" weight range for their height can be determined by calculating the

Body Mass Index, *see p.88*), parental guidance about the long-term benefits of healthier foods in maintaining a steady weight may be very helpful.

A good diet needs to be accompanied by regular exercise. Exercise tones the muscles, maintains and improves cardiovascular health, and prevents accumulation of fat. Good dietary and exercise habits established in adolescence are often continued into adulthood. In later life they may contribute significantly to a reduction in the incidence of heart disease and certain cancers.

Eating disorders

A few adolescents respond—often subconsciously—to the changes occurring in their body by drastically altering their eating habits and developing an eating disorder. The term "eating disorder" describes a condition in which someone eats much more or much less than they actually need. The most familiar of these disorders is obesity, a condition found in all age groups, in which overconsumption leads to accumulation of fat. Two other eating disorders are restricted mainly to adolescent and young women: anorexia nervosa and bulimia nervosa. Both illnesses are characterized by a desire not to gain weight, and can seriously affect normal development.

Anorexia nervosa
Anorexia affects around one in 100 adolescent girls, and one in 2,000 teenage boys. Sufferers refuse to maintain their weight at or above a normal minimum standard for their age and height, and have an intense fear of gaining weight. When looking in a mirror, an anorexic sees herself as "fat" even when she is seriously underweight and no more than "skin and bones." Anorexics eat less and less in an attempt to get rid of fat. As a result, they suffer a dramatic loss of body weight. This may be accelerated by obsessive exercising.

The first signs and symptoms of anorexia commonly appear in the mid-teens. The sufferer eats little food, often in secret, and tends to have devious eating habits, such as cutting up food into smaller and smaller pieces. As weight is lost, the girl may wear shapeless clothes to hide the fact, feel the cold more than normal, be restless, sleep badly, have dry skin, and develop fine hair on her cheeks, neck, and limbs. Once she has lost about 22 percent of her body weight, her periods will stop. If anorexia develops before the start of adolescence, the physical changes of puberty will be put on hold until a normal pattern of eating and weight gain is resumed.

The precise causes of anorexia are difficult to determine and are still being debated. Anorexics are often high achievers in school despite very high anxiety, poor self-esteem, depression, and obsessiveness. Anorexia may be an attempt to gain control of their lives by stopping the process of growing up and preventing the development of female sexual characteristics; anorexics certainly lack the fat necessary to produce a female body shape and breasts, and their menstrual cycles cease or never begin. Because many anorexics come from families that stress achievement, some researchers wonder if it is the pressure to succeed that induces the disorder. It is also possible that anorexics suffer from an abnormality in the functioning of the brain. A cultural element may be involved as well, because anorexia is only found in societies in which thinness is equated with attractiveness. Reinforcing a waiflike or childlike image is the appearance of many actresses and models in magazines, movies, and television, whose success appears to be the result of their possessing the "perfect" figure.

Whatever its cause, the sooner anorexia is identified, the better, if treatment is to stand a good chance of success. Anorexia is a mental illness that cannot be cured by family persuasion. It needs help from a specialist. The usual procedure is to attempt to get a girl back to her normal weight, while providing her with therapy to help her overcome the need to starve herself. The entire family is often involved in this therapy as well. Around three-quarters of those treated eventually make a full recovery. However, up to 50 percent of anorexics may develop bulimia *(see p.84)* during the course of treatment, and about 5 percent of anorexics die of the disorder.

Bulimia nervosa

Bulimia nervosa is characterized by bouts of excessive overeating—called binging—followed by attempts to get rid of the food by vomiting or using laxatives or purgatives. Bulimics are usually of normal weight or just under. When binging, bulimics typically eat a large amount of high-calorie foods (sugary and fatty foods) and then induce vomiting, or use high doses of laxatives, to remove the excess calories. The cycle may be repeated several times each day. In the long term, this can lead to serious damage to the digestive system, tooth decay, heart problems, urinary infections, and, in a few cases, death. Like anorexia, treatment for bulimia involves therapy and requires professional help.

Depression

Depression means having a feeling of gloom about life, and it is something that most of us experience at some point, albeit only temporarily. It is also a common but transient feature of the emotional roller-coaster of adolescence. However, some teenagers develop a feeling of deep unhappiness that stays with them and will not go away. They may lose interest in their favorite activities, stop eating properly, lose weight without dieting, lose energy, cut themselves off from friends and social life, and start getting bad grades at school. If an adolescent shows any of these signs, parents should be acutely aware of the possibility of depression.

Chronic depression can have many causes and courses. The surrounding social context is a key factor. It could be that the parents are getting divorced, there are problems at school, a relationship is ending, or the teenager is being rejected by peers. Whatever the cause, the teenager needs help to tackle her or his feelings of helplessness and confusion. A first step may be for parents to encourage their child to talk about possible problems, although this may not always succeed. A doctor may refer a teenager for counseling or therapy and, if the depression is severe and persistent, may prescribe drugs to help alleviate the problem.

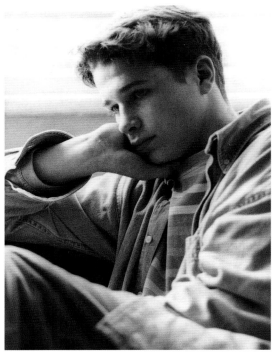

If a teenager is withdrawn and generally uninterested in life for a prolonged period it may be a sign that he is depressed. Depression may be temporary and have a particular cause—losing a girlfriend, for example—but it may be more serious and require medical help.

Teenage suicide

Although teenage suicide is rare, the number of young people killing themselves, or attempting to do so, is on the increase in Western countries. In children under 14 years old, suicide is rare, but in adolescents over 14 the annual suicide rate is 12 per 100,000 in the United States (a three-fold increase since the 1960s) and 3 per 100,000 in the United Kingdom. In the United States, twice as many boys commit suicide as girls, probably because the former choose more "final" methods of killing themselves, and because suicides are closely linked to other violent behaviors, and to alcohol and substance abuse, which are more common among males.

Why do some adolescents see suicide as an answer to their problems? Some are socially isolated, with long-term psychiatric problems. But many adolescents who think about or attempt suicide do so because in the mental upheaval that can form part of adolescence

SUBSTANCE ABUSE IN TEENAGERS

Increasingly, young people and those who care for them (teachers as well as parents) are having to make daily decisions about how they should deal with drinking, smoking, and drugs. The following questions are typical of the kind that adolescents are frequently having to ask themselves: Should I refuse to drink or take drugs even though my friends do? Should I accept a lift in a car when a friend is too drunk to drive? For the past two years I've been an increasingly heavy smoker—how can I stop? How do I explain to my parents that my recent "illnesses" are due to a drinking (or drug) problem? For parents the problem is how and when to explain to their children the dangers of drugs, alcohol, and cigarettes; how to help them resist peer pressure to take these substances; and how to help them if they become involved in substance abuse.

First, young people have to accept that whatever their experiences so far or whatever their friends say, bad things can happen to you if you take drugs, smoke, or drink. Second, it will take time, effort, and often outside help to break a drug habit. Third, it is usually easier to break your habit a step at a time rather than believing you can stop all at once. Last but not least, if possible, talk to someone you respect about your problem, don't keep it to yourself.

For their part, parents should find out for themselves about the dangers of drugs, cigarettes, and alcohol, so that they can give their children informed information and answers. They must also examine their own use of drugs (both illegal and prescribed), drink, and cigarettes; one of the best ways to help their children is to set a good example (see also p.70 and pp.126–7).

they lose their self-esteem, feel that their problems are insurmountable, see no future for themselves, or feel lonely, unloved, and inadequate—and make the tragic mistake of viewing suicide as a quick solution.

Fortunately, most adolescents who think about suicide never attempt it, and many of those who try to commit suicide fail in the attempt. Those close to adolescents, especially their parents, may be able to help avert a potential suicide if they notice clues which might indicate that she or he may be thinking about suicide. These clues can include depression and crying; a sudden personality change; isolation from friends; conflict with a boyfriend or girlfriend, or with parents; not eating food or getting enough sleep; showing self-destructive behavior by overindulging in alcohol or drugs; a decline in the quality of school or college work; problems in concentrating; or neglect of personal appearance. If an adolescent talks about suicide, discusses ways of killing themselves, or makes statements such as "I wish I was dead," these may indicate a high level of risk.

Although there may be no cause for alarm, if these signs are evident, parents should take them seriously, and should talk directly to their teenager about his or her feelings and try to provide reassurance. It is advisable also to seek medical advice. If an adolescent has attempted suicide and survived, it is important that parents come to terms with their own thoughts and emotions in order to help their teenager recover fully. Many parents, angry and upset that their child has tried to take his or her own life, are determined to discover why it has happened, and whether they are to blame. For a parent to express feelings of guilt is of little use. It is far better for the young person to be given as much love and reassurance as possible to help them recover. Therapy for the adolescent, and possibly for the whole family as well, may help resolve some of the problems that led to the suicide attempt in the first place.

It is always important for adolescents to talk about how they feel. Otherwise, nobody else can imagine what they are experiencing. More often than not, parents are there to listen, advise, and provide love—despite differences, family members are basically on the same side. If not parents, then grandparents are often good listeners; or failing that, hotline numbers can be found in telephone directories, libraries, and doctor's offices.

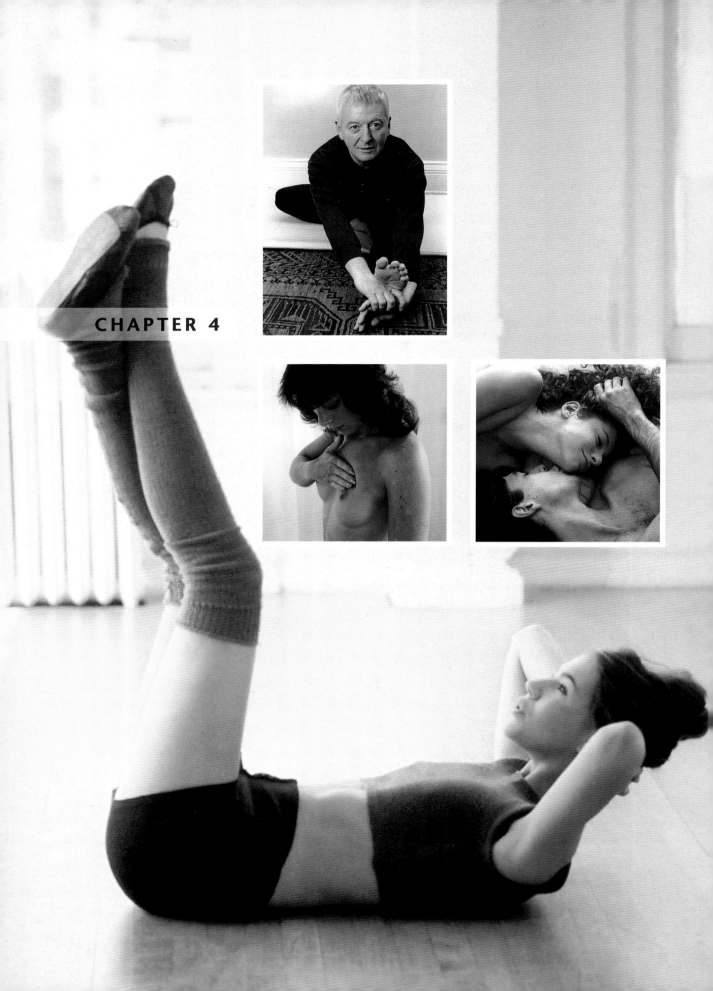

CHAPTER 4

The Healthy Body

The human body is in many ways like an expensive, finely tuned machine. If it is nurtured, used properly, and protected, the machine purrs quietly and functions efficiently. If it is battered and abused, it starts to malfunction and perform poorly.

A body that performs well is one that is properly cared for. Good performance includes being fit, looking good, being mentally active, not being stressed, and, in sexually active adults, having a good sex life. Keeping the body in good shape depends primarily on providing it with a well-balanced diet that is low in junk food and high in fresh foods; ensuring that it receives regular exercise throughout life; and making sure that it does not become unnecessarily stressed. Most people who exercise on a regular basis find that this improves the way they look and the way that they feel about themselves. A sense of self-esteem established in this way can help to make and maintain a good relationship with a partner.

Staying healthy is not just about doing exercise and eating the right foods. It is also about avoiding the many disorders that can affect the body, or if a disease develops, knowing when and how quickly to seek medical advice. Diseases are body malfunctions. Infectious diseases are caused by external agents, known collectively as germs or microorganisms, that enter the body and attempt to establish themselves there. The body's natural defenses, including its immune system, work constantly to withstand the battalions of bacteria and viruses that attempt to invade the body. Many of these infectious diseases can be transmitted from one person to another; some of them, known as sexually transmitted diseases (STDs), are transferred by sexual contact.

Non-infectious diseases are not caused by infectious microorganisms and therefore cannot be transmitted to others. These include the cancers that can affect various areas inside the body, including parts of the reproductive systems such as the prostate gland in men and the ovaries in women. Cancers are abnormal cell growths which, unless challenged by the immune system, form tumors that grow out of control and eventually cause death.

Modern medicine has developed many weapons to combat the infectious and non-infectious diseases that can affect the body. But it is important for men and women to be aware of when their body is not functioning as it should, so that they can report any symptoms to their doctor as soon as possible. The doctor, in turn, will look for signs that will, along with the patient's description of the symptoms, enable him or her to make a diagnosis, in order to suggest a cure.

BODY MASS INDEX (BMI)

Obesity is a growing problem in developed countries, and it is important for individuals to be aware when their body weight (in relation to their height) is putting them at risk. The most straightforward and accurate indication of whether a person is overweight or underweight is the BMI (Body Mass Index). Far better than just a reading from the bathroom scale, BMI relates a person's body weight to their height. Your BMI equals your weight (in kilograms) divided by your height (in meters) squared. It is calculated as follows (you will need a calculator).

1 Measure your weight:
• Find out your weight in kilograms.
• If your bathroom scale measures in pounds, convert them to kilograms by dividing by 2.2.

2 Measure your height:
• Find out your height in meters.
• Write down this measurement.
• If you have measured your height in inches, convert them to meters by dividing by 39.37.

3 Calculate your height squared:
• Multiply your height by itself. For example, if you are 1.65m tall, calculate 1.65 x 1.65.

4 Now, calculate your BMI:

Your BMI = $\dfrac{\text{your weight in kilograms} \div \text{your height in meters}^2}{\text{(the measurement from 1} \div \text{the calculation from 3)}}$

An example of BMI:
Imagine a person who weighs 60kg, and who is 1.65m tall
• Her weight is 60kg.
• Her height is 1.65m.
• Her height squared is 1.65 x 1.65, which is 2.72.
• So her BMI = 60 ÷ 2.72, which is 22. Her BMI is 22.

5 Understanding your BMI value:
Less than 20
   This means that you are underweight for your height.
20–25
   This means that you are within the recommended healthy weight range for your height.
25–30
   This means that you are overweight for your height.
Over 30
   This means that you are obese (seriously overweight) for your height; your weight is having a detrimental effect on your health.

Diet and exercise

Most authorities agree that a fit body means a better sex life. People who are in good shape look healthier and more sexually attractive. They are less likely to be stressed and therefore more likely to have a strong sex drive. And they are likely to be happier and so more able to enjoy sex.

A fit body is generally one that is fed with a balanced diet rich in fresh foods, vitamins, and minerals, and low in animal fats; that is exercised at least two or three times a week; that is not abused by drugs or excessive amounts of alcohol; that does not have cigarette smoke drawn into its lungs; and that is emotionally healthy and relatively stress-free.

Healthy eating

A balanced diet contains around 55 percent carbohydrate (from foods such as potatoes, bread, and pasta); less than 30 percent fat, with less than 10 percent being animal fats; and around 15 percent protein (from foods such as meat, fish, beans, or eggs). If the diet is balanced and contains a range of fresh foods, it should also provide all the vitamins and minerals required. In reality, diets in the developed world are too high in animal fats and too low in fresh fruit and vegetables. This imbalance leads to high rates of obesity, heart disease, and high blood pressure, as well as other conditions, including some cancers. Health authorities in these countries are advising people to consume less fat and more carbohydrates, fresh vegetables, and fruit.

The food pyramid *opposite* shows the proportions in which the main food groups should be eaten. An ideal diet contains a variety of foods—with very few from group 1, a little more from group 2, and increasing amounts from groups 3 and 4.

Exercise and fitness

A fit body is one that, taking age into consideration, can carry out everyday activities—for example, climbing stairs or running for a bus —without showing signs of distress such as breathlessness or excessive fatigue. Through maintaining a high level of fitness, a person can ensure that his or her heart is working more efficiently: a healthy heart pumps 25 percent more blood with each beat than does an unfit heart while a person is at rest. Regular exercise is the most reliable way to keep fit on a day-to-day basis, and as an insurance policy for future health in the years ahead. Ideally, exercise should be aerobic (designed to increase the amount of oxygen in the blood and strengthen the heart and lungs—for example, running, swimming, or brisk walking); should make a person sweat and become somewhat breathless; should last at least 20 minutes per session; and should take place at least three or four times a week. Anaerobic exercise, such as weight-lifting, increases strength by increasing muscle bulk but does not itself promote cardiac health. Exercise should aim to improve three elements of fitness: strength, flexibility, and stamina. Regular aerobic exercise has these benefits:

• It increases cardiovascular (heart and blood

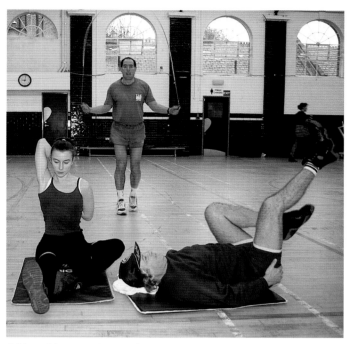

Brisk walking, running, and jumping rope are great ways to maintain fitness and stay trim. A person out of shape should start to exercise gradually, and build up slowly. Stretching exercises keep the body loose and supple, and help prevent muscle stiffness after exercise.

THE FOOD PYRAMID

Group 1 **Foods rich in oils, fats, and refined sugars and alcohol**	Alcoholic drinks Bacon Butter Cakes Candy	Chips Chocolate Cookies Fast foods (e.g., burgers)	Fatty meat cuts French fries Margarine Pastries Salami	Sausages Sugar Sugary drinks (e.g., soda) Vegetable oils
Group 2 **Protein-rich foods**	Bean curd (tofu) Chicken Cottage cheese Eggs Lean beef cuts	Lean lamb cuts Lean pork cuts Lowfat cheese Lowfat milk Nuts—in	moderation Oily fish (e.g., tuna) Pulses (e.g., beans, lentils)	Seafood (e.g., shrimp) White fish (e.g., cod, flounder) Yogurt
Group 3 **Fresh fruit and vegetables**	Apples Apricots Avocado Bananas Broccoli	Brussels sprouts Cabbage Carrots Celery Corn	Cucumbers Melons Oranges Peaches Pears	Peppers Spinach Strawberries Tomatoes Zucchini
Group 4 **Foods rich in complex carbohydrates**	Bagels Bread and rolls Breakfast cereals Buckwheat (kasha)	Bulgur Couscous Parsnips Pasta Pita bread	Polenta Potatoes Rice Semolina Sweet potatoes	Turnips Yams

vessels) fitness, making a person more active and lively, and decreasing the risk of their developing heart disease, strokes, or high blood pressure.

• Combined with a balanced diet that contains the right amount of calories (energy), exercise helps prevent obesity, which, apart from making the body look less attractive, increases the risk of high blood pressure, heart disease, and diabetes.

• It helps reduce the effects of stress in various ways. First, exercise causes the release of endorphins into the bloodstream. These are naturally occurring opiates that induce a feeling of relaxation and well-being. Second, feeling both tired and relaxed after exercise

helps a person sleep well, and regular deep sleep is essential for stress reduction. Third, having a healthy, well-toned body also makes a person feel good about themselves—so that they feel and look more sexually attractive.

• It normally (unless done in excess) boosts the immune system. People who are in good shape are probably less likely to develop infectious diseases such as colds, or non-infectious diseases such as cancers. Fitness also aids recovery if illness does strike. But it cannot guarantee protection against disease—fitness is not the same as health.

• It tones and strengthens muscles, improving body shape and enabling muscles to work more efficiently. This, in combination with avoiding obesity, can improve posture and decrease the occurrence of backache. It also strengthens bones and increases joint mobility, reducing the problem of stiff and painful joints in old age.

• For women with menstrual problems (see pp.95–8), it can help reduce the severity of some cramps.

EXERCISES FOR STRENGTH, FLEXIBILITY, AND STAMINA

This chart shows a range of popular activities and sports, and the contribution that each can make to the body's strength, flexibility, and stamina—the three components of fitness. For example, while weight-lifting promotes a high level of strength, it produces only a low level of stamina; jogging, on the other hand, is not a good strength exercise, but is an excellent way of increasing stamina. Swimming is a good exercise for strength, flexibility, and stamina, and does not put any strain on the knees. If possible, exercise should be carried out three or four times a week, for at least 20 minutes per session. Increasing the amount of weekly exercise does not necessarily mean going to a gym—it could simply be a matter of walking instead of using the car. The benefit of each activity or sport in terms of improving strength, flexibility, or stamina is indicated.

Exercise	Strength	Flexibility	Stamina
Aerobics	••	••	•••
Basketball	••	••	•••
Climbing stairs	•	•	••
Cycling	••	•	•••
Dance	••	•••	•••
Golf	•	•	•
Jogging	••	••	•••
Running	•••	••	•••
Soccer	••	••	•••
Squash	•••	••	•••
Swimming	•••	•••	•••
Tennis	••	•••	••
Walking	•	•	••
Weight-lifting	•••	••	•
Yoga	•	•••	•

• = Low benefit   •• = Medium benefit   ••• = High benefit

Personal hygiene

If it were possible to travel back in time and walk along a crowded street in the sixteenth century, one of our first sensations would probably be the smell of unwashed bodies. Nowadays, there is a much greater awareness of cleanliness and personal hygiene, and a vast range of products are available to wash, perfume, and deodorize the human body.

Cleanliness is certainly an important factor in many sexual relationships. Most people would find sharing a bed with a dirty, smelly body something of a turnoff. The reason that unwashed people develop an unpleasant body odor is because of the sweat produced by the apocrine glands of the armpits and around the genitals and anus. The sweat is odorless when first produced, but after it has been "processed" by bacteria living on the skin, it takes on a musky smell. Daily bathing or showering is not only refreshing but removes sweat and dirt from the body and minimizes the chances of developing armpit and other smells. Many people find that underarm antiperspirants and deodorants also help reduce the risk of body smells developing during the day. Of course, it is also important to keep the genitals clean.

Male genital hygiene

The penis has glands that produce natural secretions and odors, and it will also develop an unpleasant smell if not washed regularly. Genital hygiene is particularly important for men who are not circumcised. If the penis is left unwashed for a few days, the secretions of the sebaceous glands under the foreskin produce a white material called smegma. It is important during washing to pull back the foreskin and wash the glans thoroughly. Accumulation of smegma can cause balanitis —inflammation of the glans—because of the development of fungal or bacterial conditions under the unwashed foreskin.

Female genital hygiene

The vulva— the external female genitals (see pp.16–17)—also produces secretions that generate a particular odor, but provided the area is washed regularly that smell will not become unpleasant. It is best to wash the vulva from front to back, to avoid transferring any bacteria from the anus into the vagina or the urethra and reduce the risk of developing any infections. There is no need to wash inside the vagina; it is self-cleaning.

A healthy vulva smells slightly musky, a smell that may become more noticeable during sexual arousal and that may act as an attractant for a sexual partner. The use of vaginal deodorants and scented panty liners has become more prevalent, but these only serve, in a clean woman, to mask natural, pleasing scents produced by the body. In addition, some of the chemicals contained in the products may cause irritation leading to vaginitis (see p.116) and increase sensitivity to spermicides and lubricants used for condoms.

Emotional health

Feeling happy, relaxed, and confident about oneself plays an important part in having and maintaining a successful relationship, and in experiencing a good sex life. Worries, fears, and anxieties can inhibit a person's sex life, and even bring it to a halt. Yet the pace of modern life causes many people to feel anxious so that they cannot enjoy life to the fullest. One word serves to encapsulate all these worries and fears, and that is "stress."

Stress

Stress is now recognized as a major health issue that reduces our quality of life, makes us more prone to disease, and, if prolonged, shortens our life span. It also makes us feel less sexual. Fortunately, stress can be managed and even avoided.

The most common signs and symptoms of stress include breathlessness, nausea, loss of appetite, insomnia, fatigue, tearfulness, constipation or diarrhea, headaches, dizziness, backache, and trembling. Stress also reduces the effectiveness of the immune system, so that people who are stressed are much more likely to become ill.

Stress affects a person's sexuality, too. Both men and women who are stressed may lose

---

DO HUMAN PHEROMONES EXIST?

Pheromones are chemicals released by many animal species that change the behavior—often the sexual behavior—of other members of the same species. The classic example of this is the pheromone released by a female moth (Bombyx mori) to advertise her sexual receptivity. The pheromone attracts male moths from miles around to mate with her. It has been suggested that female humans who are feeling sexually receptive release a pheromone that elicits a sexual response from males. However, there is no hard evidence that human pheromones exist, or that they cause the "switching on" of stereotyped patterns of sexual behavior in men. It appears that the mechanism of sexual attraction between men and women is far more complex and subtle than it is between moths!

interest in sex altogether, thereby putting a strain on their relationships. Men who are stressed are more likely to lose an erection, or not have an erection at all. Women who suffer long-term stress may develop irregular periods or may stop having periods altogether.

Worrying about sexual problems can make them worse, and lead to more stress and a risk of more serious illness. To break this vicious circle it is important to talk to your partner about difficulties and/or to seek outside help. In the long term, stress can lead to more serious conditions such as anxiety disorders, or a "nervous breakdown," where a person is unable to cope on a day-to-day basis because of the state of their emotional health.

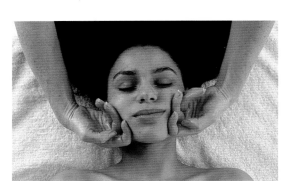

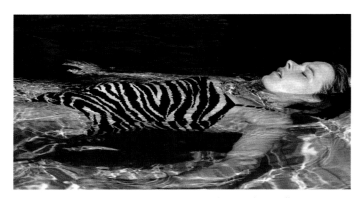

Making time for yourself, so that you can forget about all your worries by relaxing completely, is one of the most effective ways of beating stress. Everyone has their own ways of relaxing. Getting a massage and swimming are both excellent ways of managing stress.

Managing stress

To manage stress effectively, some or all of the following changes can be implemented.
• Identify the factors that are probably causing stress and talk them over with a partner or with colleagues at work in order to eliminate them or reduce their impact.
• Set realistic goals on a daily basis to avoid getting behind and letting work pile up.
• Avoid pressure by not taking on too many commitments.
• Take regular breaks during working hours and during the break concentrate on something else other than work.
• Exercise on a regular basis.
• Learn to relax completely and forget problems. This may involve regular exercise or other kinds of relaxation, such as reading or meditation.
• Take regular short vacations away from home in order to experience a complete change of scene.
• Avoid too many lifestyle changes at once.
• Adopt a more positive attitude to life, focusing on the present and not worrying too much about the future.

CAUSES OF STRESS

There are many possible causes of stress. Those listed below are life events that are likely to cause stress, listed in decreasing order of their effect. Being aware of what is likely to cause stress can often help to make its management easier and more realistic:
• bereavement—death of a spouse or partner
• divorce
• death of a parent, sibling, or child

• getting married
• losing a job or fear of losing a job
• starting a new job
• illness
• retirement
• illness in the family
• pregnancy and birth
• sexual problems
• verbal or physical abuse at home or in the workplace
• sexual or racial harassment
• coping with small children

• coping with elderly or dependent relatives
• death of a close friend
• excessive noise from neighbors
• financial difficulties
• change in work patterns or problems at work
• starting or finishing a close relationship
• moving home
• children leaving home
• going on vacation.

• Avoid using alcohol, or other drugs, for relaxation. They simply put off decision-making and interrupt sleep patterns, making stress even worse in the long term.

• If necessary, seek medical help to break the vicious cycles of stress.

Female health

Women are probably more aware of the workings of their reproductive organs than men are of theirs because of the monthly sequence of events that occurs during the fertile years and culminates in menstruation. Sometimes the internal mechanism controlling the menstrual cycle can go wrong and a woman suffers menstrual problems. Other parts of her reproductive system, such as the ovaries or breasts, may also be affected by disorders. Fortunately, women today have a greater chance than ever before of successful treatment of reproductive-system disorders. But they should be aware of the signs and symptoms that could give them early warning of possible disorders of their reproductive organs, so that they can seek medical advice as soon as possible.

Menstruation

Menstruation is a normal, healthy event that happens about once a month for many years of a woman's life. It marks the end of one menstrual cycle and the beginning of the next. Each menstrual cycle includes the release of an egg from an ovary, and the preparation of the uterus to receive a fertilized egg. If an egg has not been fertilized, the thickened uterine lining breaks down and is shed, with some blood, through the vagina. This is menstruation, or the period, which normally lasts about five days, but may last as little as two days or longer than a week *(menstrual cycles are described in detail on p.22-3)*.

More than any other biological function, menstruation has been, and may still be, misunderstood and surrounded by superstition. In certain cultures women are still regarded as "unclean" during their periods. And even in the "sophisticated" developed world, the belief still persists among many men that any changes in behavior only confirm that women are the "weaker" sex. Premenstrual syndrome (PMS), the term used to describe a woman's feelings of anxiety or discomfort during or before menstruation, has been adopted these men to describe any "irrational" behavior in a woman. Thankfully, attitudes are changing, periods are becoming recognized as a natural part of a woman's life, and PMS is now accepted as a clinical phenomenon, caused by hormonal fluctuations.

Menstrual protection
Tampons

A tampon is a tight roll of cotton or rayon that is inserted into the vagina, where it expands to fit and absorbs the menstrual flow. At one end is a string with which to remove it. Some tampons come with an applicator to aid insertion, others are inserted into the vagina using a finger. Tampons are available in a range of sizes and absorbencies to suit different menstrual flows. The advantage of tampons is that they are inconspicuous, and they can be worn during swimming and other forms of exercise. However, they may cause leakage if the flow is particularly heavy, in which case some women may prefer to use a pad as well. Tampons should be changed every four to six hours, for the sake of cleanliness and also because of the increased risk of toxic shock syndrome *(see box, p.95)*. Some women prefer to use sanitary pads for overnight protection, rather than leaving a tampon in place for that length of time.

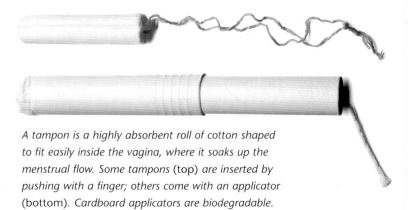

A tampon is a highly absorbent roll of cotton shaped to fit easily inside the vagina, where it soaks up the menstrual flow. Some tampons (top) *are inserted by pushing with a finger; others come with an applicator* (bottom). *Cardboard applicators are biodegradable.*

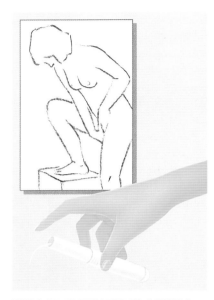

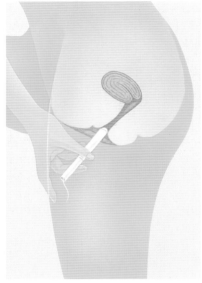

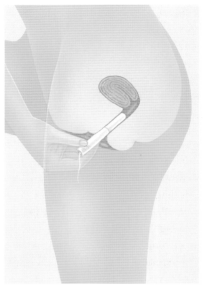

USING AN APPLICATOR TO INSERT A TAMPON

1 *Some women prefer to use tampons that have a disposable applicator. This consists of two hollow tubes: one surrounding the tampon, and a narrower tube that pushes the tampon into its correct position.*

2 *Get into a comfortable position in which the vagina will be more open. Some women prefer to raise one leg, by putting one foot on a raised surface; others favor squatting. Hold the outer tube of the applicator between your thumb and fingers and introduce it carefully into the vaginal opening.*

3 *Still holding the outer tube, put your index finger over the end of the narrower tube—the one that has the string emerging from it. Use the index finger to push the narrow inner tube inside the outer tube as far as it will go so that it acts like a plunger, pushing the tampon into your vagina.*

QUESTIONS AND ANSWERS: USING TAMPONS

Q. Is it safe to use tampons throughout the month to stop any vaginal discharges from staining underwear?
A. This is not a good idea. Normal vaginal discharges help clean the vagina and keep it healthy. Using a tampon throughout the month will soak up these secretions, dry the wall of the vagina, and possibly increase the chance of developing vaginal conditions such as yeast infections (*see p.116*). Use panty liners for this purpose instead.

Q. Can tampons get "lost" inside?
A. Tampons cannot get lost in the vagina, although sometimes a woman may forget to remove one at the end of her period or, rarely, a small fragment of tampon may remain in the vagina. In both instances this may lead to irritation of the vagina and a smelly discharge, the cause of which may only be discovered when the woman sees her doctor.

Q. I have tried tampons, but I don't find them very effective. What else can I use?
A. You may need a more absorbent tampon. Most brands are available in various absorbencies, labeled regular, super, and super plus. Perhaps you need to move from regular to super; or try another brand that expands differently. Alternatively, you could use panty liners or pads with tampons.

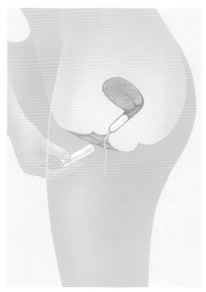

4 *Once the tampon is in place, remove the applicator from the vaginal entrance and dispose of it properly. You can check that the tampon is in the right position in your vagina by inserting a finger. Use the string to remove the tampon after four to six hours.*

SEX DURING MENSTRUATION

Whether or not a couple makes love during a woman's period depends totally on their own shared views and feelings. If a woman feels sexually receptive during her period and both she and her partner feel comfortable about having sex, then there is no reason why they should not enjoy sex at this time. Some women find that they become aroused more easily during their period and experience more intense feelings during intercourse or masturbation than at other times of the month. Orgasm may also help relieve menstrual cramps. Women who use a diaphragm *(see pp.137–40)* find that it temporarily holds back the menstrual flow during sex. Other couples prefer to abstain from sex during menstruation. This may be because the woman is not interested in sex during her period; because her partner is not comfortable about having sex at this time; or because the couple have religious or cultural objections to menstrual sex. There is no right or wrong attitude in this matter.

TOXIC SHOCK SYNDROME

Toxic shock syndrome, or TSS, is a very rare but serious condition that has affected a few tampon users. Research has linked incidence of TSS to the use of a particular type of super-absorbent tampon, which has now been withdrawn from the market. As a consequence, the incidence of TSS has decreased significantly. TSS is caused by a bacterium called *Staphylococcus aureus* that can live harmlessly on the skin's surface but which, when introduced into the vagina on a tampon, may multiply uncontrollably and release toxins that are absorbed into the bloodstream. The main symptoms of TSS are fairly nonspecific. Typically they include sudden high temperature, vomiting and diarrhea, weakness and dizziness, a sore throat, muscle aches, and a sunburnlike rash. If a woman experiences these symptoms, she should remove her tampon immediately and see a doctor as soon as possible, although there is a good chance that she is not suffering from TSS. To minimize the risk, use the lowest absorbency tampon suitable for your menstrual flow.

Sanitary pads

These are soft cotton pads that are absorbent on one side and waterproof on the other. They are worn inside the underpants so that the absorbent part absorbs blood as it leaves the vagina. Modern pads are increasingly streamlined and absorbent, with a "press-on" adhesive panel to attach them firmly to the underpants. Like tampons, pads vary in absorbency, to provide for women's differing needs. And like tampons, pads should be changed regularly for reasons of cleanliness and to avoid the risk of odors.

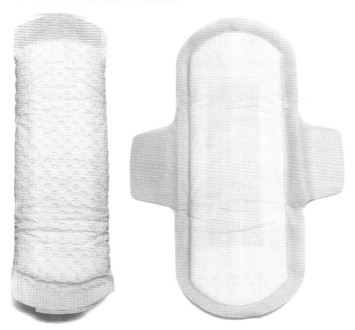

A standard sanitary pad (left) *contrasts with a slightly wider, flatter design* (right), *which in this case has "wings" that serve both to hold it in place more firmly and to cut down on leakage at the sides.*

Menstrual problems

Many women have years of menstrual cycles and periods that cause few if any problems. But the complexity of the internal mechanism that controls menstruation does cause problems for some women. These may be very mild, or they may be so painful and disruptive that they upset a woman's life for at least part of each month.

Although some women may well conform to the "ideal" 28-day menstrual cycle, with a period that lasts five days and presents no problems, many do not. Some suffer from emotional and physical symptoms before their periods start, or pains and cramps during their periods; others have very heavy periods, or irregular periods, or miss periods altogether. All or most of these conditions are treatable, either using medications that modify the hormonal mechanism that controls the menstrual cycle, or by self-help techniques, such as switching to a better diet and doing more exercise.

A woman of any age who is concerned in any way about menstrual problems should consult her doctor.

Premenstrual syndrome (PMS)

In the week or two weeks leading up to their period, many women notice certain physical and emotional changes which indicate that another menstrual cycle is reaching completion. Collectively, the symptoms that women may experience are known as premenstrual syndrome or PMS. They are probably related to fluctuations in the levels of the hormones estrogen and progesterone, and possibly also to levels of prostaglandins, in the latter part of the menstrual cycle, which have an effect on the brain.

A woman may experience one or more of these symptoms:
- depression and irritability
- mood swings
- headache
- fatigue
- dizziness or disturbances of vision
- nausea
- breast tenderness
- water retention (feeling bloated), resulting in a temporary increase in weight
- a feeling of clumsiness
- a low tolerance to alcohol
- a craving for sweets
- back pain
- breathlessness

Symptoms of PMS often first appear when a woman is in her twenties or thirties. There is no cure as such, but the following precautions may provide relief from the symptoms. Each woman is different, however, and a method

WHEN TO SEE THE DOCTOR

Women who have menstrual problems should consult their doctor if they experience any of the following:
- heavy menstrual flow that lasts for more than seven days
- irregularity in the menstrual cycle that cannot be attributed to long-distance travel, excessive weight loss or illness
- intervals between periods of fewer than 21 days or more than 60
- bleeding at any other times during the menstrual cycle apart from during the period
- severe cramps or pain at times during the menstrual cycle other than at the start of a period or, briefly, around ovulation (see p.21–2). One or more of these symptoms may indicate a disorder such as endometriosis, PID (pelvic inflammatory disease), or fibroids (see p.106), or may be caused simply by the nature of a woman's own particular menstrual cycle. Either way, it is important to get a medical opinion so that a serious disorder, if present, can be treated.

that works well for one individual may not be at all effective for another:
- getting regular exercise
- changing to a healthier diet, with more fiber
- eating less salt, to reduce fluid retention
- reducing caffeine and alcohol intake
- taking the pill (see pp.142–7), which is prescribed by doctors for some PMS sufferers because it creates an artificial menstrual cycle
- taking diuretic drugs (with prescription) to relieve water retention
- taking vitamins B6 and E.

Alternative therapies include:
- yoga and/or meditation
- taking evening primrose oil (which contains an essential fatty acid, gamma-linolenic acid)
- aromatherapy involving adding oils of lemon grass or lavender to bath water
- the Alexander technique.

Painful periods

Dysmenorrhea, or painful periods, is the most common of all menstrual disorders. Most women, at some time in their lives, experience

MENSTRUAL EXERCISES TO INCREASE BLOOD FLOW TO THE UTERUS AND PELVIS

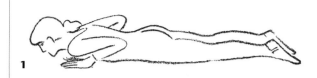

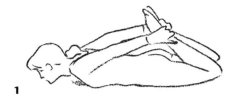

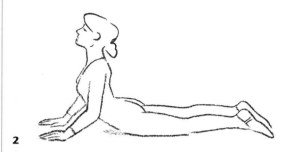

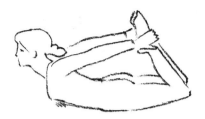

PELVIC PRESS

Lying flat on the floor, slowly push your upper body off the ground until your arms are stretched. Lower yourself back to the floor, and relax. Repeat the exercise several times.

PELVIC ROCK

Lying on the floor, stretch your arms behind you to grasp your ankles. Pull your legs, head, and shoulders off the floor, and rock gently back and forth several times.

menstrual pain or cramps in the lower abdomen and sometimes lower back, just before or during the first couple of days of their period. There are two forms of dysmenorrhea: primary and secondary.

Primary dysmenorrhea

Most women who experience menstrual pain are suffering from primary dysmenorrhea. Typically this starts some two or three years after a girl's first period, and is most frequent in the 17–25 age group. By their late twenties, or after having children, many women who previously suffered from painful periods no longer experience any menstrual pain.

Secondary dysmenorrhea

This is menstrual pain that begins during adult life and is the result of some other disorder such as PID (pelvic inflammatory disease, *see pp.124–5*), endometriosis, or fibroids *(see p.106)*. Conditions like these need to be diagnosed and treated by a doctor.

While many women experience menstrual pains as a mild ache, one in 10 finds the pain so severe that it interferes with their life. The

pains are believed to be caused by prostaglandins, substances that, among other effects, cause contraction of the muscles in the wall of the uterus, most notably during childbirth. Excessive secretion of prostaglandins results in a tightening of these muscles, which squeezes their blood vessels, temporarily cuts off their supply of blood and oxygen, and results in cramping pains.

In dealing with cramps, it is worth trying different remedies to see which is effective:
• aspirin, ibuprofen, or other antiprostaglandin pain medications
• exercises *(see above)* that increase blood flow to the pelvis and uterus
• back massage
• resting with a heating pad on the lower abdomen
• taking evening primrose oil
• masturbating to orgasm—which also increases blood flow to the uterus
• in more severe cases, a doctor may prescribe an oral contraceptive *(see pp.142–7)*, which relieves symptoms by suppressing ovulation.

Very heavy periods (menorrhagia)

Menorrhagia, or heavy menstrual bleeding, occurs in some women who regularly lose more than the "average" amount of blood during their periods. Menorrhagia can have various causes. In some women, an imbalance of the hormones estrogen and progesterone produces a thicker-than-normal endometrium (lining of the uterus), thus increasing the menstrual flow during a period. In others, uterine disorders such as fibroids or polyps *(see p.106)* may cause excessive bleeding. An investigation of the uterus called a dilation and curettage (D and C) may be used to determine the cause of menorrhagia *(see p.106)*. If there are no uterine problems, and the heavy bleeding does not cause anemia (or if it causes anemia mild enough to be counteracted by regular iron supplements), the condition may be left untreated. In cases that require treatment, there are several possibilities. For younger women, especially those who wish to have children in the future, hormones may be used to control bleeding. Laser treatment or cauterization can also be used to treat the endometrium. In cases of severe and persistent menorrhagia in older women, a hysterectomy *(see pp.108–9)* may be considered.

Menorrhagia may also occur in some women who use an IUD for contraception *(see pp.152–5)*. If the bleeding is not much heavier than usual, this should cause no problems, but if it is severe, a woman may wish to consider a different form of contraception.

Irregular periods

Women who do not experience the "normal" pattern of menstruation are said to be suffering from irregular periods. This can take one of three forms.

• A woman may experience considerable differences in the amount of blood she loses from one period to the next.

• A woman may find that the duration of bleeding varies greatly from one period to the next, so that, for example, one period lasts for one day, and another period for 10 days.

• A woman may notice that the time between one period and the next is very variable, sometimes lasting for months and at other times for weeks.

Irregular periods can have various causes. They are common, and natural, in teenage girls whose periods have just started and in older women approaching menopause. If a woman is not ovulating regularly because of hormonal problems, this may cause her periods to be both late and heavy, and she should consult her doctor. Other causes of irregular periods include stress, frequent travel across time zones, and, sometimes, disorders of the uterus.

Absence of periods

If a woman's periods have never started, or if they are interrupted for more than three months, she is suffering from amenorrhea, or absence of periods. There are two types of amenorrhea: primary and secondary.

IRREGULAR VAGINAL BLEEDING

The most common cause of vaginal bleeding is during a period, when the lining of the uterus is shed though the vagina. But if vaginal bleeding is irregular, it may be caused by a disorder that requires medical attention.

• Tiny spots of blood appearing in the panties or on toilet paper between periods—known as spotting—can be the result of using an IUD as a contraceptive, or taking certain types of contraceptive pills. Normally it is harmless, but a woman may want to discuss this with her doctor.

• Bleeding after intercourse may be a sign of erosion of the cervix *(see p.107)*, or another condition affecting the neck of the uterus, which should be reported to a doctor immediately.

• If a woman is past menopause, and has not had a period for six months, and she has vaginal bleeding, she should see her doctor: it might indicate a cancer of the uterus or cervix. However, the bleeding may be due simply to the vagina itself becoming dry and losing a little blood, a condition that may be helped by using a hormonal cream *(see p.274)*.

• If a woman has spotting during pregnancy she should see her doctor, especially in the later stages, when it may indicate a problem.

Primary amenorrhea

This condition occurs in young women who have never had a period. This may be because late menarche (the onset of menstruation) runs in the family, in which case it is a matter of waiting. It may result from a girl being underweight if, for example, she undertakes intensive athletic training or has an eating disorder such as anorexia nervosa (see p.83). Alternatively, it may be caused by a hormonal problem. If a girl has not started her periods by the age of 16, her parents should seek medical help.

Secondary amenorrhea

This describes a condition in which a woman has had at least one period before menstruation ceases for three months or more. The most common causes of secondary amenorrhea are pregnancy—which should be eliminated as a cause before treatment for any other conditions is implemented—and breastfeeding. Periods may also cease if a woman is stressed or depressed; if she does the type of frequent exercise that results in excessive weight loss; if she suffers from anorexia nervosa and has too little body fat; if she has a hormonal imbalance; or if she has been using certain types of drugs over long periods. Obviously, treatment of amenorrhea depends on its particular cause. In the case of pregnancy and breastfeeding, periods should start when these cease. The causes of stress and depression or the need to exercise excessively may be alleviated through counseling or support groups. The other conditions mentioned above require medical assistance.

Breast health

Breast disorders cause great anxiety for many women, although the better informed they are about the signs and symptoms of these disorders, the more likelihood there is of successful treatment. Common breast disorders include breast pain and tenderness, usually just before a period, which normally requires no treatment; and breast lumps, which as many as half of all women experience at some time during their life. In a minority of cases, a lump may be cancerous, requiring treatment by

BREAST TENDERNESS
There are several ways in which a woman can alleviate breast pain or tenderness. • Wear a supportive, properly fitting bra. • Wear a bra at night to support the breasts when asleep. • Take a mild pain medication, such as aspirin or ibuprofen. • Take vitamin B6. • Take evening primrose oil. If the breast tenderness is severe and does not respond to any of the above treatments, a doctor may prescribe a low-dose hormonal contraceptive to alleviate symptoms, or a diuretic drug that relieves water retention in breast tissue.

surgery. The sooner it is discovered, the greater the chance of a successful cure. This is why it is recommended that women over 20 examine their breasts monthly and report significant changes to their doctor.

Breast pain

Around three-quarters of women experience breast pain or tenderness (mastalgia) at some time in their lives. For one quarter of breast pain sufferers, the pain is severe enough to affect their lives. It may stop them from sleeping; inhibit their normal relationship with a partner because they cannot bear their breasts being touched; prevent them from enjoying sports; or make them worry all the time that people will bump into them accidentally and cause them pain. Most women find that breast pain is cyclical, occurring in the week or so before their period. Cyclical breast pain is probably caused by hormonal fluctuations that are taking place at this point in the menstrual cycle. These cause the breasts to retain excess fluid, making them feel full and sore. Some women find that breast pain happens at any time during the month. However, neither form of breast pain is likely to be caused by any serious disorder. Tenderness may also occur during early pregnancy, and during breastfeeding. And while some contraceptive pills make breast pain worse, it has been found that some low-dose contraceptive pills *(see pp.146–7)* reduce breast tenderness. There is always the worry that breast pain means breast cancer. In fact, breast cancer is normally painless and not connected with breast tenderness. But if a woman is concerned about breast pain, or if it is severe and persistent, it is advisable to see a doctor.

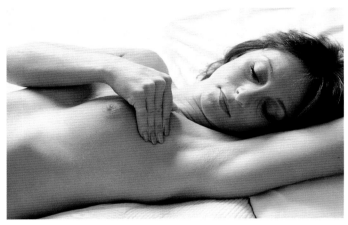

Monthly breast examination helps detect any changes or lumps that may indicate the presence of breast cancer, and is recommended for all women. With early detection, breast cancer can be beaten.

Breast self-examination

Every woman should regularly examine her breasts for any changes or irregularities. This way she becomes so familiar with their usual texture that she can rapidly identify anything abnormal. Her doctor, on the other hand, may detect only relatively large breast lumps.

The best time for women to examine their breasts is two or three days after their period finishes, when the breasts are usually at their least tender. Breasts are also less lumpy at this time because any cyclical breast lumpiness has subsided by this time of the month. After menopause, women can examine their breasts on the same day each month.

Most women who examine their breasts do so by following this sequence:
• visual inspection in front of a mirror to look for any changes in breast size or shape; also, visual inspection with the arms raised to look for dimpling of breast tissue
• manual inspection of all of both breasts while lying down
Some women feel their breasts in the bath or

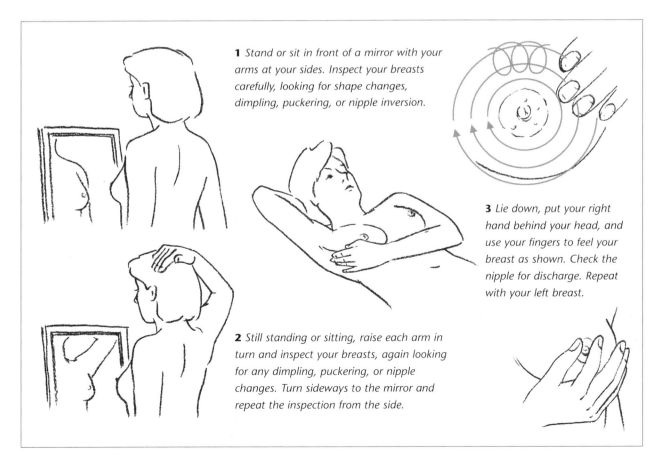

1 *Stand or sit in front of a mirror with your arms at your sides. Inspect your breasts carefully, looking for shape changes, dimpling, puckering, or nipple inversion.*

2 *Still standing or sitting, raise each arm in turn and inspect your breasts, again looking for any dimpling, puckering, or nipple changes. Turn sideways to the mirror and repeat the inspection from the side.*

3 *Lie down, put your right hand behind your head, and use your fingers to feel your breast as shown. Check the nipple for discharge. Repeat with your left breast.*

shower, because lubrication by soap enables the fingers to slide easily over the breasts.

When a woman is carrying out breast self-examination she should watch for any of the following changes or irregularities that might indicate a breast disorder:

• any lumps or bumps in the breast or armpit —remembering that in many women, soft, sore lumps appear and disappear just before their period every month, and also that 80–90 percent of unusual lumps are subsequently found to be benign

• any changes in the shape of the breasts, especially bulges on the surface

• the appearance of "orange peel" skin

• any swelling in the upper arm or armpit

• any discharge or bleeding from a nipple

• inversion (turning inward) of a nipple, if it normally projects outward

• recurrent eczema near the nipple

• any dimpling or other changes to the areola.

If a woman does notice something unusual, or is concerned with anything to do with breast health, she should get in touch with her doctor immediately. He or she may recommend further investigation using mammography or a biopsy *(see below)*.

Mammography

Mammography is a simple diagnostic technique used to check a woman's breast health. It involves exposing the breasts to low doses of X-rays in order to produce a mammogram —an X-ray photograph of the breast's tissues. It may be recommended for two reasons: either as part of a preventive screening program or to investigate a lump discovered during self-examination.

This technique can detect breast tumors as small as ⅓ inch across—the size of a small pea —which are too small to be felt during self-examination. At this size, if a tumor is cancerous, the cancer is much less likely to have spread to other parts of the body. Early detection of cancerous tumors by mammography significantly increases the chance of successful treatment, and probably minimizes the extent of treatment required.

Mammography is performed using a special X-ray machine. A radiographer positions the patient so that her breast is placed on the machine and gently "sandwiched" between an upper plastic cover and the lower X-ray plate, which contains the film. This may feel somewhat uncomfortable, but it does not take very long, and flattening the breast produces a better image.

If a breast contains a tumor, it will show up on the mammogram in about 85 percent of

QUESTIONS AND ANSWERS: BREAST HEALTH

Q. If I have inverted nipples, does it mean that I am more likely to get breast cancer?
A. If your nipples have always turned inward, it does not mean that you are more, or less, likely to develop breast cancer. But if your nipples have recently turned inward, you should see your doctor as soon as possible in case there is a problem.

Q. If a woman takes the pill, will it increase the risk of her developing breast cancer?
A. Overall, there seems to be no increased risk of breast cancer for woman who take the pill. However, recent studies suggest that one group of women—those who started taking the pill in their teens—may have a slightly increased risk. Using pills with a lower estrogen dose may minimize this increased risk.

Q. My daughter has large breasts. Does this mean that she is more likely to get breast cancer than someone with small breasts?
A. No. Breast size does not increase the risk. However, she will have an increased risk if you or other close relatives have had breast cancer.

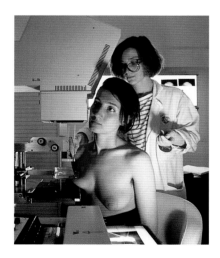

This special type of X-ray machine is used to produce a mammogram —an image of the inside of the breast. The resulting mammograms are examined for any growths too small to detect by touch that may be cancerous. Treatment of breast cancer at this early stage has a much greater chance of success.

cases. In these cases, the doctor will carry out a biopsy to determine whether the tumor is malignant (cancerous) or not. If the tumor is smaller than ⅓ inch in diameter, it will probably not show up on the mammogram.

Screening by mammography

In the United States, mammography is recommended from the age of 40: every one to two years for 40–49-year-olds, and every year for the over-50s. In other Western countries, it is felt that regular mammographies for younger women do not significantly reduce the death rate from breast cancer, and regular mammography is recommended only for women over 50. A woman's doctor should be able to give informed advice. Younger women whose immediate female relatives have had breast cancer, and who are therefore at greater risk, are recommended to have regular mammography even before they reach 40.

Breast lumps

If a woman discovers a lump, she should not panic—only a small percentage of breast lumps turn out to be cancerous—but she should seek medical advice immediately in order to get a diagnosis as soon as possible. Most breast lumps are benign (not malignant)

and are caused by one of the following three common conditions.

Fibrocystic breast disease
Also known as fibroadenosis, this is an increase in the glandular and fibrous tissue of the breast, possibly due to fluctuating hormone levels. It results in breast tenderness, pain, swelling and, occasionally, cysts.

Breast cysts
Cysts are fluid-filled lumps. Usually they are drained by needle aspiration, and the fluid is tested to check that no cancerous cells are present if the cysts remain.

Fibroadenomas
These are benign breast tumors, most common in women under 30. They are firm, round, painless lumps usually ½–2 inches in diameter, and can be moved under the skin.

Biopsy

If a woman has discovered a lump in her breast, or if a growth is shown on a mammogram, and her doctor suspects that it might be malignant, he or she will refer the patient for a breast biopsy to see whether the growth is benign or malignant. A biopsy is a diagnostic test that involves removing a small sample of tissue from the area, and examining it for cancerous cells. If a tumor is found to be malignant, the doctor can discuss the best course of action with her or his patient.

Breast cancer

Breast cancer is the most common type of cancer among women, affecting around 1 in 20 women in Western Europe, North America, and Australia. It is rare in women under 30, and more common in women over 50. This age distribution should not mean that younger women can feel complacent and not examine their breasts regularly. Women who are believed to be at a higher risk of developing breast cancer include:
• women with close female relatives who developed breast cancer
• women who have never had children, or had their first child in their thirties or forties
• women whose periods began early, and/or whose menopause was late
• women whose diet is high in animal fats.

DISCOVERING THAT YOU HAVE BREAST CANCER

However kind and sympathetic a doctor may be, the news that a breast biopsy indicates the presence of malignant cells, and therefore the presence of breast cancer, usually comes as a devastating shock. In the days following diagnosis, most women will experience fears of a premature death, of being "mutilated" by possible breast removal, of losing part of themselves and their sexuality—and their partner's reaction to that—and of being out of control of their lives. Such fears are understandable, and yet modern treatments mean that many more women are surviving breast cancer, and more of those who are treated do not necessarily have a complete mastectomy or breast removal. Probably the best strategy for a woman with breast cancer to adopt is to talk about her fears, and to find out more about the disease and possible treatments. Talk and help may come from family and friends, or from local support groups; more information may be provided by trained nurses or counselors who are affiliated with hospital oncology departments.

Studies have indicated that there is a direct relationship between the low incidence of breast cancer in Japan, Thailand, and the Philippines and the low levels of animal fats found in the diets of these countries.

Breast cancer usually starts as a single lump in the breast, most commonly in the upper, outer part of the breast (closest to the armpit). Other signs and symptoms include swelling and dimpling of the breast and discharge from the nipple. If a lump is found to be cancerous, further tests—blood tests, X-rays, and bone scans—are carried out to see if the cancer has spread, in order to determine what kind of treatment would be best. If her cancer is treated at an early stage, the patient's long-term survival chances are good.

The initial treatment for breast cancer is the removal of part or all of the breast. In the past, the entire breast was removed as a matter of routine; today, less extensive and less disfiguring surgery is often just as effective. The type of surgery depends on the type of cancer, whether it has spread to other parts of the body, and the age of the woman. Following surgery, she may also receive radiology treatments and/or chemotherapy to destroy any cancerous cells that may remain. Surgeons generally remove as little of the breast as possible.

Lumpectomy
If the tumor is discovered in its early stages, most surgeons will perform a lumpectomy. This involves removing the tumor and its surrounding tissues, and some of the underarm lymph glands, to leave a small scar and depression in the breast.

Partial mastectomy
This procedure removes the segment of breast tissue containing the tumor, leaving a visible scar and the breast smaller than before.

Simple mastectomy
Here, the whole breast is removed but the lymph glands and underlying chest muscles are left in place. The breast may be reconstructed later by a procedure known as mammoplasty.

Subcutaneous mastectomy
Subcutaneous mastectomy involves removing the inner tissue of the breast but leaving the

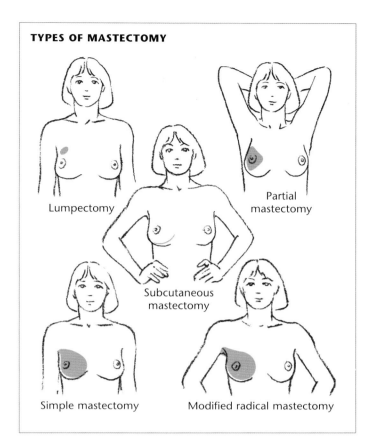

TYPES OF MASTECTOMY

Lumpectomy

Partial mastectomy

Subcutaneous mastectomy

Simple mastectomy

Modified radical mastectomy

Breast cancer is treated by surgery, but the type of the surgery depends on the size of the tumor inside the breast and the extent of the spread of the cancer. When the cancer is detected early, only the lump is removed. In more severe cases, part or all of the breast tissue is removed.

skin and the nipple intact. A silicone implant is then inserted under the skin in order to give the impression of a complete breast.

Modified radical mastectomy
This is usually the most extensive form of surgery. The whole breast and associated armpit lymph glands are removed in one piece. Like a simple mastectomy, it leaves a scar across the chest. Some women may opt for breast reconstruction at the same time as, or after, the operation, in which case the breast is "rebuilt" and a saline implant is inserted under the skin.

Living with breast surgery
After surgery, women are generally given radiology treatments (in which radiation kills or slows down the development of the cancerous cells) or chemotherapy with anti-cancer drugs

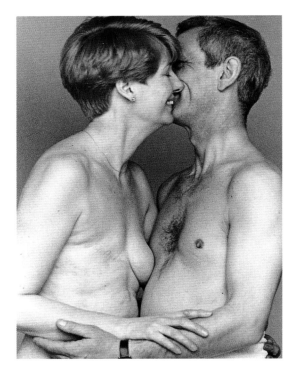

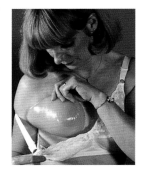

Loss of part or all of a breast can have a devastating effect on a woman emotionally, but the support of a loving partner can help restore her self-esteem and sexual confidence. A prosthesis (right) also helps boost confidence.

Implants, reconstruction, and prostheses

Breast surgery need not necessarily mean that a woman loses her breast shape, even though part of the breast has been removed.

Implants and reconstruction

A breast implant is a floppy bag containing saline (just like those used to increase breast size). The surgeon uses skin and fat from a site near the removed breast to rebuild the breast, inserting the implant to give it shape.

Prostheses

After their mastectomy, many women are offered an artificial breast or prosthesis that fits into their bra and balances the remaining breast. It can give a woman confidence after her operation, because there is no external sign that she has had a mastectomy; and, by balancing the other breast it prevents shoulder and back pain produced by compensating for less weight on one side of the body.

Disorders of the ovaries

The ovaries are the primary female sex organs. Between a woman's puberty and her menopause, they release eggs and female hormones *(see pp.20–3)*. The location of the ovaries deep in the abdominal cavity means that any ovarian disorders tend to be "silent" initially, without obvious signs or symptoms. The main conditions affecting the ovaries are ovarian cysts and, less commonly, cancer.

Ovarian cysts

Ovarian cysts are common; they are abnormal swellings of the ovary. Inside a woman's ovary each month, an egg develops within its bag-like follicle. In the middle of the menstrual cycle, the follicle bursts, and the egg starts on its journey toward the uterus. Sometimes a follicle fails to rupture, and this is the most common cause of cysts.

The vast majority of cysts are benign rather than malignant. However, some enlarge and become solid, and may cause disturbances in the menstrual cycle, unfamiliar pains and discomfort in the abdomen (which may also become swollen), and possibly pain during intercourse. If a woman has any of these symptoms, she should see her doctor.

in order to destroy any remaining cancers. Women who have major breast surgery may find it difficult to come to terms with the fact that they have lost all or most of one of their breasts. However, the better the counseling they receive before and after the operation, and the more they are kept informed, the less likely women are to experience feelings of depression or despair. Where a whole breast has been removed, some women choose to use an external prosthesis that slips inside the bra. Alternatively, some women opt for breast reconstruction. Many women may also worry that their cancer might return. They may be helped by counseling or by self-help groups. Some doctors also recommend alterations in diet and other lifestyle changes.

Cysts are usually discovered by pelvic examination, when the doctor feels the area around the ovaries and uterus, and are confirmed by ultrasound or laparoscopy (examination through a viewing tube). Although some cysts disappear on their own, it may be necessary for a doctor to remove the cyst or, if it is very large, the entire ovary *(see oophorectomy, below)*.

Polycystic ovarian syndrome (PCOS)

Also known as Stein-Leventhal syndrome, PCOS is caused by an imbalance in the hormones released by the pituitary gland that cause the development of eggs inside the ovary. This results in a thickening in the outer layer of the ovary, and the formation of tiny cysts around its outside. Women with PCOS may not know anything is wrong until they try to get pregnant. However, the syndrome is often characterized by irregular periods, and other symptoms may include excessive hair growth, acne, oily skin, and obesity. PCOS can be treated with drugs that restore the normal hormonal balance, although the specific treatment depends on whether or not a woman wants to become pregnant.

Ovarian cancer

Cancer of the ovary is comparatively rare, but it kills more women than cancers of the uterus and cervix combined, mainly because it is difficult to detect in its early stages. However, if it is diagnosed early, the outlook is optimistic.

Women are more likely to develop ovarian cancer after menopause. It also appears that the risk is increased if a woman has never had children; if there is a history of ovarian cancer in her close family; if she has a history of cancer of the breast or uterus, or of the rectum; and if she is overweight. Breastfeeding and taking the pill appear to lower the risk.

Ovarian cancer can develop in one or both ovaries. Typically, there are few signs or symptoms initially. In later stages of development, when the cancer is more widespread, a woman may suffer from an upset stomach, abdominal pain, and flatulence, and may have abnormal bleeding from the vagina or abdominal swelling. These symptoms may, of course,

be due to another condition, so a woman needs to visit her doctor.

If a pelvic examination reveals a swelling, a laparoscopy (using a viewing instrument to look inside the abdomen), or laparotomy (opening up the abdomen) can be used to make a diagnosis. If confirmed, ovarian cancer in its early stages can be treated by oophorectomy; or by the removal of the ovaries, fallopian tubes, and uterus (hysterectomy—*see pp.108–9*), if at a later stage. After surgery, a woman is usually given a course of radiation or anticancer drugs to help ensure the cancer is completely removed.

Oophorectomy

This is the surgical removal of one or both of the ovaries, usually because of ovarian cancer, but sometimes because of a large ovarian cyst *(see above)*, and also sometimes as part of hysterectomy.

For younger women, especially if they want to have children, the prospect of having both ovaries removed can be particularly upsetting because it means that menopause comes early. Where possible, surgeons attempt to perform a partial oophorectomy in women of this age group so that normal ovarian function is maintained. If just a small part of one ovary is left behind inside the body, a woman of reproductive age may well continue to have periods and be able to become pregnant. However, if both ovaries have to be removed, younger women will experience a premature menopause. They can be given hormone replacement therapy to mimic the effects of hormones released by the ovary *(see pp.271–5)* and thereby minimize the symptoms of menopause, but of course this will not restore their ability to have children.

Disorders of the uterus

Disorders of the uterus (womb) are among the most common reasons for women to consult their doctor. Apart from menstrual disorders *(see pp.95–9)*, other conditions that affect the uterus include growths that may be benign or cancerous. In the past, hysterectomy (removal of the uterus) was commonly used as a cure for many uterine complaints, but today a wider range of less drastic treatments are used where hysterectomy is not deemed necessary.

Fibroids

Fibroids are rounded, benign tumors that develop in the muscular wall of the uterus of over 20 percent of women over the age of 35. The most common type of tumor found inside the human body, fibroids vary from pea to tennis-ball sized, although in some cases they can become as big as a grapefruit. Small fibroids produce no symptoms, but as they grow they sometimes cause heavy periods *(see p.98)*. If fibroids are large they may distort the uterus; they can cause back pain, abdominal discomfort, and frequent urination; and they may, in some women, cause infertility.

Fibroids are diagnosed by pelvic examination and ultrasound. Small fibroids require no treatment, but larger ones can be removed so that they do not cause infertility. In severe cases, where the fibroids are large and numerous, a hysterectomy *(see pp.108–9)* may be required. Medical therapy that suppresses estrogen production may also be used as an alternative means of treating fibroids.

Polyps

These are small, benign growths from the wall of the uterus that protrude into its inner cavity. Most common among women in their late thirties or forties, polyps can result in cramps and irregular periods *(see p.98)*. If they cause

DILATION AND CURETTAGE

Also known as D and C, this is a routine procedure used to investigate disorders of the uterus, including heavy bleeding *(see p.98)*. The D and C is normally carried out under local or general anesthetic. The gynecologist scrapes away all or part of the endometrium (the lining of the uterus). In order to do this, the opening of the cervix is carefully dilated (widened), using metal rods known as dilators. Then a curette, a spoon-shaped instrument with a sharp end, is inserted through the cervix and into the uterus in order to scrape out the endometrium. The D and C is often carried out with the help of a hysteroscope, a viewing instrument used to examine the inside of the uterus. Samples of endometrium can then be examined to help diagnose the disorder.

problems they are usually investigated and removed by dilation and curettage *(see box)*.

Endometriosis

Normally, during a menstrual period, the endometrium passes out of a woman's body through her vagina. But in some cases it seems that fragments of the endometrium pass in the "wrong" direction along the fallopian tubes and into the pelvic cavity, causing the condition known as endometriosis. The small fragments of endometrium form cysts. Each month, during the menstrual cycle, these cysts respond to changes in hormone levels by increasing in size and bleeding, as if they were still inside the uterus. But blood cannot escape from the cysts, and as they slowly enlarge, they cause inflammation and pain.

Endometriosis occurs most commonly in women between the ages of 25 and 40, and in women who are childless. Between 30 and 40 percent of women with endometriosis experience infertility. The most common symptoms of endometriosis are heavy and extremely painful periods, back pain, diarrhea, and blood in the feces. If cysts are located behind the uterus, sexual intercourse may be painful.

How endometriosis is treated depends on how severe it is, and the age of the patient. Hormonal treatment may be used to suppress normal menstruation so that the cysts shrink away. If a woman becomes pregnant, that may have the same effect. In more severe cases, the cysts may be removed surgically.

Uterine prolapse

A prolapsed uterus sags downward into the vagina, and sometimes protrudes out of it. Prolapse happens when the ligaments and pelvic muscles holding the uterus in place are stretched by childbirth or become weakened after menopause. Women often first notice the condition because they experience the sensation of something falling out of the vagina.

If symptoms become annoying, and the cervix has not descended too far into the vagina, a rubber device can be fitted around the cervix to support the uterus. In some cases an operation may be carried out to repair stretched tissues. If the prolapse is severe, and the uterus is protruding from the vagina, a hysterectomy may be considered.

The risk of prolapse can be diminished by activities such as pelvic floor exercises *(see p.221)* to strengthen the muscles that support the uterus; avoiding obesity; and stopping smoking, because a chronic cough can aggravate the situation.

Cancer of the uterus—endometrial cancer

Cancer can occur in two parts of the uterus: the endometrium or the cervix. However, the term "cancer of the uterus" usually refers to endometrial cancer.

Endometrial cancer is most common in women who have been through menopause. The risk of developing the cancer appears to be greater in women who are overweight, have high blood pressure, have never had children, and have experienced a delayed menopause. Before menopause, the risk of developing endometrial cancer is less in women who are taking the pill.

The most common symptom of endometrial cancer in women whose periods have stopped is irregular vaginal bleeding, and any woman who experiences this after menopause should consult her doctor as soon as possible. In younger women, it may be indicated by heavy periods, bleeding between periods, or bleeding after intercourse, although there may well be other causes of these symptoms.

This cancer is usually treated by hysterectomy and removal of associated lymph glands. Radiation, chemotherapy, or hormonal therapy may also be used to ensure that all traces of cancer are destroyed. The outlook for women with endometrial cancer is generally good, if it is treated early.

Cervical cancer

Cervical cancer is the most common cancer of the female reproductive system, and one of the most common cancers affecting women worldwide. But it develops relatively slowly and, if detected at an early stage, has a good chance of being completely cured. Screening programs for cervical cancer have reduced the death rate from the disease even though its overall incidence has increased.

Before cervical cancer appears, and before a woman notices any symptoms, the cells on the surface of the cervix undergo changes that make them appear increasingly abnormal. These are known as precancerous ("before cancer") changes, and it is these that can be detected by a Pap smear.

If these precancerous stages remain untreated, there is a risk of cancer developing: the greater the severity of these abnormal changes *(see box, below)*, the greater risk there is of developing cancer. In its early stages, cancer may cause an unusual vaginal discharge or a discharge containing blood in mid-menstrual cycle or after the menopause. In its later stages, it can cause pelvic pain and pain in the back and legs, as well as a bloody discharge or bleeding.

Pap smears

A Pap smear is a simple procedure used to take a small sample of cells from the cervix. In order to take a smear, the doctor or nurse inserts a speculum into the vagina, to hold it open so that the cervix can be seen. A small spatula is then used to scrape a few cells from the cervix. This cell sample is smeared onto a microscope slide and sent to a laboratory to be examined under a microscope. If abnormal cells are found on her cervix, a woman will usually be referred for further investigation.

Women are now recommended to have their first Pap smear six months after first sexual intercourse, then another after one year, and subsequently every one to three years for the rest of their life.

CIN GRADING

Normal cervical cells have a characteristic appearance that changes if a type of abnormal cell growth called cervical intraepithelial neoplasia (CIN) takes place on the surface of the cervix. If changes are seen, they are given a low or high CIN grading, according to the severity of the abnormal cell growth. The higher the grade of CIN, the greater the risk of developing cancer. But the presence of CIN does not mean that cancer is inevitable. Many cases of low-grade CIN show a spontaneous reversal to a normal condition. The reason for this is that low-grade CIN may be the result of cell changes that will not necessarily lead to cancer.

Colposcopy

If a cervical smear shows unusual cells, a doctor will examine the cervix for abnormalities using a viewing instrument called a colposcope. A small sample of tissue may also be taken for investigation—a biopsy. If the biopsy confirms precancerous change, this area of the cervix may be treated by laser, freezing, heating, or removal of the tissue with an electric cutting wire (loop excision).

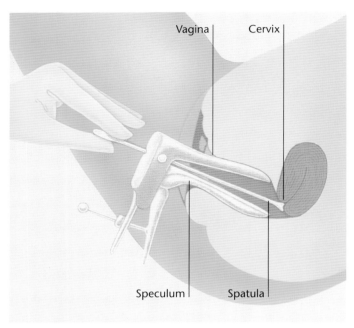

Vagina | Cervix

Speculum | Spatula

For a Pap smear, a woman lies on her back with her legs apart, and the doctor inserts a speculum into the vagina. The speculum is then opened, to hold the vaginal walls apart, and a small spatula is used to scrape a sample of cells from the surface of the cervix.

RISK FACTORS FOR CERVICAL CANCER

The single most important risk factor in the development of cervical cancer is infection with the human papilloma virus (HPV) that causes genital warts *(see p.123)*. A woman is at risk of infection with HPV if she has sexual intercourse with a man who has genital warts. Over 90 percent of women with cervical cancer are infected with HPV. The other factors listed below can increase the risk of developing cervical cancer:

• becoming sexually active at an early age
• having a sexual partner who is not circumcised
• being infected with herpes *(see pp.122–3)*
• having many sexual partners
• smoking, probably because carcinogens (cancer-causing chemicals) absorbed from cigarette smoke are excreted in fluid produced by the cervix.

Cone biopsy

If the colposcopy indicates that precancerous changes extend into the cervical canal, or the severity is difficult to ascertain, the doctor will perform a cone biopsy. This involves using a laser or scalpel to cut a cone-shaped piece of tissue from the cervix, which can then be examined to see how far the precancerous changes have spread. In 90 percent of cases, cone biopsy removes all affected tissue.

Treatment of cancer of the cervix

If cancer of the cervix is diagnosed, treatment will depend on the age of the patient and how far the cancer has spread. Some patients are treated with radiation, while in others a total hysterectomy is carried out; in severe cases, a radical hysterectomy may be performed, along with removal of the lymph glands.

Hysterectomy

Hysterectomy is the removal of the uterus, performed to treat serious uterine disorders. It is the most common major operation for women in developed countries, but is increasingly being replaced by less drastic treatments.

Conditions for which a hysterectomy is usually considered include cancer of the endometrium or cervix, severe and prolonged heavy uterine bleeding (including menorrhagia), severe fibroids, severe uterine prolapse, and extensive, painful endometriosis.

A hysterectomy is carried out either through the abdomen or through the vagina.

Total hysterectomy

This involves removing the uterus and cervix—and, if necessary, the ovaries and fallopian tubes (oophorectomy—*see p.105*).

Radical hysterectomy

Radical hysterectomy—often performed to treat cancer—involves removing the uterus, cervix, surrounding tissues, lymph glands, and part of the vagina. If necessary, the fallopian tubes and ovaries are removed as well.

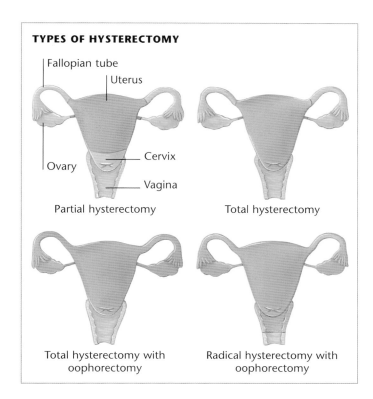

TYPES OF HYSTERECTOMY

Fallopian tube
Uterus
Ovary
Cervix
Vagina

Partial hysterectomy

Total hysterectomy

Total hysterectomy with oophorectomy

Radical hysterectomy with oophorectomy

Hysterectomy is the surgical removal of part or all of the uterus. Four types of hysterectomy are shown (left)*: the red area shows how much of the uterus is removed in each instance. In some cases, the ovaries are also removed (oophorectomy), along with the woman's fallopian tubes.*

Partial hysterectomy

More rarely, a surgeon will remove the body of the uterus but leave the cervix. Some women prefer this because they feel it retains fuller sexual sensation.

After a hysterectomy

Following her operation, a woman will remain in hospital for a few days. Full recovery usually takes up to six weeks; during this time she should avoid overexertion, but gentle exercise such as walking will help her recover her strength. She can expect light bleeding from her vagina at first and, if her ovaries were removed, she may have hot flashes because of the reduction in estrogen—if the ovaries have been removed, she is now effectively past menopause *(see Chapter 10)*. After four to six weeks, she should return to hospital for a checkup. If she and her partner wish, she can then resume sexual activity.

In cases where symptoms such as heavy bleeding or pain were debilitating, a hysterectomy can leave a woman revitalized and more able to enjoy her sex life. But many find that after hysterectomy they suffer for a while from depression and/or lack of interest in sex.

To some extent, this may be caused by the sudden hormonal changes resulting from removal of the ovaries. However, removing the uterus alone, or uterus plus one ovary, will not cause these changes; and if both ovaries have to be removed, hormone replacement therapy (HRT—*see pp.271–5*) should help.

Alternatively, depression may be due to anxiety about the effects of hysterectomy. Common worries include:
• Fear of aging rapidly and/or becoming "unfeminine." This is very unlikely if the ovaries are left in place. Again, if the ovaries have to be removed, HRT is generally found to be highly effective.
• Fear of losing enjoyment of sex. In fact, after a recovery period, a woman should be able to enjoy sex as much as she did before.
• Fear of putting on weight and becoming obese. There is no direct link between hysterectomy and obesity.

Counseling before and after hysterectomy may help to assuage such fears. If the woman and her doctor or doctors have fully discussed the extent and possible consequences of the operation beforehand, post-operative problems are likely to be greatly reduced.

Male health

Major disorders of the male reproductive system mainly concern two organs—the testes and the prostate gland—and tend to occur in two particular phases of the life span. Cancer of the testis, although rare, is most common in younger men. Enlargement of the prostate gland and cancer of the prostate are more prevalent among older men. As with cancer of the breast or the cervix, the sooner testicular and prostate cancer are detected, and the quicker they are treated, the greater the chance that they will be cured. There are also a number of other male reproductive disorders requiring medical attention that may affect the male reproductive organs.

Cancer of the testis

Although comparatively rare, cancer of the testis is the most common form of cancer in young men between the ages of 15 and 35. If detected early—usually by self-examination of the testes—there is a very good chance of a complete cure. The risk of developing testicular cancer is much higher in men who have or have had an undescended testicle—one that is still located in the abdomen during adolescence or adulthood. However, if the testicle is surgically brought down into the scrotum during early childhood, the risk of developing testicular cancer is minimized. Testicular cancer also appears to occur more frequently in men of Caucasian origin than it does among other ethnic groups.

Testicular cancer usually appears first as a hard, painless swelling on the side of the testicle. This can usually be detected by self-examination if a man feels his testes on a regular basis and is therefore familiar with their normal state. In later stages of the disease, there may be pain.

If a man goes to his doctor with a lump in the testis, the doctor will first ensure that it is not due to any other disorder of the testis. If cancer is confirmed, a surgeon will remove the affected testis under general anesthetic—orchidectomy—examining the other testis at the same time to make sure it is healthy. Radiation and anticancer drugs may also be used. Some surgeons insert a testicular prosthesis—a firm but flexible ball—into the scrotum to restore its normal appearance. If the cancer has been detected early, there is a survival rate of almost 100 percent over a five-year period.

Self-examination of the testis

The first symptoms of testicular cancer are most likely to be discovered by men themselves. And if discovered early, testicular cancer can be completely cured in the vast majority of cases.

These two statements underpin the importance of carrying out regular self-examination

---

MEN AND THEIR SEXUAL HEALTH

Many men are reluctant to see doctors when they experience symptoms—especially those symptoms that affect their reproductive systems. Unfortunately, in the case of cancers of the testis and prostate, the later the reporting and treatment of the disease, the less likelihood there is of a cure. Early detection generally means more treatment options and higher survival rates. It is in men's best interests to be aware of what their bodies are telling them, and not to be afraid to consult a doctor if they have worries about any symptoms. Partners can certainly help by persuading men to seek help as soon as possible if something appears to be wrong. And of course men, like women, will also benefit from a general checkup on a regular basis in order to assess and monitor all the various aspects of their health.

HEALTH PROBLEMS WITH THE TESTES

Q. If a man has one of his testes removed because of cancer, does this mean that he will not be able to be a father or, if he is a father already, to have any more children?
A. In most cases, the removal of one testis does not affect a man's ability to become a father because the remaining testis will produce a sufficient quantity of sperm.
Q. I can feel a firm area running around part of each of my testes. Do I have cancer?
A. If this area curves around the back of each testis, and feels quite rubbery, then it is the epididymis, which is a normal part of the testis. If not, consult your doctor.

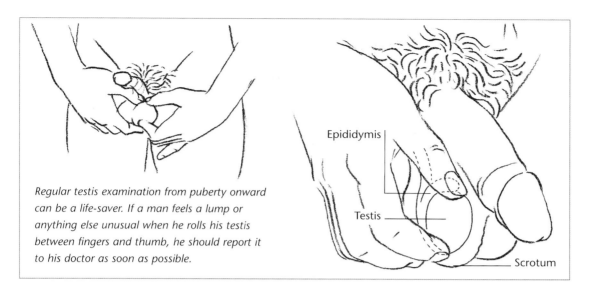

Regular testis examination from puberty onward can be a life-saver. If a man feels a lump or anything else unusual when he rolls his testis between fingers and thumb, he should report it to his doctor as soon as possible.

Epididymis

Testis

Scrotum

of the testes from puberty onward. Each testis should be examined in turn, using the fingers of both hands, to feel for any changes in size, shape, or texture. The best time to do this is after a bath or shower, when the scrotum is soft and relaxed. By gently rolling each testis between thumb and fingers, the entire surface can be felt for any hard lumps or bumps. If present, these commonly occur on the side or front of the testis. These bumps should not be confused with the epididymis, a rubbery band that runs down the back of the testis *(see p.23)*, and the vas deferens, the tube that carries sperm away from the testis *(see p.24)*; these are perfectly normal parts of the body. If there is any suspicion of a lump or anything unusual, a man should see his doctor as soon as possible.

Prostate problems

The prostate gland is a part of the male reproductive system that may often cause health problems in later life. The size and shape of a walnut, the prostate is located at the base of the bladder, surrounding the urethra, the tube which carries urine from the bladder to the outside of the body through the penis. The prostate may become swollen and inflamed by bacterial infection, a condition known as prostatitis. But the major disorders affecting this gland are enlarged prostate and cancer of the prostate.

Enlarged prostate

Enlargement of the prostate gland, also known as benign prostatic hypertrophy (BPH), is common in men aged 50 years or over. It is not the same as cancer of the prostate. As the prostate gets bigger it presses on the urethra and interrupts the flow of urine, producing its main symptoms: a frequent need to urinate, especially annoying at night; difficulty in starting to urinate; and a weak urinary stream, sometimes just a few drops at a time. If a man notices he has these symptoms he should consult his doctor immediately. An enlarged prostate is detected by rectal examination. If it causes urinary problems, an enlarged prostate gland requires treatment, most commonly by surgery to remove all or part of the prostate. Newer treatments include introducing a narrow balloonlike device into the penis, then inflating it to widen the urethra where it passes through the prostate; using lasers to remove excess prostate tissue; and using drugs that shrink the prostate.

Cancer of the prostate

The incidence of prostate cancer increases with age, and over 80 percent of cases occur in men aged 55 years or older. If prostate cancer is identified in its early stages, the outlook for the patient is good. Symptoms of prostate cancer are similar to those experienced by someone with an enlarged prostate and should be investigated by a rectal examination. In addition, a sample of blood can be screened for prostate-specific antigen (PSA), high levels of which may indicate the presence of prostate cancer. If the prostate feels hard when examined, or the PSA screening is positive, the doctor will take a biopsy to confirm whether or not there are cancerous cells present, and may also do a blood test to seek further confirmation. Because prostate cancer can spread to the bones, the doctor may also perform a bone scan.

Routine examinations of the prostate and PSA screening are important for older men. They can increase the chances of detecting a possibly cancerous prostate in its early stages before the man notices any symptoms himself.

Prostate cancer is treated by surgery to remove all or part of the prostate gland, or by radiation to destroy the cancer. It appears that the male hormone testosterone encourages spread of the cancer. If the cancer spreads to other parts of the body, drugs may be given to inhibit the release of testosterone from the testes; female hormones may be given; or, in some cases, the testes may be removed, in order to shrink the tumor.

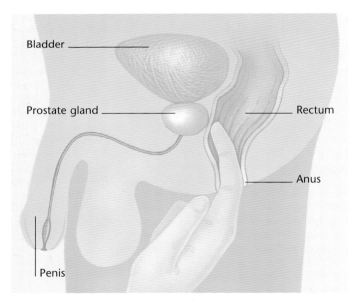

Bladder

Prostate gland

Rectum

Anus

Penis

A frequently used test for prostate enlargement is a digital prostate examination. The doctor feels the shape and size of the prostate gland through the front wall of the rectum using a gloved, lubricated finger pushed into the rectum through the anus.

Examination of the prostate gland

Prostate problems are discovered or confirmed by a manual examination. The doctor inserts a finger—gloved and lubricated—into the rectum, to determine the size, shape, and texture of the gland. A healthy prostate is smooth and rubbery; an enlarged prostate is, obviously, larger than would be expected; and a cancerous prostate feels hard and knobbly.

Prostate surgery

Prostate surgery usually takes one of two forms. Transurethral resectoscopy (TUR) involves putting a type of endoscope (viewing tube) called a resectoscope into the urethra, through the tip of the penis, then using a heated wire on the end of the resectoscope to cut away part of the prostate, and washing out the pieces through the resectoscope. Retropubic prostactomy involves making an incision in the abdomen and removing the prostate, neck of the bladder, seminal vesicles, and nearby lymph nodes. Both types of surgery require general anesthetic.

In most cases, a result of prostate surgery is retrograde ejaculation, which means that semen shoots backward into the bladder

---

HEALTH PROBLEMS WITH THE PROSTATE

Q. My father died of cancer of the prostate. Does this mean that I have a greater chance of developing the disease?
A. It is true that some cancers, such as breast cancer, run in families. However, there is no evidence that this is true for prostate cancer.

Q. I have an enlarged prostate and am soon to receive treatment to reduce it. I am worried that this may make me impotent—a friend of mine has had treatment and has had some sexual difficulties since the operation.
A. The occurrence of sexual problems after prostate surgery has decreased dramatically with the introduction of new methods. However, it would be best to discuss with your doctor the nature of your operation and what aftereffects you might experience. The likelihood of having sexual problems will be much reduced if you know precisely what, if any, changes to expect.

DYSFUNCTION AFTER PROSTATE SURGERY

Many men fear that they may lose the ability to have an erection after their prostate operation, or lose interest in sex itself. These fears are probably based on the more radical surgical procedures used in the past to treat enlarged prostate and cancer of the prostate, which commonly destroyed the nerve pathways that controlled sexual functions such as erection. Today, erectile problems or loss of libido affect only a small percentage of men who have retropubic prostatectomy, and a smaller percentage who have TUR. It is important for the surgeon and patient to discuss such issues before the operation, as research has shown that patients who have been reassured that they will continue to become sexually aroused and achieve erections after the operation very rarely have sexual problems following surgery.

during ejaculation instead of coming out through the penis. This is harmless, as the semen passes out during urination.

Other disorders of the testes

Hydrocele
This is a painless swelling of the scrotum that is common in middle-aged and older men, produced by fluid accumulating in the space around the testis. Sometimes this is caused by an injury, although other causes include inflammation or infection. If the swelling becomes uncomfortable or painful, the fluid can be drawn off under local anesthetic.

Orchitis
Orchitis—inflammation of a testis, causing swelling, pain, and fever—is normally treated with painkillers and bed rest for several days until the swelling has gone down; antibiotics may be prescribed if an infection is suspected. Orchitis also occurs in around one in four men who develop mumps after puberty.

Epididymal cyst
A fluid-filled "bag" may sometimes form inside the scrotum. These are generally harm-

less, although if a man detects an unusual growth when examining his testes, he should report it to his doctor.

Torsion (twisting) of the testis
This is severe swelling and pain in the testis caused by the testis turning so that its blood vessels become twisted and obstructed. Deprived of its blood supply, the testis soon becomes painful, and there may be pain in the abdomen and nausea. If these symptoms appear, immediate medical attention is required. The doctor may try to manipulate the testis back into position. If that fails, the scrotum is opened to untwist the testis, which is then anchored with stitches to prevent it from twisting again. Without treatment, the testis may be permanently damaged and need to be removed. Torsion of the testis is most common during puberty, although it may occur in younger boys and in young adults.

Disorders of the penis

Balanitis
This is an inflammation of the glans of the penis and, if present, the foreskin. It may be caused by a condition such as a yeast infection (see p.116); poor hygiene through failing to wash the penis, especially under the foreskin in uncircumcised men; irritation from spermicides, particularly those used in condoms; rubbing against clothes; excessive washing or use of antiseptics; or having a tight foreskin. Treatment involves washing the penis regularly and, if prescribed, taking a course of antibiotics. If balanitis is caused by using condoms lubricated with spermicide, a man can try using nonlubricated condoms instead.

Blood in the semen
This is a rare condition caused by the rupture of tiny blood vessels in the urethra during an erection. It should heal rapidly, but if it recurs the man should consult his doctor.

Tight foreskin
The foreskin is often tight in young boys and should not be forced back. However, if it continues to be tight into adulthood, a condition

known as phimosis, it may make erection painful and sexual activities impossible. It may also cause balanitis because the glans cannot be washed. If this is the case, circumcision (see p.26) is usually recommended.

Priapism

Priapism is a rare condition in which an erect penis remains, often painfully, erect, instead of softening. Erection is produced when blood accumulates in the spongy tissues of the penis; when excess blood drains from these tissues the penis softens. In the case of priapism this natural drainage does not occur, and the condition must be treated immediately to ensure that the penis is not permanently damaged. Priapsim is usually found as a side effect of drugs given to men with erectile problems or in men who have sickle-cell disease, an inherited disorder of red blood cells.

Cancer of the penis

This is an extremely rare form of cancer, most prevalent among uncircumcised men whose genital hygiene is poor. Initial symptoms include a wartlike lump on the foreskin or glans or a painful sore on the glans. A man who has these symptoms should consult his doctor immediately, although these symptoms are more likely to be caused by a sexually transmitted disease (see pp.117-26). As with other cancers, the earlier it is detected the greater the chance of a cure.

Sexual infections

Everyone suffers from diseases during their lives. A disease is an abnormality in the way the body functions. It can be non-infectious (such as the cancers described in this chapter) or infectious (such as the common cold) and caused by microorganisms, such as bacteria and viruses. These disease-causing microorganisms (known commonly as germs) usually enter the body through openings, or cuts in the skin, and multiply rapidly until destroyed by the body's defense system or by drugs.

The term "sexual infections" in this chapter is used to describe some common infectious diseases that affect the organs of the male and female reproductive systems, and sometimes the female urinary system. Some of these are not usually passed on by sexual contact, and are described under nonsexually transmitted diseases. Those infections that are passed on by sexual contact are described later in this chapter under the heading sexually transmitted diseases.

Unfortunately, many people feel unnecessarily confused and ashamed if they develop a sexual infection and may be too embarrassed to consult a doctor. The description of sexual infections that follows is not intended to be a guide to self-diagnosis. If you or your partner show signs or symptoms of a sexual infection or irritation, you should consult your doctor or visit a hospital as soon as possible to obtain an accurate diagnosis. Doctors and nurses who treat sexual diseases are used to seeing people who have—or turn out not to have—these infections. They will not be embarrassed, patronizing, or judgmental. Their job is to treat a patient with a sexual infection in the same way that an orthopedist would treat someone with a broken leg. Ignoring a sexual infection or irritation will not make it go away. Nor will it do any good to blame a partner for passing on a disease that may not even be present. It may well be the case that the infection has not been passed on sexually or that it is non-infectious.

Nonsexually transmitted diseases

These are sexual infections that are not generally transmitted by sexual contact and that mainly affect women (usually in the urinary tract). So what causes them? On the skin, and inside certain body openings—such as the mouth, vagina, rectum, and anus—a community of microorganisms including bacteria and fungi live quite harmlessly, keeping each other in check and stopping any one type of microorganism from taking over. This is much like a cultivated garden where different types of plants coexist but prevent any one variety from dominating. In fact, the community of bacteria and fungi on or in the body is often described as "flora." But sometimes things go wrong. Bacteria that are harmless in the rectum, for example, might be accidentally transferred to the vagina, where they cause infection. Alternatively, the vaginal flora might be disrupted so that one microorganism grows out of control and causes an infection.

Nonsexually transmitted diseases can occur in women of all ages, who may or may not be sexually active. Vaginal and urinary infections cause discomfort to many women, and are among the most common gynecological complaints that women consult their doctors about.

Acute urethral syndrome

This is a condition that affects the urethra (the tube that carries urine from the bladder) in women. Common symptoms include a frequent urge to urinate, a feeling of discomfort in the lower part of the stomach, and pain around the vulva. It may be caused by infection of the urethra by bacteria from the large intestine, in which case it can be treated with antibiotics and by drinking plenty of water. Alternatively it may, in women who have gone through menopause, be caused by an inflammation of the vulva that can be treated with hormonal creams (see p.274). However, in a large proportion of women the cause is unknown.

Bacterial vaginosis

Bacterial vaginosis (BV) is an infection of the vagina that occurs in sexually active women. The main symptoms are the presence of a grayish white, often frothy vaginal discharge that has a fishy odor, and sometimes mild irritation and burning in the vagina and vulva. BV is caused by a disturbance in the vaginal flora: naturally protective bacteria decrease in number, while others undergo a "population explosion" that produces the symptoms of vaginosis. This bacterial imbalance is believed to be caused by sexual activity, but is not sexually transmitted. BV is treated by antibiotics, either taken by mouth or introduced in cream or gel form into the vagina.

Cystitis

Cystitis is an inflammation of the bladder, normally caused by bacterial infection. It is common in women of all ages and can be irritating and annoying, especially if it lasts for long periods. The main symptoms are a frequent urge to urinate, although only releasing a small amount of urine each time; and a burning or stinging feeling during urination. This happens because the inflammation of the bladder's interior prevents the complete emptying of the bladder during urination, allowing infective bacteria to multiply in the urine stagnating in the bladder and urethra.

The bladder and urethra are normally free of any microorganisms. The bacteria that cause cystitis are unwanted invaders either from the vagina or from the rectum via the anus. They are accidentally introduced into the entrance of the urethra from the vulva, where there may be various bacteria present, and travel up to the bladder. Cystitis is much more common in women than men because the female urethra is much shorter than the male's, so bacteria do not have far to travel to the bladder. Movement of bacteria into the urethra may be assisted by sexual intercourse.

Cystitis can often disappear on its own. If symptoms persist beyond 48 hours, or if they are severe—especially if the urine is foul-smelling or tinged with blood, or if a woman has chills or a fever—she should consult her

"HONEYMOON" CYSTITIS

Some women find that if they are starting a new relationship, or are sexually active after a prolonged period of celibacy, they develop symptoms of cystitis, including a burning feeling on urination. This condition is commonly referred to as honeymoon cystitis because traditionally it was found in brides who had never had any sexual experience until their wedding night. The cause of honeymoon cystitis is believed to be friction between the walls of the urethra caused by the penis thrusting inside the vagina during sexual intercourse. Apart from irritating the urethra, it may also allow harmful bacteria to enter this sterile area and infect it. Treatment is the same as for cystitis.

doctor. If bacterial cystitis has been confirmed —by taking a urine sample—a doctor will prescribe antibiotics to remove the infective bacteria. If left untreated, the bacteria may spread to the kidneys and cause pyelonephritis, an inflammation of the kidneys, which is far more serious.

Self-help remedies for cystitis include drinking plenty of water to flush out the urinary system, and drinking cranberry juice and over-the-counter preparations of potassium citrate. Women who are sexually active and prone to cystitis may find it helpful to urinate before and after intercourse to flush out any bacteria. Some women find that using the diaphragm *(see pp.137–40)* as a contraceptive method makes them prone to cystitis.

Yeast infections

Also known as candidiasis, yeast infections affect the vagina. Like cystitis, they can occur in women of all ages, sexually active or not.

Symptoms typically include a thick, white vaginal discharge, almost like cottage cheese, which has a yeasty smell; vaginal irritation and itching; and, possibly, a burning feeling in the vagina during sexual intercourse. The condition is caused by a yeastlike fungus, called *Candida albicans*, found in the vagina, vulva, rectum, and mouth, and on the skin. As part of the natural vaginal flora, *C. albicans* is normally prevented from spreading excessively by vaginal bacteria. But sometimes the vaginal flora is disrupted and the fungus grows uncontrollably to produce the symptoms of a yeast infection. Often this happens because the vaginal environment is altered—for example, by taking an antibiotic to control a bacterial infection that also kills vaginal bacteria; by using certain types of combined oral contraceptive pill; or by becoming pregnant.

Yeast infections may also occur where the body's immune system is weakened by stress; by long-term use of corticosteroid drugs; or in people with AIDS or diabetes. Occasionally, men develop yeast infections after intercourse with an infected partner, as indicated by inflammation of the glans of the penis.

Treatment involves the use of an antifungal drug. For women, this usually takes the form of a suppository or cream to be inserted into the vagina, and possibly as a cream to be applied to the vulva. Doctors may also prescribe a cream for a male partner to apply to his penis to prevent possible reinfection.

A natural remedy that may help to treat yeast infections is the use of plain yogurt containing live bacteria, *Lactobacillus acidophilus*. Some should be applied inside the vagina and left for at least two hours.

During infection it is preferable to refrain from intercourse—this may be painful in any case—or to use a condom. Yeast infections can grow in the mouth, so oral sex should also be avoided until treatment is completed.

Vaginitis

Vaginitis is a general term that describes the uncomfortable, irritating, and sometimes painful condition caused by inflammation of the vagina, which may also produce an abnormal and excessive vaginal discharge. It may be caused by yeast infections or by a sexually transmitted disease called trichomoniasis, both conditions that require medical treatment. Alternatively, vaginitis can be a non-infectious disease, resulting from an allergy to a spermicide, irritation by soaps or bath oils, or the use of vaginal deodorants. In all these cases, alleviation of symptoms can be achieved by avoiding particular products.

Preventing vaginal and urinary infections

Practical ways for women to reduce the risk of vaginal and urinary infections are as follows:
• When using toilet paper, wipe from front to back, so that intestinal bacteria are not

---

QUESTIONS AND ANSWERS: YEAST INFECTION/CYSTITIS

Q. I have recently had a yeast infection for the first time. Was it passed on to me by my sexual partner?
A. This is unlikely. The fungus that causes yeast infection lives naturally in the vagina, and it is more likely that something— such as taking antibiotics or going on the pill—changed conditions in your vagina, causing a yeast infection to develop.
Q. If a women has had cystitis several times in the past, will it affect the fetus if she becomes pregnant?
A. No. Cystitis will not affect the fetus, but medical attention should be sought if cystitis occurs during pregnancy.

carried from the anus to the vagina or urethra.
• Urinate when you need; do not hold back.
• Avoid "feminine hygiene" products that
may irritate the vagina.
• Avoid unprotected sexual intercourse.
• Wear underwear made from cotton, rather
than nylon or other synthetics which make the
vulva warmer and moister than normal, so
providing a perfect environment for microorganisms to infect the vagina or urethra.
• Avoid douching—flushing out the vagina
with water or deodorant solutions. Douching
may upset healthy bacteria normally found in
the vagina by destroying beneficial bacteria,
thus allowing potentially harmful bacteria to
thrive and cause infection. It may also introduce infection into the vagina, or spread
vaginal infection into the uterus. For the same
reason, it is also advisable to avoid hot baths.

Sexually transmitted diseases

Infectious diseases are passed on in a variety
of ways, depending on the type of disease.
Cold viruses are inhaled in droplets from the
air; food poisoning bacteria are swallowed
with contaminated food and water; and
malaria is transmitted by bites from infected
mosquitoes. Sexually transmitted diseases
(STDs) are passed from one person to another
by sexual contact. Specifically, an STD may be
passed on to someone if they are exposed to
infected body fluids (such as semen or vaginal
fluid, and sometimes blood) during vaginal
intercourse, anal intercourse, and sometimes
during oral sex.

STDs have traditionally been regarded as
unmentionable and something shameful
because of the generally negative attitude to
sexual matters found in most societies. There
has often been an assumption that infection
with an STD implies that a person is promiscuous and deserves to get an infection because
of their immoral behavior. This sort of attitude has been seen recently in extremist
descriptions of AIDS as a "gay plague," as if it
were a punishment for homosexual behavior.

The reality is, however, that STDs are diseases like any others. They simply happen to
be passed on by sexual activity. Some STDs
are more infectious than others, although
anyone—regardless of sex, class, age, ethnic
background, or wealth—may develop an STD
if he or she has sexual contact with a partner
and is not protected by the use of, for
example, a condom.

Like many other diseases, an STD requires
medical treatment. Left untreated, STDs may
cause further complications. Unfortunately,
some STDs can be present, especially in
women, without causing symptoms. This is
why it is important for people with STD
symptoms to let their partners know, so that
they can get treatment as well. If a man or
woman thinks they may have an STD, they
should visit a doctor or a clinic that specializes
in reproductive health and STDs. These are
normally found at hospitals. Trained staff will
make a diagnosis—it may not be an STD—
and prescribe a course of treatment that
should clear up the infection. They will also
help the patient psychologically and enable
their partner (sometimes referred to as their
"contact") or partners to be traced and, if
necessary, tested and treated. This is all done
in a confidential and discreet manner. To
reduce the risk of contracting STDs—apart
from complete abstinence—it is advisable
always to practice safe sex by using a condom (and using it correctly—*see pp.132–7*).
This applies as much to long-term relationships as it does to casual sex. People do get
STDs in long-term relationships even with
both partners claiming to be monogamous.

Considered first in this section is HIV, a
virus that can be transmitted sexually, and
which eventually causes AIDS. The rest of the
section deals with common STDs.

HIV and AIDS

HIV (human immunodeficiency virus) is a
virus that attacks the immune system and can
eventually cause AIDS (acquired immune deficiency syndrome), a syndrome that was first
identified in 1981. HIV, recognized as the
causative agent in 1983, is commonly passed

on by sexual intercourse through body fluids such as blood, semen, and vaginal secretions. In addition, HIV can be passed on by injecting equipment (needles and unsterilized syringes) shared by drug users, infected blood in transfusions, from infected mothers to newborn babies, and (less commonly) by blood contact through open cuts.

At present HIV appears to be incurable and, over time, causes the body's natural defense system to stop functioning so that the carrier becomes prey to one or more opportunistic diseases that eventually cause death (although new therapies are allowing people with HIV to live much longer). If a person has HIV and one or more of these diseases, they are diagnosed as having AIDS. The most encouraging aspect is that people can considerably reduce the risk of contracting HIV and developing AIDS by altering their sexual behavior and practicing "safe sex." It has to be remembered, however, that once a person has HIV, he or she may pass it on to another person at any time if they have unsafe sex.

Initially, AIDS in Europe and North America appeared to be confined mainly to homosexual and bisexual men and intravenous drug users. But the number of men and women who have contracted HIV through heterosexual sex has increased in Europe and North America, and AIDS has become a major cause of death among young people in their twenties and thirties. Anyone of any age or sexual orientation can contract HIV through unprotected sex. (In Africa, HIV has from the start spread mainly through the heterosexual population, probably because the predominant HIV sub-type in this part of the world is different.) By the end of 1994, the WHO (World Health Organization) estimated that worldwide about 4.5 million people had developed AIDS.

With no cure in sight at present, it has become clear that people must be educated to be aware that they are at risk of developing an HIV infection if they have unprotected sex. This is a point that parents and teachers should raise with children when they talk to them about HIV and AIDS, and about sexually transmitted diseases in general.

What causes AIDS?

AIDS is caused by HIV (human immunodeficiency virus), which can be transmitted in body fluids—primarily blood, semen, and vaginal secretions—that enter the body during sexual contact, through small cuts or lesions in the skin, or via the tissue lining the internal parts of the reproductive system. The chances of contracting HIV are much higher through

HOW HIV IS SPREAD

There is often confusion about the ways in which HIV can, or cannot, be passed from one person to another. Ignorance about the means of transmission can be particularly unhelpful in a home or workplace where someone is HIV-positive. It can provoke unnecessary fears among relatives or colleagues, and may result in cruel and ignorant comments being made to or about the infected person.

HIV may be passed on:
• by unprotected sexual contact involving the exchange of body fluids (blood, semen, or vaginal secretions) with a person who already has an HIV infection
• by sharing hypodermic needles and syringes used to inject intravenous drugs with someone who has an HIV infection

• from an infected mother to her fetus during pregnancy or childbirth. (This is not inevitable, but occurs in about one in seven cases in which the mother has the HIV virus; the risk to the child increases with breastfeeding.)

HIV cannot be acquired from casual contact or:
• blood-sucking insects, such as mosquitoes
• swimming pools
• toilet seats
• doorknobs
• sharing glasses, cutlery, or plates
• shaking hands
• dry or cheek-to-cheek kissing
• embracing
• sharing towels
• coughs, sneezes, or contact with sweat, such as from a floor mat in a gym.

unprotected anal intercourse—where delicate tissues are more likely to tear—than through vaginal intercourse. The risk is also greater if other STDs that cause breaks in the skin, such as herpes, are already present.

To understand how HIV infects the body, and how AIDS develops, it helps to understand, in simple terms, the workings of the body's immune system. Throughout its life, the human body faces an onslaught of disease-causing microorganisms, including bacteria and viruses, attempting to enter the body. Those that penetrate the first line of defenses —such as the skin—are then detected and destroyed by the immune system. This system consists of billions of cells that enable us to fight off infections. Some, called macrophages, roam through the bloodstream and tissues searching for invading microorganisms and destroying them. Macrophages also "inform" other cells of the immune system that there are invaders inside the body. First on the scene are the helper T-cells, which alert the entire immune system to launch an all-out attack on the specific invader. This includes production of "killer chemicals," called antibodies, which help wipe out microorganisms.

This is what normally happens when infections threaten, but when HIV invades the body things go wrong. All viruses need to enter living cells in order to reproduce. The cells that HIV selects for invasion are the helper T-cells, key elements in the immune response. HIV viruses take over the genetic material of these cells and replicate themselves, destroying the helper T-cell in the process. Although the body produces antibodies to combat the growing HIV menace, the immune system is gradually worn down over the years as the number of key helper T-cells decreases. This is the stage at which AIDS develops. Lacking its normal defenses, the body is vulnerable to infection by opportunistic diseases that would normally be repelled by a healthy immune system. Eventually, one or more of these diseases completely overwhelms the body, leading to the death of the AIDS sufferer.

The stages of HIV infection

As yet, there is no conclusive proof that all people infected with HIV will necessarily go on to develop AIDS. Because the disease was only identified relatively recently, long-term studies have not yet been able to identify which of the people who are HIV-positive will not develop AIDS. However, men and women who are infected with HIV, and who do develop AIDS, typically progress through four noticeable stages.

REDUCING THE RISK OF PASSING ON THE HIV INFECTION

People can minimize the risk of passing on HIV infection by adopting safer sex practices. These are forms of sexual activity that avoid the exchange of bodily fluids between the sexual partners. Examples of various sexual activities are graded here, from safe and risk-free to unsafe and high-risk.

Safe, risk-free sexual activities:
• all sexual activities between partners who are both uninfected
• self-masturbation; touching or stroking a partner's genitals
• fellatio (oral–genital sex by a woman or man on a man's penis) with a latex condom on the penis

• dry or cheek-to-cheek kissing
• cuddling, hugging, massaging

Low-risk sexual activities:
• all sexual activities between partners who both have low-risk sexual histories
• French (wet) kissing with no cracked lips, broken skin, or ulcers
• vaginal intercourse using a latex condom (only a risk if condom tears —almost always due to putting it on incorrectly)
• anal intercourse using a latex condom (only a risk if condom tears)
• contact between mouth and anus
• contact between genitals without penetration

• fellatio without a condom, without ejaculation taking place in the mouth
• cunnilingus (oral–genital sex by a man or woman on a woman's vulva), if the woman does not have a period

Unsafe, high-risk sexual activities:
• vaginal or anal intercourse without a latex condom
• sharing sex toys, such as vibrators, inserted into the vagina or anus
• fellatio without a condom if ejaculation takes place in the mouth
• cunnilingus when the woman has her period
• sexual activities that cause bleeding, as the blood may enter the other person's bloodstream

Stage 1—Initial acute infection

Up to a quarter of people show initial symptoms between two and five weeks after infection with HIV. These symptoms can include general body aches, sore throat, fever, chills, widespread rash, oral and genital ulceration, and swollen lymph glands. However, it is very important to realize that these are non-specific symptoms that could indicate other mild viral infections apart from HIV.

Stage 2—Asymptomatic HIV infection

During the asymptomatic (without symptoms) phase, which lasts on average up to 10 years or longer, a person looks and feels completely healthy, although the virus is actively replicating inside the body. But he or she may suffer from lymphadenopathy: swelling of the lymph nodes (or glands)—centers for fighting infections—found in the neck, armpits, and groin. During this phase a person is infective and may pass on the virus to other people without realizing that he or she is infected. Why this phase varies in length among different individuals is not yet clear, although it probably depends on a number of factors, including age, lifestyle, and the presence of other infections. Some people—known as non-progressors—have remained symptom-free for many years, and only time will tell if they will ever develop AIDS. If they do not, it may be the result of their particular lifestyle, the type of HIV they were infected with, or the potency of their individual immune system.

Stage 3—Symptomatic HIV infection

The onset of this symptomatic (with symptoms) phase indicates that the immune system is weakening under the HIV onslaught, making the body more susceptible to diseases that would normally be controlled. These include yeast infections, or thrush (candidiasis), in the mouth—in healthy women this is a common infection of the vagina (see p.116). Other common symptoms are skin complaints, weight loss, bouts of tiredness, diarrhea, and sweating. Men or women may pass on the infection unknowingly at this stage, unaware that they are infected.

Stage 4—Advanced symptoms: AIDS

As the immune system weakens further, the symptoms of AIDS develop. There is a fixed set of symptoms and diseases that characterize the syndrome. Some are worsening of the symptoms experienced during symptomatic HIV infection: fevers and night sweats, and progressive weight loss. Opportunistic infections, such as *Pneumocystis carinii pneumonia* (PCP), extensive herpes, tuberculosis, or encephalitis, which eventually prove fatal, are also AIDS-defining. HIV may infect brain cells, too, causing dementia. Once a person

SUPPORT FOR PEOPLE WITH AIDS

AIDS is a devastating disease, but much can be done to provide constructive help and support for a relative or friend who is suffering from it. It is all to easy to assume that one individual is powerless to help someone else whose life has been shortened, yet it may be possible to make a positive difference during the last months or years of someone's life by helping to improve their life in some way. But be sensitive to the person's feelings. Overprotection can be as bad as ignoring someone. Ask if your help is actually wanted. Support for a person with AIDS could include:

• being honest about the situation and talking about the disease in realistic terms

• touching and hugging to provide reassurance (if they wish!)

• helping with planning and implementing future activities

• making contact with other friends or relatives to ensure that there are regular visitors

• visiting someone in a hospital or hospice

• dropping by to see someone or spending an afternoon finding out how they are

• doing tiring chores like shopping or cleaning

QUESTIONS & ANSWERS: AIDS

Q. We are both 17, both virgins and want to start having a sexual relationship. Will we get AIDS if we don't use a condom?

A. It is very unlikely, unless you have ever injected drugs (and provided you both really are virgins), that either of you has HIV. And AIDS cannot be "created" by sexual contact.

Q. Can you tell if someone has HIV or AIDS?

A. It is impossible to tell if someone is infected with HIV simply by looking at them. The only way to know is by getting a blood test.

has AIDS—with one or more of these specific conditions and HIV—it will probably prove fatal at some time in the next four years.

Testing for HIV

If someone is worried that they may have been infected with HIV, there are a number of people to talk to. There is no point in waiting and worrying needlessly. A helpline might be the first stop. At a clinic that specializes in STDs or an HIV/AIDS advice center there is always a counselor or doctor with whom to talk through the issues, discuss the possible advantages and disadvantages of testing, and enable someone to come to an informed decision as to whether or not to take a test to see whether they have an HIV infection. It may help to talk to a friend or relative, if they are sympathetic and can be trusted to keep a confidence.

If a man or woman does decide to be tested, a blood sample is taken and sent to a laboratory for testing. The blood test identifies the presence or absence of antibodies against HIV. If the test is negative it means that the person is probably not infected with HIV, although antibodies can take some time to appear in the blood (more than six weeks) and another, later blood test may be suggested. If the test is positive, it will be repeated with a more sensitive test to check that it is correct before the patient is informed of the result. If the more sensitive test is also positive this means that the person is infected with HIV—they are HIV-positive.

Once the test result comes through, a doctor or counselor at the clinic will inform the patient in person whether the test was positive or negative. Not surprisingly, many people react with shock and despair when they discover they are HIV-positive. Usually, clinic staff will refer them to suitable counselors and support groups. If an individual has told his or her trustworthy friends or relatives, they can be of great help in providing support, and helping to plan for the future, although unfortunately some people have a more hostile reaction. People with HIV can lead normal working and social lives, and may well appear healthy for a number of years.

Treating HIV and AIDS

At the time of writing there is no cure for HIV infection or AIDS, although treatments have been used to alleviate the effects of both. Since the late 1980s, the drug AZT has been used to slow the progression of HIV infection, although recent research has shown that its benefits may be limited when used alone. However, many centers use AZT as part of a cocktail of drugs (combination therapy) employed to inhibit the development of HIV infection. Patients also receive antibiotics to prevent AIDS-related infections. People with symptomatic HIV or with full-blown AIDS are given specific treatment according to the condition, although there comes a time when the infections are no longer treatable.

Common sexually transmitted diseases

Chlamydia

This is the general name for infections caused by the bacteria-like organism *Chlamydia trachomatis*. Chlamydial infections occur in both men and women and are transmitted mainly by vaginal intercourse, or less commonly by anal intercourse or oral sex. *C. trachomatis* is the main infective agent in mucopurulent cervicitis (MPC) in women and non-gonococcal urethritis (NGU) in men. A high proportion of women with chlamydia do not have MPC or any of its symptoms.

Mucopurulent cervicitis (MPC)

This is an inflammation of the cervix caused most often by *Chlamydia trachomatis*, but it can also be caused by *Neisseria gonorrhoeae* (the bacterium that causes gonorrhea). The main symptom of MPC is a discharge from the cervix, although many women do not notice that it is any different from a normal vaginal discharge. If MPC is diagnosed (by seeing a red cervix and pus discharge), it can be treated with antibiotics. Untreated, *C. trachomatis* and other microorganisms that cause MPC can spread to other parts of the reproductive system and may cause pelvic inflammatory disease (PID).

Non-gonococcal urethritis (NGU)

NGU, one of the most common male STDs, is

an inflammation of the male urethra produced by microorganisms other than the bacterium that causes gonorrhea. Over 50 percent of cases of NGU are caused by *Chlamydia trachomatis*. Symptoms of NGU include a clear or pus-like discharge from the penis and pain or a burning feeling when urinating. Some men, however, have very mild symptoms or none at all. NGU is usually treated by antibiotics, although the type of treatment depends on what type of agent has caused the disease. Female partners should also be treated, as transmission of NGU may cause MPC or PID, and the couple should refrain from sexual contact until both of them are cured. Untreated, NGU can cause painful inflammation of the epididymis (part of the testis) or a urethral stricture, a narrowing of the urethra.

Genital herpes

This sexually transmitted disease produces sporadic outbreaks of painful blisters on the genitals. It is caused mainly by the herpes simplex type two virus. Once a person has become infected by herpes simplex, the virus stays inside the body for life, although it may remain inactive for much or all of that time, and some infected people never show any symptoms at all.

Genital herpes is highly infectious. Usually a person contracts the disease through sexual contact with a partner who has the blisters on his or her genitals. However, it appears that the virus may sometimes be passed on by someone who is infected but shows no outward signs of infection. Oral sex may sometimes cause infection if the person performing the act has cold sores, as may use of infected sex toys, such as vibrators.

Some three to six days after infection, a person who develops symptoms of herpes first feels irritation or burning in the genitals

before small, clear blisters appear on the penis or vulva. These blisters burst open to leave painful ulcers that will heal within 10–21 days. This first episode of herpes is often accompanied by high temperature, headaches, and muscle pains. Sufferers may experience a burning feeling during urination and women may have a discharge.

After this first occurrence of herpes, one third of sufferers have no more flare-ups, another third have a few more episodes, and the remaining third have frequent attacks—more than three times a year. Recurrences may be triggered by sunbathing, stress, or sometimes sexual intercourse. A tingling feeling in the genitals is often an early warning sign that an attack is about to start. Subsequent attacks may be less painful than the first because the body starts to build up some resistance, but men and women who experience repeated occurrences of genital herpes commonly find the condition both distressing and painful.

There is no "cure" for genital herpes because the virus cannot be eliminated. If a sex partner has been diagnosed as having genital herpes, condoms should always be used to prevent infection of the other partner. However, the antiviral drug acyclovir is very effective in reducing the pain and duration of the first attack. In patients with frequent, long-term attacks, the use of acyclovir will reduce or abolish the attacks while the drug is taken. Genital herpes passed from a mother to her newborn child can cause severe illness and possibly death. For this reason, mothers who suffer an attack when they are about to give birth may be delivered by cesarean section and acyclovir given to the infant.

Several self-help strategies may help alleviate the effects of an attack of genital herpes.
• Avoid sexual contact during an attack and until two or three days after blisters have healed completely.
• Wear loose-fitting cotton underwear.
• Take aspirin or ibuprofen to reduce pain.
• Wash the genitals regularly during an infection and pat them dry with a towel—it should be washed afterward.
• Wash hands carefully after touching the

QUESTION AND ANSWER: VASECTOMY

Q. My boyfriend has had a vasectomy. Do we still have to practice safe sex?
A. A man who has had a vasectomy cannot make you pregnant, but he can still pass on sexually transmitted diseases, including HIV.

affected area, in order to avoid spreading the infection to other parts of the body.
• After swimming, do not sit around wearing a damp swimsuit.

Genital warts

Warts are skin growths that commonly appear on the hands and often disappear without treatment. Genital warts, however, appear on the genitals or around the anus and must be treated medically. Soft and generally painless, genital warts range in form from individual small, flat bumps to pink or grayish white growths that resemble tiny cauliflowers and can form an extensive covering. Genital warts are caused by certain types of the human papilloma virus (HPV) that can be transmitted by sexual contact.

Over 60 percent of partners of individuals who have genital warts will develop the disease. However, it may take weeks, months, or even years before signs and symptoms appear, and even before they do, the virus can be passed on to a new partner. Sufferers may experience embarrassment about their warts, and possibly discomfort. They should, however, seek treatment as soon as possible. In addition, women should seek diagnosis if their partner has genital warts because, even if they themselves show no signs of infection, the warts may be concealed inside the vagina or on the cervix.

Various types of treatment are available, including application of podophyllin, a caustic chemical that erodes the warts (not to be used for pregnant women); liquid nitrogen, which is used to freeze the warts; or laser treatment to burn away the warts. However, no treatment can remove the virus from the body; it remains inactive within body tissues, but it may reactivate and genital warts may recur. In addition to seeking treatment, a woman who has had genital warts—or whose partner has had them—should also have regular Pap smears *(see pp.107–8)* because there is evidence that women infected with certain types of HPV have an increased risk of developing cervical cancer *(see p.107)*. If either sexual partner has genital warts, they should use a condom to prevent infection.

Gonorrhea

Also known as "the clap," gonorrhea is one of the most common STDs worldwide, although it is becoming uncommon in most Western countries. It is a highly infectious disease caused by the bacterium *Neisseria gonorrhoeae*, which affects more men than women and is more prevalent among teenagers and young adults, especially those with numerous sexual partners. It is usually passed on by anal, vaginal, or oral sex.

Symptoms of gonorrhea, when they occur, appear within two days to two weeks of getting the infection. Male symptoms include a burning sensation during urination, followed by a milky discharge from the penis, which becomes thicker over time. However, some 10 percent of men and 50 percent of women show no initial symptoms.

Untreated, gonorrhea may spread to the prostate gland or the epididymis of the testis, causing inflammation and, possibly in the latter case, permanent sterility, although this is now rare. Women infected with gonorrhea may also feel burning when urinating, although the most usual symptoms are vaginal discharge, dyspareunia (painful sexual intercourse), and pelvic pain. But about half of all women infected with gonorrhea show no symptoms, or have symptoms so mild that they ignore them.

Even when symptoms are present, they are so nonspecific that they could be confused with other infections such as cystitis. The problem is that, left untreated, the bacteria that cause gonorrhea can travel through the reproductive system and cause PID *(see overleaf)*, which can have serious consequences, including infertility. For this reason it is vital that, should a man discover he has gonorrhea, he must tell his female partner that she may have the infection, because it

SAFE SEX PRACTICES

Safe sex practices reduce the risk of acquiring an STD. They include:
• abstaining from sex if one partner has symptoms of an STD
• using a latex condom during vaginal intercourse
• using a latex condom during anal intercourse
• using a latex condom during fellatio

may remain hidden inside her body and cause further damage.

Once diagnosed by taking a smear of discharge for microscopic examination, gonorrhea is treated with a course of antibiotics. Women may also be given antibiotics that eliminate any chlamydia infection *(see p.121)* —around a quarter of people with gonorrhea also have chlamydia.

Hepatitis B
Although it does not affect the sexual organs, hepatitis B is frequently passed on by sexual contact. Hepatitis is an inflammation of the liver caused by a number of different viruses. Hepatitis B is a form of the disease caused by the hepatitis B virus (HBV). A person infected with hepatitis may show no symptoms, but if symptoms do develop they usually include a flulike illness, fever, loss of appetite, nausea, possibly jaundice (a yellowing of the skin and eyes), and a feeling of tenderness in the upper abdomen. Usually the illness subsides after about three weeks and the liver returns to normal functioning within a few months.

One of the major routes of transmission of hepatitis B is through sexual activity, including oral sex and kissing. It can also be transmitted via blood, shared needles, unsterile tattooing, and ear piercing, as well as from a mother to her newborn infant via her milk. The reason for this is that the HBV can be found in most of the bodily fluids of an infected person, including semen, saliva, and vaginal secretions, and it is highly infectious. The HBV can also be passed on from mother to fetus. Hepatitis B was once more common among male homosexuals, although it appears that heterosexual intercourse is now the main route for the sexual transmission of HBV, with having many partners the main risk factor. If a doctor suspects that a patient may have hepatitis B, he or she will confirm it by means of a blood test.

There is no specific treatment for hepatitis B, although rest, a good diet, and avoiding alcohol should aid recovery. Vaccination against hepatitis B is available, but at present it is targeted at those most at risk, such as doctors, nurses, people with multiple sexual partners such as prostitutes, and intravenous drug users. In 5–10 percent of cases, the HBV persists and the person becomes a carrier, able to pass on the disease but not showing any symptoms. Carriers may also risk developing other liver disease, such as cancer, which may lead to death, although a treatment is now available that will cure a huge proportion of chronic carriers.

Mucopurulent cervicitis (MPC) and non-gonococcal urethritis (NGU)
See chlamydia (p.121).

Pelvic inflammatory disease (PID)
Pelvic inflammatory disease (PID) is an inflammation of the female reproductive organs, especially the ovaries, fallopian tubes, and uterus, and is a common cause of lower abdominal pain in women. It is most common in younger, sexually active women, and it has a higher incidence in women who use the IUD as a contraceptive *(see pp.152–5).*

PID is often caused by a sexually transmitted disease (such as chlamydia or gonorrhea —*see above*) that has not been treated, often because it has shown no symptoms. Women with PID may have pain in the abdominal or pelvic regions, especially during or just after sex. They may also develop a fever or backache and have irregular periods. However, many women with PID show no symptoms.

Once diagnosed, PID is treated immediately with antibiotics; specific antibiotics can be prescribed once the microorganism(s) causing the infection have been identified.

PID AND STERILITY

If pelvic inflammatory disease (PID) remains untreated, it may lead to scarring of the fallopian tubes, the ducts that link the ovaries to the uterus and carry eggs to the uterus following their release from the ovaries. Scarred fallopian tubes may become blocked so that sperm cannot reach an egg to fertilize it, and the egg cannot make its way to the uterus. This leads to infertility in up to 10 percent of women with chronic PID, and the risk of infertility increases with each recurrence of PID.

Present and past sexual partners should also be treated to prevent further cases of infection. In more serious cases of PID, women are often admitted to hospital for treatment. Left untreated, PID can cause infertility *(see box)*, or increase the risk of ectopic pregnancy—a pregnancy occurring inside the fallopian tube that has to be terminated to avoid harming the mother *(see p.230–1)*.

Pubic lice

Many parents are familiar with head lice—tiny insects that bite into the scalp and feed on blood—either because their children have had them or because they themselves had them as children. Another species of these tiny insects lives on and among the pubic hair of adults, feeding on blood and causing irritation and itching. These pubic lice are also known as crab lice or crabs because they have "claws," which they use to grip the shafts of pubic hair in order to avoid being dislodged.

Pubic lice are usually transmitted by sexual contact—they simply move from one person's pubic hair to his or her partner's—although they may also be spread by infected sheets or towels. Infection can be confirmed by inspecting the pubic hair. If the pinhead-sized lice cannot be seen, their white eggs—called nits —may be visible, attached to the pubic hairs. Normal bathing or showering will not remove lice or their eggs. A special shampoo that contains insecticide is needed to do this. Sheets and towels should be washed in very hot water to prevent reinfection. It is also advisable to visit a doctor or clinic for treatment and have a checkup, as other STDs may have been picked up at the same time.

Syphilis

Once a widespread and much-feared disease, syphilis is now less common because of effective treatment, although it is still a serious illness. In recent times, localized outbreaks of the disease have occurred among some groups of drug users who have turned to prostitution on a large scale to finance their habit. Primary and secondary syphilis are highly infectious and can be transmitted by most forms of sexual contact with an infected person,

THE POX

The pox, as syphilis was once known, was first recorded as a major epidemic in Europe at the end of the 15th century. It may have arisen as a more virulent form of a disease already present, or it may have been a temperate modification of a tropical disease brought back from the Caribbean by Christopher Columbus and his sailors. Many celebrated men and women in history—including King Henry VIII of England and Czar Ivan the Terrible of Russia—suffered from syphilis. In the 16th century it was discovered that a mercury ointment provided relief from symptoms, but at some cost because mercury is a poison that causes many side effects. This led to the expression that "a night with Venus [the goddess of love] means a lifetime with mercury!" The discovery of salvarsan by the German Paul Ehrlich in 1910 provided a cure for syphilis, albeit a painful one. It took the later discovery of penicillin to significantly reduce the number of syphilis cases.

including oral sex and kissing. Syphilis can also be transmitted across the placenta from mother to fetus, although this is now less common because of routine testing for syphilis during pregnancy.

Syphilis is caused by the bacterium *Treponema pallidum*, which remains in the body indefinitely if not treated, causing a disease that follows three distinct stages. The symptom of primary syphilis, which appears between 10 and 90 days after infection, is a painless ulcer that appears at the site of exposure—either on the genitals or around the anus or mouth—and heals within 6–10 weeks. In the following weeks, secondary syphilis develops. Its symptoms can include skin rashes, headache, sore throat, enlarged lymph nodes, mild fever, hair loss, and flattened, wartlike growths that occur on moist areas around the genitals and anus. These symptoms disappear within a few weeks or months, and a person moves into the latent, symptomless phase of the disease.

Some years after infection, some untreated people develop the tertiary, and most destructive, stage of the disease. Its effects include damage to the brain and nervous system, and to the cardiovascular (blood) system, which may cause mental disorders or even death. Progression to the latent and tertiary phases is unusual, however. If syphilis is diagnosed—by a blood test—in its primary, secondary, or latent stages, the disease can be treated effectively with the antibiotic penicillin.

Trichomoniasis

Trichomoniasis is one of the causes of vaginitis *(see p.116)*, the inflammation of the vagina. It is caused by *Trichomonas vaginalis*, which belongs to a group of microorganisms known as protists.

Symptoms of trichomoniasis include painful irritation of the vulva and vagina; an excessive, yellow, frothy discharge, with a foul smell; and possibly painful urination. Some women show no symptoms of the disease, and *T. vaginalis* may live inside the vagina for some time without causing infection and then suddenly flare up and produce trichomoniasis symptoms. Although the disease is sexually transmitted, men rarely show symptoms. So a man may unwittingly pass on the disease, picked up months or years previously, to a new female partner, and she might erroneously think he has been unfaithful. Some men, however, develop NGU *(see pp.121–2)* as a result of infection. Once diagnosed, trichomoniasis is treated with antibiotics.

STD clinics

STD clinics, also sometimes known as special clinics, provide expert advice, diagnosis, and treatment for suspected sexually transmitted diseases. Typically, they do not require referral of a patient from another doctor; the patient simply goes directly to the clinic.

Attitudes toward STDs and their treatment have been transformed in recent years. Today, with far less stigma attached to them, a more enlightened attitude is taken toward STDs, and this is reflected in the workings of STD clinics. The welcoming, relaxed atmosphere found in the majority of STD clinics puts most people at ease. Information about individual patients is always totally confidential, and in some cases clinic staff refer to patients by a number or by a code name rather than their own name in order to preserve their anonymity. Health advisers and psychologists are available to help patients deal with the psychological aspects of sexual infections such as HIV and genital herpes.

After an initial examination by a doctor who specializes in STDs, the patient is given a full set of tests to screen for a number of different STDs. This is because, even when a patient only appears to have symptoms of one particular STD, that STD may be accompanied by others even though the symptoms of any other STDs may not be clear. Testing may involve taking a sample from inside the vagina or from the cervix, or just inside the male urethra (the tube that tuns inside the penis). Or it may require a urine sample or a blood test. If an STD is diagnosed, then treatment can begin. This often takes the form of antibiotics, but again, it depends on the particular disease. A doctor will also ask about an individual's sexual history to ascertain whether he or she is at risk of further infections, or whether they have a sexual partner or partners who will also need treatment to prevent the disease spreading further.

Drugs, addiction, and sex

Drugs are substances taken into the body that affect the way in which it functions. There are hundreds of different drugs available to us. We take some—including alcohol, cigarettes, caffeine (in coffee and tea), and even marijuana and other "soft" drugs—to help us relax or to relieve stress; these all have some sort of physiological effect.

We take other drugs—including tranquillizers, sleeping pills, and numerous other prescribed drugs—to help relieve pain, or to cure or relieve the symptoms of an illness or disease. Unknown to many people, a number of prescription drugs may affect their sex lives (for instance, by reducing their desire for sex, reducing a woman's vaginal lubrication, or making it difficult for a man to get an erection), especially if the drugs are taken over a prolonged period. If a prescribed drug seems to be affecting one's sex drive or performance, it is wise to consult a doctor to find out whether a different medication can be prescribed.

All of us are aware that some drugs can damage our health in either a general or specific way. Unfortunately, there is so much ignorance and fear surrounding the question of drugs and how they can affect different individuals or groups of people that many people are unaware—or, alternatively, exaggerate—how a drug can affect their health. Although it is impossible to generalize about either drugs or drug users, there are some helpful guidelines that can be followed in regard to the most common drugs and their effect on our sexual health.

Alcohol

One of the most common legal drugs in use and abuse is ethanol, better known as alcohol and found in a number of forms, including wine, beer, and whisky. Physiologically, alcohol is a depressant of the central nervous system, the body's control and coordination center. Initially the effect is one of relaxation, but as the amount of alcohol in the blood increases, a person typically becomes more uninhibited and starts to lose motor (movement) control, until, if they get very drunk, they suffer memory loss and blackouts and may even finally fall into a coma.

What physiological effects does alcohol consumption have on sex? As the gatekeeper in Shakespeare's *Macbeth* explained so clearly, alcohol "provoketh the desire but taketh away the performance:" it is believed to be a sexual stimulant but in fact has the opposite effect. Drinking may make people believe that they "feel" more sexual and are more ready to take part in sexual acts, but it makes them physiologically less sexual. In men, alcohol suppresses erections and causes retarded (late) ejaculation; when copious amounts of alcohol have been consumed, there may be—despite the desire—no erection at all. Many women apparently feel sexier the more they drink, despite the fact that physiologically the opposite seems to be occurring: alcohol reduces blood flow to the vagina and vulva, delays orgasms, makes the orgasm less intense, and interferes with vaginal lubrication.

Chronic alcohol use and alcohol addiction can cause all types of sexual problems. In men it can cause loss of erection, failure to ejaculate, and loss of libido (sex drive), possibly as a result of the testes shrinking and production of the male hormone testosterone decreasing. Women may similarly lose interest in sex and have problems reaching orgasm. In addition, chronic drinkers of both sexes may find that they wake up with a partner they do not remember going to bed with; forget to use any form of contraception; pick up a sexually transmitted disease through promiscuity; or show violent behavior toward their husbands, wives, or partners.

Nicotine

Nicotine, the principal active agent in tobacco, is a highly addictive drug. Apart from significantly increasing the risk of lung cancer and fatal heart disease, cigarette smoking causes a wide range of other harmful effects on the body, including some that affect an individual's sex life.
- Heavy smokers generally smell and taste of cigarette smoke and are therefore less attractive in terms of basic cleanliness.
- Women smokers have an increased risk of developing cervical cancer.
- Women smokers who are on the pill and are overweight are more likely to develop a thrombosis (a blood clot in a blood vessel).
- Women smokers may experience earlier menopause as a result of smoking.
- Women smokers who are pregnant may adversely affect the health of their developing child.
- Smoking makes skin age more rapidly.
- Men who smoke heavily may find it difficult to attain or maintain an erection.

Illegal drugs

Although many illegal drugs are often thought to have an aphrodisiac effect, the opposite is often true. Long-term use may lead to a decrease in desire and the ability to enjoy sex.

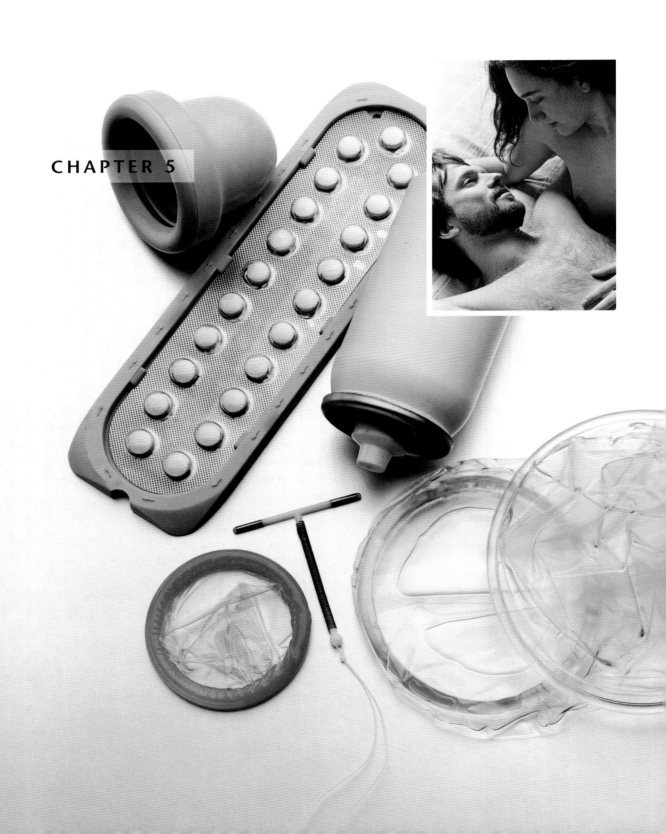

CHAPTER 5

Contraception

Contraception (or birth control) is prevention of pregnancy. It literally means "against conception:" the union of sperm and egg to form an embryo. A contraceptive is any device or medication that achieves this. Some contraceptive methods prevent fertilization, while others permit fertilization but prevent implantation of a fertilized egg in the lining of the uterus. (Abortion, in contrast, is not a form of contraception but the termination of a pregnancy after implantation.)

Most sexually active people have access to a range of different contraceptive methods that enable them to enjoy sexual intercourse without fear of unwanted pregnancy. The various methods of contraception described in this chapter are:

• barrier methods, such as the condom and diaphragm, which form simple obstructions to stop the sperm and egg from meeting
• hormonal methods, such as the pill, which prevent an egg from being released by the woman's ovary or, in some cases, prevent sperm from reaching the egg
• the intrauterine device, or IUD, which sits like a sentry inside the uterus, primarily acting by halting the progress of sperm on their way to the fallopian tubes
• natural methods, which require couples to abstain from intercourse on the days when the woman is fertile and likely to conceive
• sterilization, which offers a permanent surgical means of preventing pregnancy.

Contraception enables people to view lovemaking as an enjoyable activity rather than a purely procreative one. It allows them to have an active sex life as well as controlling whether and when they have children.

How risky is sex without contraception? The likelihood of a woman becoming pregnant if she has regular sexual intercourse but no contraception depends on a number of factors, especially her age, because a woman's fertility decreases over time, after peaking in her late teens and early twenties. This means that 85 percent of women aged 25 are likely to become pregnant within one year if they have regular unprotected sex. ("Regular" is taken to mean an average of about twice a week, with corresponding likelihood of having sex around her fertile days.) For women aged 40 the figure drops to 45 percent, and by the age of 50 it is down to less than 5 percent.

Contraception has another important benefit: some contraceptives can help to reduce the risk of contracting a sexually transmitted disease (STD). Male and female latex condoms offer effective all-around protection; diaphragms and cervical caps protect against bacterial STDs but not against viruses. Protection against STDs is particularly important for men and women who are not in a long-term relationship and have a number of different partners each year, as they are at higher risk of contracting an STD, including the HIV virus that leads to AIDS. With the spread of AIDS, this issue has become even more crucial, and condoms, which had shown signs of fading popularity in the face of more sophisticated contraceptive techniques, are again playing a vital role. Doctors recommend anyone not in a mutually faithful, HIV-free relationship always to use a condom, even if they use another method of contraception at the same time. The best protection against infection (other than abstinence) is consistent, correct use of condoms (see pp.132–7).

Where to get contraception

Where to go for contraception depends on the contraceptive method you choose.
- Male condoms are available from drugstores, supermarkets, other retail outlets, and vending machines, and also from family planning clinics.
- Female condoms, along with spermicidal creams, foams, and suppositories, can be bought at pharmacies.
- Diaphragms, cervical caps, IUDs, and hormonal contraceptives require a prescription from a doctor or family planning clinic.
- For sterilization you need to visit a family planning clinic or hospital, where a trained doctor will carry out the surgical technique.

MYTHS ABOUT CONCEPTION AND CONTRACEPTION

There are many popular myths about conception and contraception, which seem to be passed from generation to generation, regardless of improvements in sex education and the increasing coverage of sexual topics in magazines and books. The basic truth is this: if a woman is of childbearing age (between puberty and menopause), she is at the fertile time of her monthly cycle (the few days before and after an egg is released from one of her ovaries), and she has sexual intercourse without any sort of contraceptive protection, there is a reasonable chance that she will become pregnant. Here are a few of the more common myths.

A woman cannot get pregnant the first time she has sex.
This is a common myth among teenagers. She can get pregnant. There is no trial offer with sex.

A woman cannot get pregnant during her period.
Although the chance of becoming pregnant at this point in the menstrual cycle is small, the risk does still exist for some women.

If a man masturbates to ejaculation shortly before having intercourse he reduces his sperm count sufficiently to prevent conception.
No. There will still be sufficient numbers of sperm to make conception possible.

If a woman jumps up and down after intercourse she will not get pregnant.
Neither jumping up and down nor any other type of physical activity will reduce the risk of becoming pregnant after unprotected intercourse. Sperm will reach her cervix, the entrance to the uterus, within 90 seconds of her partner ejaculating, whether she is lying down or standing up.

If a woman has a hot bath before sex she reduces the risk of pregnancy.
Hot baths have no contraceptive effect at all.

A woman has to have an orgasm during intercourse to get pregnant.
No. A woman can get pregnant during unprotected intercourse whether she has an orgasm or not.

A woman can get pregnant by swallowing semen during oral sex.
Not true. There is no way sperm can reach the uterus if they are swallowed.

A woman cannot get pregnant without full penetration—that is, if her partner ejaculates on her vulva rather than inside her vagina.
Not true. There is a chance that sperm will swim into her vagina and on to the uterus.

Douching—washing out the vagina with liquids such as water, soap, or warm cola—after intercourse washes out sperm and stops a woman getting pregnant.
Douching is not an effective contraception. It can also cause infections in the vagina.

A girl cannot get pregnant before her periods have started.
She could become pregnant. During puberty, girls may ovulate before they have their first period.

If a woman urinates just after her partner ejaculates inside her she will not get pregnant.
It will make no difference. Urine leaves her body through a tube called the urethra, which lies in front of the vagina, so it will not wash away the sperm.

How to choose the right contraceptive

It is important to choose a contraceptive method which you and your partner both feel comfortable with. The right contraceptive will depend on a number of factors: your age, lifestyle, relationship, health, and safe sex plan. What might be a suitable contraceptive method for a young, fit, sexually active woman of 24 may not be appropriate for her contemporary who smokes and has a history of high blood pressure, nor for her mother, aged 45, who is in a long-term relationship and has completed her family. Who should or should not use a particular contraceptive method is discussed in the description of each contraceptive later in this chapter.

Unfortunately, there is no perfect contraceptive method currently available. You and your partner must choose a contraceptive method that provides maximum protection from pregnancy, but also gives you the freedom to enjoy sex without adversely affecting your health. It is usually recommended that the decision be made by both partners, if necessary in consultation with a doctor or family planning adviser. The contraceptive checklist (p.169) summarizes the pros and cons of each method.

When to reassess your contraception

• When you are planning to have sex for the first time. Some methods are not suitable for couples and/or women if they have never had sexual intercourse. IUDs are not usually prescribed for women who haven't had children, while the rhythm method and withdrawal are generally too unreliable. Most young couples are therefore advised to use condoms, a diaphragm, or the pill.

• When you change sexual partners. Medical experts recommend that you use condoms early in a relationship to minimize the risk of contracting a sexually transmitted disease (STD), and continue using them until you are sure that neither of you has an STD. It can take up to six months for infection by HIV to show up in a blood test.

• When you settle down with one person. If you and your partner are mutually monogamous (and neither has an STD), you may want to stop using condoms and find an alternative method of preventing pregnancy that suits you both.

• Before pregnancy. Most physicians advise women to stop taking the pill two to three months before attempting to conceive, to allow their natural cycles to settle down (users of the Depo-Provera contraceptive injection may find it takes up to a year for their cycles to stabilize). Fertility should return right away once an IUD has been removed or when you stop using condoms, cervical caps, or diaphragms.

• After childbirth. Many women are more prone to vaginal infections in the first few months following childbirth, so it may be a good idea to use condoms. During breast-feeding, doctors will probably advise you to avoid the combined pill (which may affect the composition and quantity of milk).

• When you have completed your family. Some couples choose sterilization as a permanent means of preventing pregnancy. For long-term but reversible contraceptive methods, you could consider hormonal implants, injections, or an IUD.

• If you develop a medical disorder. Women with high blood pressure, sickle cell anemia or cardiovascular disease, or diabetics with complications, or where the diabetic is over 35, are advised to avoid the combined pill or any other birth control method containing synthetic estrogen.

• When you have a problem with your current method. If you suffer from side effects from your present method, or you are tired of interrupting your lovemaking to look for a condom, or you keep forgetting to take the pill, you may want to reconsider your choice of contraception method.

THE IDEAL CONTRACEPTIVE?

As yet, the perfect contraceptive does not exist, but these are some of the characteristics that it should have:

• 100 percent effectiveness in preventing pregnancy
• completely safe, without side effects
• completely reversible
• does not interrupt sex
• not capable of being forgotten
• inexpensive
• easy to obtain
• does not require a prescription
• protects against sexually transmitted diseases.

Barrier Methods

When a man ejaculates inside a woman's vagina during sexual intercourse, millions of sperm start their energetic effort to reach her fallopian tubes. For centuries, however, people have known that pregnancy can be prevented by using some sort of barrier to stop the sperm from swimming into the uterus and onward to their goal—the unfertilized egg. Nowadays, such barrier methods are the most universally familiar forms of contraception. They include:

- condoms for men or women
- diaphragms and cervical caps
- spermicidal (sperm-killing) products.

Condoms

Condoms are balloon-like tubes, closed at one end, and usually made of latex. They act as a physical barrier against conception, trapping sperm at the point of ejaculation so they can't reach the egg. They also help protect against cancer of the cervix and reduce the risk of catching STDs, including HIV. The most familiar type is the male condom—also known as a sheath, rubber, protection, or glove—which has been in use for hundreds of years, although the modern version came into being only with the discovery of latex rubber in the nineteenth century. The female condom is a much more recent invention. Many brands of condoms are lubricated for ease of use. This lubrication often contains the spermicide nonoxynol-9, but in such small amounts that there is no evidence that it has a contraceptive effect on any sperm that leak out from the condom. For additional contraceptive protection, couples are advised also to use spermicidal foam, cream, suppositories, or contraceptive film inserted into the vagina *(see p.141)*. Vaginal spermicides have the additional benefit of killing many of the microorganisms that cause STDs.

Reliability of condoms

Both male and female condoms have a 2–4 percent failure rate if used properly, although this figure can increase to between 12 and 15 percent for "typical use" of male condoms, and current data suggests a similar efficacy for female condoms in "typical use." There is evidence that the failure rate for male condoms could be reduced more if they are used consistently and correctly and with a vaginal spermicide.

Where to buy condoms

Both male and female condoms are readily available in drugstores; male condoms can also be bought in many supermarkets and smaller stores, through mail-order outlets, and from vending machines. Both types may also be available free of charge from family planning clinics and some doctors.

The male condom

This is the primary form of contraception currently used by men, apart from the surgical procedure of vasectomy *(see male sterilization, pp.164–7)* and the less effective withdrawal method. The condom fits snugly over a man's erect penis, so that when he ejaculates inside his partner's vagina the sperm are trapped in the space at the tip of the condom.

Male condoms come in many types, including different colors, flavors, and shapes. They are usually made in one size and individually wrapped, although some manufacturers make condoms in different sizes—usually called large, magnum, or jumbo, but never small (probably so they won't dent their purchasers' egos!). Some men find one type more comfortable than another, so it's worth experimenting with different brands until you find one you like. All condoms sold in the United States have met performance standards established by the American Society for Testing and Materials, and have been approved by the Food and Drug Administration.

How to use a condom

Using condoms is straightforward, although it may be a little awkward the first few times. It can be helpful for a man to practice on his own, or for both partners to go through the procedure together before they actually have intercourse. A substitute penis, such as a banana, can prove useful when practicing.

It is important that the condom is put on the penis as soon as it becomes erect and before any contact takes place between the penis and vagina because, as a man becomes aroused, a tiny amount of semen may seep out of his penis before ejaculation—and it only takes one sperm to fertilize an egg.

Avoiding problems with male condoms

• Occasionally things can go wrong with condoms. They can slip off inside the vagina, for example, or split. If a mishap does occur, ask your doctor for emergency contraception *(see pp.167–8)*.

• Never use oil-based products such as body oils, Vaseline, butter, suntan lotion, or any other oil-based lubricant as a lubricant with condoms because these will damage the latex and make the condom leak. Use a water-based lubricating gel or cream, such as K-Y Jelly.

• Follow instructions on the pack. Avoid tearing the pack open with your teeth. Make sure your fingernails are not sharp or jagged and you are not wearing sharp jewelry. Teeth, nails, and metal can all tear condoms. Unroll the condom over the penis—do not pull it on.

• Use a new condom every time you have sexual intercourse.

• Always check the expiration date on the packet.

HOW CONDOMS PROTECT AGAINST STDs

The reason latex and plastic condoms are so effective at stopping the spread of STDs and reducing the incidence of cervical cancer is that they are waterproof. This means that if there are any pores in the condom, they are too small to allow even water molecules through. Water molecules are far smaller than viruses such as HIV or the human papilloma viruses implicated in causing cervical cancer; they are also minute in comparison with the bacteria that cause gonorrhoea and syphilis; and they are over 2,000 times smaller than a sperm. If water molecules cannot escape through the condom, nothing can.

BEING PREPARED OR BEING EASY?

Male condoms may be worn by men, but women not only buy male condoms but also carry them. More often than not, a woman who carries condoms does so in order to be responsible and prepared, not—as some men appear to mistakenly imagine—to advertise herself as "easy" and available for sex. Condoms are doubly useful because they make for safe sex by preventing the spread of HIV and other sexually transmitted diseases, as well as preventing pregnancy.

Fresh from its packet, a male condom (top) *is rolled up, making it easier to put on the erect penis. Once unrolled* (below), *the condom is long enough to enclose most of the penis.*

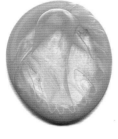

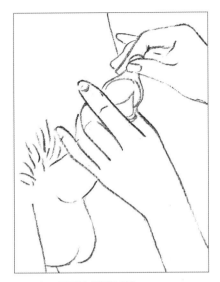

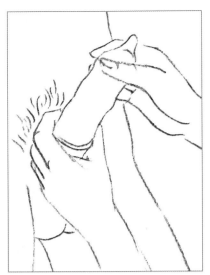

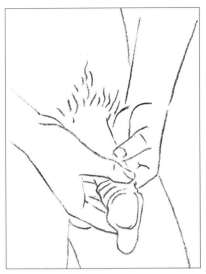

USING A MALE CONDOM

1 *Putting on a male condom can be done by either partner and can be fun, rather than a chore, if it forms part of sexual play and does not interrupt sex. Here it is being put on by the partner. Squeeze the tip of the condom between your thumb and finger, to get rid of the air inside, and with your other hand start to unroll it over the erect penis.*

2 *Still holding the tip, completely unroll the condom over the penis until its rim is near the bottom of the penis shaft. Don't pull at the condom or you may tear it. If the condom refuses to unroll, turn it over; it is probably upside down. If you need to use a lubricant, make sure it is a water-based one (such as K-Y Jelly): oil-based lubricants can damage a condom.*

3 *After the man ejaculates, his penis starts to become limp. Before this happens, he or his partner should hold the condom tightly around its rim, at the base of the penis, and pull the penis carefully out of the vagina. This will ensure that the condom does not slip off as the penis loses its stiffness, which might allow semen to be released accidentally into the vagina.*

• Store your condoms where they cannot be damaged by heat, light, or dampness.

• Avoid flushing used condoms down the toilet; they cannot be broken down in the sewage system. Wrap them in a tissue and put them in the trash.

• To increase a condom's effectiveness, also use an application of spermicide in the vagina.

Do male condoms affect lovemaking?

Male condoms can add to or detract from the pleasures of sex, depending on the attitude of the couple using them. Many couples, for example, incorporate putting on a condom into their foreplay. Also, by reducing the intensity of sensation felt via the penis, condoms can prolong intercourse and enhance pleasure for both women and men. Condoms reduce the mess after ejaculation as well.

On the minus side, they can interrupt the spontaneity of sex, and may mean that men feel less intense pleasure during intercourse. Also, some condoms taste unpleasant.

Who are male condoms suitable for?

Male condoms are suitable for most men, provided they are prepared to take an active role in contraception and are sufficiently motivated to ensure that condoms are used properly during sex—that is, they put the condom on correctly (without tearing or splitting it) before any sexual contact takes place; they remove it immediately after intercourse, and wash their penis before any further sexual contact; and a new condom is used every time a couple have sex.

Some men and women show an allergic response—indicated by a sore penis or vagina—after using a condom. There are various reasons for this. They may be sensitive to nonoxynol-9, the spermicidal lubricant used in many condoms. If this is the case, they could switch to condoms with a different lubricant, or brands that don't use a spermicidal lubricant. They may be allergic to the coloring or flavoring used in "fun" condoms; the solution to this problem is to use a more conventional condom. They may be allergic to latex; the alternative is to use natural condoms made from lambs' intestines—although these offer less effective protection against pregnancy and sexually transmitted diseases, including HIV—or the new polyurethane condoms, which are currently being tested and are believed to be effective against HIV.

Advantages of male condoms

- They are widely available without prescription, and are fairly inexpensive.
- They are easy to use and require no instruction from a doctor or nurse.
- They have minimal medical side effects.
- Used correctly and consistently, they have a low failure rate.
- Latex condoms (and female condoms) offer a greater degree of protection against sexually transmitted diseases, including HIV, than any other form of contraception.
- They may reduce the risk of cervical cancer.
- They do not affect or delay fertility in men or women.
- They offer men direct responsibility for birth control.
- They can help delay orgasm for men who regularly experience premature ejaculation.

Disadvantages of male condoms

- Condoms require some planning: you have to know intercourse is going to take place and have a condom on hand.
- They usually interrupt sex.
- They can tear or slip off if not used properly.
- They may leak sperm if the man does not withdraw immediately after he has ejaculated.
- Although rare, some people are allergic to latex rubber.
- They may reduce sensation for the man, leading to loss of erection, or at least less pleasure.
- They have an unattractive appearance and smell.
- They may be embarrassing to buy, talk to a partner about, put on, take off, and/or dispose of.

ON CONDOMS...

A slogan from California used to promote the use of condoms:
"Use a condom and you will learn
No deposit
No return."

The female condom

The newly developed female condom is larger than its male counterpart, and is made of a very thin plastic, polyurethane. It works in much the same way as the male condom except that it fits inside the vagina. It is closed at one end and contains a flexible ring to keep it in place. The ring at the open end lies just outside the vulva and holds the condom open. When the man ejaculates, his sperm-carrying semen stays inside the condom, which is then removed and disposed of. However, female condoms are currently quite expensive.

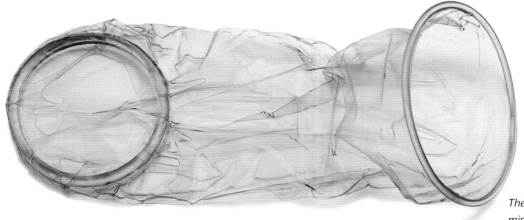

The female condom mirrors the action of the male condom, fitting inside the vagina instead of over the penis.

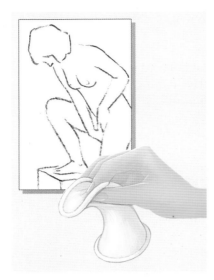

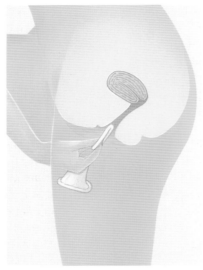

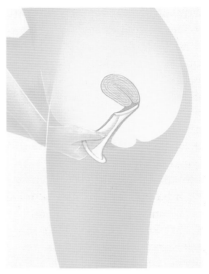

USING A FEMALE CONDOM

1 *Open the packet carefully; clumsy handling of a condom, especially if you have long fingernails or sharp jewelry, can tear it and render it useless. Get into a comfortable position—squatting, lying down, or with one foot on a chair, whichever feels easiest for you.*

2 *Use the fingers of one hand to compress the inner ring at the closed end of the condom. Use the other hand to hold apart the lips of your vulva. Push the squeezed closed end of the condom as far as you can into your vagina and "hook" it under your pubic bone (much like inserting a diaphragm).*

3 *Put your index or middle finger inside the condom and gently push upward to ensure that the condom is right inside the vagina. The ring at the open end of the condom should be lying close to the vulva and not dangling down.*

How to use a female condom

Using the female condom is reasonably easy with some practice. It can be put in the vagina at any time before sexual contact. Some men and women complain that it makes a rustling noise during intercourse, but many other couples are satisfied with it.

Avoiding problems with female condoms

• Follow the instructions carefully, and make sure your fingernails are not sharp or jagged: torn condoms are ineffective.
• Use a new condom every time you have sexual intercourse.
• Check the expiration date on the packet.
• Store condoms where they cannot be damaged by heat, light, or dampness.
• Avoid flushing used condoms down the toilet; they cannot be broken down in the sewage system. Wrap them in a tissue and put them in the trash.
• If your partner ejaculates inside the vagina but outside the female condom, ask a doctor to give you emergency contraception *(see pp.167–8).*

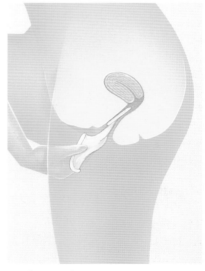

4 *When you have intercourse, it may be wise to guide your partner's penis inside the condom to make sure that it is not inserted outside the condom. After your partner has ejaculated, twist the outer end of the condom to prevent the semen from getting out, gently pull the condom down and out of your vagina, and dispose of it in a trash can.*

Advantages of female condoms

- The female condom has many of the same advantages as the male condom, but it seems to be free of any allergic problems because it is made of plastic and does not contain any potentially allergenic spermicidal lubricants.
- It can be inserted before intercourse and removed any time after.
- Oil-based products can be used with the female condom.

Disadvantages of female condoms

- Like male condoms, you have to be prepared, with a condom on hand.
- The penis may accidentally be inserted between the condom and the vagina wall.
- It protrudes from the vagina, and may make rustling noises, both of which can be off-putting during foreplay or intercourse.
- They are currently quite expensive.

The diaphragm and the cervical cap

While condoms act as barriers to sperm by trapping the semen ejaculated from the penis during intercourse, diaphragms and cervical caps—with the aid of sperm-killing chemicals called spermicides—form barriers by acting as gatekeepers to the uterus, denying access to any sperm. Both diaphragms and cervical caps must be fitted by a medical professional and require a prescription.

The diaphragm

The diaphragm is a circular dome made of rubber, kept in shape by a thin piece of rubber-covered metal that forms the rim. It fits over the cervix to stop sperm from getting into the uterus. This is not a tight fit, however, and movement may take place during intercourse. For that reason, spermicidal cream must be squeezed onto the inside of the diaphragm before it is inserted, to destroy any sperm that get past the rubber barrier.

The first sight of a diaphragm often causes some consternation because it looks too big to fit inside a vagina. However, insertion is easy with practice (squeeze the sides of the cap together and it forms a long thin shape that slides comfortably inside the vagina: *see p.139*) and once it is inserted, the woman shouldn't be aware of it at all.

There are three types of diaphragms, which differ in the type of metal spring found in their rims. A doctor (or nurse) will decide which is the best type to use.

The flat-spring diaphragm has a firm watch spring and is usually the first choice because it is easiest to use. The coil-spring diaphragm is softer and is recommended for women who are sensitive to the pressure exerted by the flat-spring diaphragm. The arcing-spring diaphragm has a firm double metal spring that exerts a strong pressure, making it suitable for women with weak vaginal muscular support. It forms an arc when compressed, and is therefore easier to insert for women who have a retroverted uterus *(see p.16)* or a long cervix.

Reliability of the diaphragm

Used properly, with spermicides, the diaphragm has a failure rate of 4–8 percent,

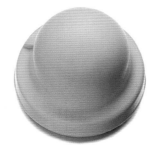
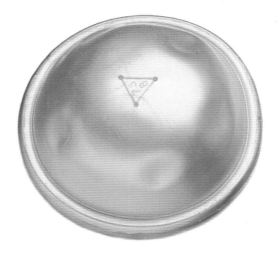

The cervical cap (left) and diaphragm (below) cover the cervix to stop sperm from entering the uterus. For maximum efficiency, both need the addition of spermicidal cream or gel.

but this rises to between 15 and 18 percent with less careful use.

Where to get a diaphragm

Diaphragms, like clothes, have to be the right size to fit. A visit to the doctor or family planning clinic is needed to find out what size diaphragm a woman requires. The doctor or nurse will also describe how to insert it, and how to use it effectively. Women are sometimes given a diaphragm to practice with at home and asked to return to the clinic a week later with the diaphragm in place, so that the doctor or nurse can check that it has been inserted correctly and is the right size.

Following pregnancy or a weight loss or gain of more than 10 pounds, women are advised to return to the doctor or clinic to have the fitting of their diaphragm checked, because a different size may now be required.

How to use a diaphragm

The diaphragm can be inserted several hours before sex takes place, although couples will need to add extra spermicide if more than three hours elapse between inserting the diaphragm and having intercourse, or if they have intercourse more than once. The diaphragm should not be removed to do this: simply use some more cream or spermicidal foam or suppositories (see p.141). Some couples incorporate the addition of more spermicide as part of their lovemaking.

After intercourse, the diaphragm must be left in place for at least six hours, to ensure there are no stray sperm left waiting to complete the journey to the fallopian tubes. The diaphragm should not be left in for more than 24 hours because of the risk of local abrasions or (very rarely) toxic shock syndrome (see p.95). After use, the diaphragm is removed by hooking it out with one finger (see opposite), then washed in warm water with mild soap, rinsed, dried, and returned to its storage box. It should be checked regularly for holes by holding it up to the light.

Avoiding problems with diaphragms

• After inserting a diaphragm, always check that it is covering the cervix properly.

• Take care with sharp fingernails when removing a diaphragm.
• Be sure to have a checkup once a year.

Do diaphragms affect lovemaking?

A diaphragm can be inserted a few hours before intercourse, so that it doesn't interfere with sex itself; and it doesn't cause any loss of sensation for either partner. On the other hand, in practice, putting in a diaphragm often does mean interrupting sex; spermicide can make sex messy and may interfere with oral sex because of its taste; the woman may be able to feel the diaphragm in certain positions (for example, if she is on top), although this may indicate she has not inserted it properly; and her partner may be able to feel it in the vagina with his fingers or penis.

Who are diaphragms suitable for?

Diaphragms are recommended for couples who want to use a barrier method—but not condoms—and find other contraceptive methods unsuitable; for women who are committed to using contraception but do not want to take the pill; and for women who want to be in control of their contraception and use it only when it is needed.

The diaphragm may not be suitable for women who do not feel comfortable touching their genital area; women who have anatomical problems that preclude the insertion and proper positioning of the diaphragm; women with poor muscle tone in the vaginal walls, so that the diaphragm does not stay in place; women who are unable to learn the correct insertion/removal procedure; women who lack the facilities for private and hygienic insertion of the diaphragm, and its cleaning and storage after use; women who are allergic to rubber or the spermicides used with the diaphragm; and women who have never had sexual intercourse, although tampon users may be able to insert a small diaphragm. In many cases, the diaphragm proves unsuitable when couples find it means interrupting sexual intercourse to put in the diaphragm—it has been said that the primary reason for diaphragm failure is the distance from the bedroom to the bathroom!

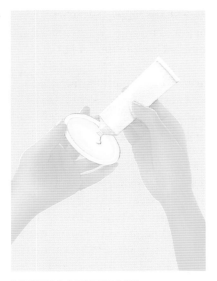

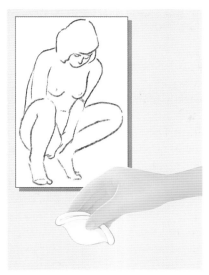

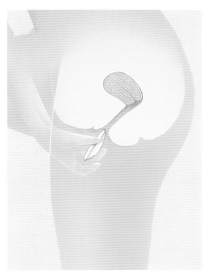

INSERTING A DIAPHRAGM

1 *First wash your hands, and then remove the diaphragm from its container. Smear spermicidal cream or gel on each side of the diaphragm, and spread it all around the rim, too.*

2 *Get into a comfortable position for inserting the diaphragm—lying down, or squatting, or with one leg up on a chair, bed, or bath. Squeeze the diaphragm between your thumb and index finger, using the other fingers to stop it from slipping out of your hand.*

3 *Push the squeezed diaphragm upward and backward into the top of the vagina as far as it will go, so that the back lies behind the cervix, and the front is behind the pubic bone.*

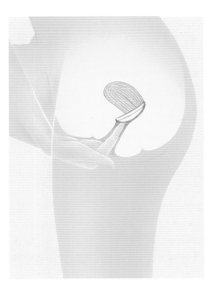

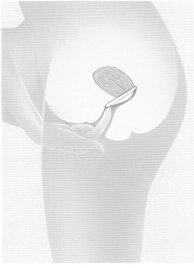

4 *Let go of the diaphragm so that it opens up to cover the cervix. Check that it is in position by feeling for the cervix—it feels a bit like a nose with one nostril—through the rubber of the diaphragm. If the cervix is not fully covered, or if the diaphragm moves when you squat and bear down, remove it and try again.*

5 *To remove the diaphragm, hook one finger over its rim and pull downward. But remember to leave it in place for at least six hours after you last have intercourse.*

QUESTION AND ANSWER: THE DIAPHRAGM

Q. Before I had a baby, I used the diaphragm for contraception. Now that I've had my baby, can I use the same diaphragm, or do I need to see my doctor to get a new one?

A. You should see your doctor to have a new diaphragm fitted, as being pregnant and giving birth will have changed the dimensions of your cervix and vagina so that the old diaphragm will no longer fit properly and may not provide adequate protection. In addition, refitting of the diaphragm is also required if a woman who is not pregnant has lost or gained more than 10 pounds in weight. Diaphragms should be replaced routinely every year or so, or as soon as they show any signs of damage.

Advantages of the diaphragm
- It has few side effects.
- It does not affect fertility.
- It reduces the risk of cervical cancer and of catching some STDs.
- Lovemaking is not necessarily interrupted.

Disadvantages of the diaphragm
- It requires some anticipation of whether and when sex is going to occur.
- It can be messy.
- It has to be fitted initially by a trained doctor or nurse.
- It can increase the chances of urinary infections such as cystitis in some women.
- It does not protect against certain STDs, such as HIV and herpes.

The cervical cap

The cervical cap is thimble-shaped and smaller than the diaphragm. Like the diaphragm, it must be fitted by a doctor or nurse. The cap fits snugly over the cervix and is held in place by suction. To be effective, the cap requires a squirt of spermicidal cream, which should be directed into the cup of the cap (it should be about half full—2 teaspoons or so) rather than onto the rim, as this might prevent suction. The cap is inserted by being pushed into the vagina, and upward onto the cervix, with the fingertips. Once in place, more spermicide is added to the dome of the

cap using an applicator. Instructions for use, removal, and cleaning of the cap are the same as for the diaphragm.

Fewer women use the cap than use the diaphragm, partly because it appears to be less effective in younger, more fertile, and more sexually active women, and partly because the shape of the cervix in some women is unsuitable for a cap.

Reliability of the cervical cap
The cap is fairly effective, with a failure rate of 9–11 percent when used properly, increasing to up to 18 percent in "typical use."

Do cervical caps affect lovemaking?
Caps can be inserted well in advance and left in place (even while taking a bath) for up to 48 hours—for example, they can be put in on a Friday night to give all-weekend protection—so they do not affect sexual spontaneity. They need only one small application of spermicide before insertion. They cannot be felt during sexual intercourse, so do not affect vaginal sensitivity. They are comfortable to use and there is no smell of spermicide (unlike the diaphragm).

Advantages of the cervical cap
- It has very few side effects.
- It does not affect fertility.
- It reduces the risk of catching some STDs (but not HIV or herpes) and of developing cervical cancer.
- It does not affect lovemaking.

Disadvantages of the cervical cap
- It requires some anticipation of when and whether sex is going to occur.
- It has to be fitted by a doctor or nurse and requires accurate selection of cap size to ensure it is not displaced during intercourse.
- Women must have a cervix that accommodates a cervical cap—not all do.
- Women with particularly long vaginas find inserting and removing the cap difficult.
- Even well-fitting caps may be dislodged during sex. This may have something to do with intercourse positions or with the changes in vaginal and cervical size and shape during

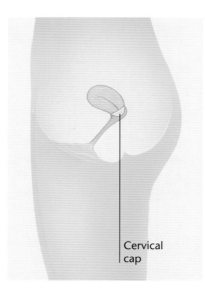

Smaller than the diaphragm, the thimble-shaped cervical cap guards the entrance to the uterus against the entry of sperm by fitting snugly over the cervix, the neck of the uterus.

Cervical cap

sexual arousal. If it becomes dislodged—you can check after intercourse—postcoital contraception *(see pp.167–8)* may be advisable.
• Insertion and removal can be more difficult than with a diaphragm.
• An unpleasant odor may develop if the cap is left in place for more than a day or two.
• In some women, using the cervical cap can increase the chances of developing urinary infections such as cystitis.
• It does not protect against certain STDs, such as HIV and herpes.

THE CONTRACEPTIVE SPONGE

The vaginal contraceptive sponge is a circular piece of foam saturated with spermicide that a woman inserts into her vagina. It releases spermicide, acts as a barrier, and absorbs sperm, but its failure rate can be as high as 25 percent. It was widely available in the late 1980s, but is no longer marketed in the United States.

Spermicidal creams, foams, suppositories, and films

Spermicides create a chemical, sperm-killing barrier in the vagina. They come in various forms, all of which should be deposited as close to the cervix as possible: foam that is squirted into the vagina; suppositories, creams, and film that are melted by body heat inside the vagina; and creams that can be squeezed into the vagina with a special applicator or used with diaphragms and caps. On their own, however, none of these types of spermicide is very effective as a contraceptive. To be reliable, spermicides must be used in conjunction with some other form of contraception, such as a condom. Always remember to check the expiration date on spermicide packages: after this date the spermicide will be ineffective and should be disposed of.

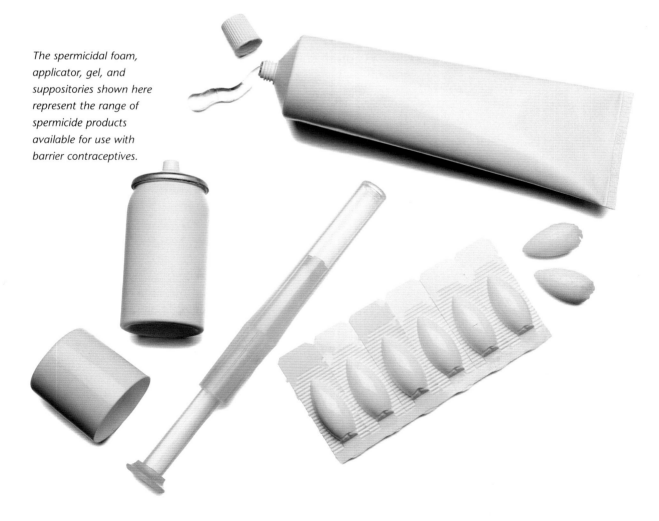

The spermicidal foam, applicator, gel, and suppositories shown here represent the range of spermicide products available for use with barrier contraceptives.

Hormonal methods

Hormonal methods of family planning alter a woman's menstrual cycle to prevent fertilization. There are several different types of hormonal contraceptive:

- the combined pill
- the progestin-only pill or minipill
- injectable contraceptives
- hormonal implants
- the vaginal ring (not yet available in the US)
- IUDs that release progestin

How do hormonal contraceptives work?

Every month, a regular cycle of changes occurs within a woman's reproductive system. The monthly ovarian and menstrual cycles, experienced by all women between menarche and menopause, prepare the body for possible pregnancy by releasing an egg, ripe for fertilization, and thickening the lining of the uterus in readiness for receiving the egg should it be fertilized. Both cycles are controlled by chemical messengers called hormones.

The hormonal sequence goes like this: the pituitary gland underneath the brain releases follicle-stimulating hormone (FSH), which stimulates one of the egg-containing follicles in the ovary to develop. This causes the ovary to release estrogen, which stimulates the uterine lining to thicken, makes the pituitary gland slow down its release of FSH, and encourages the gland to release luteinizing hormone (LH). When LH levels reach a peak, around day 14 of the cycle, the ripe follicle bursts, releasing its egg into the fallopian tube, where it may be fertilized if the woman has had intercourse. The burst follicle seals itself up and starts to produce the hormone progesterone, which encourages the uterine lining to thicken more, and also begins to thicken the mucus produced by the cervix, making it impenetrable to sperm. If there is no pregnancy, the uterine wall breaks down, a woman has her period, and the cycles repeat themselves (see also the female reproductive cycle, pp.20–3).

Hormonal contraceptives work by disrupting the normal operation of the reproductive cycles. They contain synthetic estrogen and/or progestin (a synthetic form of progesterone). These trick the body into altering the amounts of natural hormones in the bloodstream. As a result, an egg is not usually released, cervical mucus is permanently thickened and impenetrable, and the lining of the uterus does not thicken in readiness to receive the fertilized egg.

Most commonly prescribed are oral contraceptives, taken in pill form by mouth. When they are swallowed, the hormones inside them are absorbed into the bloodstream. Recently, however, longer-lasting methods of delivering hormones into a woman's body have been introduced. These include the injectable contraceptive, implants, and the intrauterine system (a type of IUD that releases progestin).

Where to get hormonal contraceptives

Only a doctor, nurse, or physician's associate can prescribe hormonal methods of contraception, so a visit to a doctor or a family planning clinic is required. Any doctor who is thinking of prescribing hormonal contraceptives must consider his or her patient's medical situation carefully, because certain illnesses or drugs may make such contraceptives unsuitable. Women using hormonal contraceptives are recommended to have regular checkups to monitor their weight and blood pressure, and regular Pap smears.

The combined oral contraceptive pill

The combined oral contraceptive pill, better known simply as the pill, is the most widely used of all hormonal contraceptive methods. It contains a combination of synthetic estrogen and progestin that together suppress the release of FSH and LH by the pituitary gland, thereby inhibiting ovulation. The uterine lining and cervical mucus are also affected, as described above. In fact, the pill is, in effect, making a woman's body believe that she is pregnant.

There are various types of combined pills, with varying levels of estrogen and progestin. (Estrogen levels in the pill have dropped considerably since it was introduced in the 1960s,

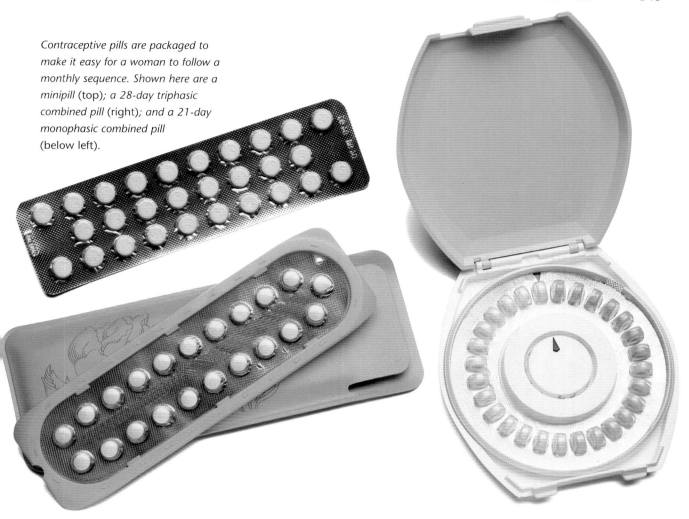

Contraceptive pills are packaged to make it easy for a woman to follow a monthly sequence. Shown here are a minipill (top); a 28-day triphasic combined pill (right); and a 21-day monophasic combined pill (below left).

in response to fears that high levels could have serious side effects in some women, such as deep-vein thrombosis, strokes, and heart attacks.)

Some combined pills are taken for 21 days, after which the user has a seven-day break when she experiences withdrawal bleeding—similar to a light period—before she starts the next pack of pills. Others are taken every day, without a break; however, seven of the pills in the pack are hormone-free, so that a woman taking these also experiences withdrawal bleeding. Both 21-day and everyday pills are commonly monophasic—that is, each pill contains the same level of hormone, although with everyday pills seven are hormone-free.

Triphasic (three-phase) pills, in contrast, contain three different levels of hormones. These are taken in sequence for the first 21 days of the month, producing a variation in

the levels of synthetic hormones that apparently reflects more closely the woman's natural hormonal fluctuations. A pack of triphasic pills may also include seven hormone-free pills.

Reliability of the combined pill

Tests have shown that—provided it is taken correctly—the combined pill is almost 100 percent effective. With less careful use, the actual failure rate is between 2 and 4 percent. Vomiting or severe diarrhea can stop the combined pill from working, so if you have an upset stomach—or forget a pill—refer to the flow chart *(see p.145)*.

Does the combined pill affect lovemaking?

Some women find not having to worry about pregnancy very liberating, enabling them to

HOW THE COMBINED PILL WORKS

Normally, two hormones released by the pituitary gland, FSH and LH, stimulate the ovaries to release eggs. But if a woman takes the pill, its synthetic hormones are released into her bloodstream, and act on the pituitary gland, causing a reduction in production of FSH and LH, and preventing ovulation and the possibility of pregnancy.

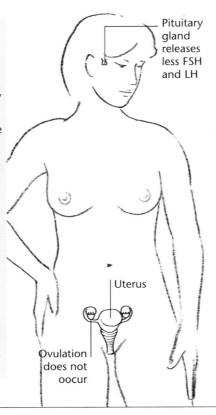

Pituitary gland releases less FSH and LH

Uterus

Ovulation does not oocur

enjoy sex more. Taking the pill certainly does not interrupt sex. On the down side, some women report a loss of libido (sex drive, *see pp.172–3*), while others find their vaginal secretions decrease and it becomes necessary to use a lubricant such as K-Y Jelly to facilitate intercourse. Also, the pill does not protect against STDs, so women who change partners regularly (or who have a partner who changes partners) will need to use condoms or another barrier method in addition to the pill.

After how many years should a woman stop taking the pill?

In theory, women could continue taking modern low-dose combined pills up to age 50–55, provided they are in good health, not very overweight, nonsmokers, and do not show any of the accepted contraindications. However, because a woman's fertility decreases with age, she does not need such an effective form of contraceptive in her later years; and given that she may not want to take hormones for a prolonged period, she may wish to switch to a nonhormonal method

HOW TO TAKE THE COMBINED PILL

Although all combined pills work in the same way, there are different types of combined pill. Some are taken for 21 days, with a seven-day gap, while others are taken every day.

21-DAY PILL:
• Take your first pill—one marked with the correct day of the week, from any part of the pack—on the first day of your period. This will give you immediate protection. (If you start any later, you will not be protected for the first seven days, during which time you should use another method of contraception as well.)
• Take the next 20 pills at about the same time each day.

Once the pack is finished, stop for seven days. You will probably bleed for a few days. You will still be protected.
• After seven pill-free days, start your next pack (whether or not you are still bleeding). You will always start a new pack on the same day of the week.

EVERYDAY PILL:
• Seven of the pills contain no hormones, so it is important to take the pills in the right order.
• Start on the first day of your period with the first pill from the pack. Then follow the package directions, taking one pill every day until you finish the pack. You will not be protected for the first 7 or 14

days (depending on the exact pill used) of the first pack, so you will need to use another method of contraception.
• When you finish all 28 pills, start another pack the next day.

TRIPHASIC (21-DAY OR 28-DAY):
• Start with pill number one on the first day of your period. You will be protected at once. Be sure to take the pills in the correct order. Once you have finished a 21-day pack, stop for seven days, during which you may bleed. You will still be protected. In a 28-day pack the last seven pills are placebos.
• Start a new pack on the day following the seven-day break or the 28th pill.

by her mid-thirties. The latest IUDs may be a possible alternative if a woman has had children and is therefore less concerned about the risk of pelvic inflammatory disease (PID), which may cause infertility *(see pp.124–5)*.

Who should not use the combined pill?
- Heavy smokers (over 35 a day), or smokers who are over 35 and/or overweight.
- Women who have past or present circulatory disease, e.g. thrombosis, ischemic heart disease or angina, clotting problems, focal migraine, or major heart-valve disease.
- Women with high blood pressure, liver disease, or breast cancer.
- Women who are or may be pregnant.
- Women who have long-term diseases that require treatment with drugs that interfere with the action of combined pills.
- Women who travel to high altitudes (over 10,000 feet) and are likely to suffer from altitude sickness.
- Women with complications of diabetes or those over 35 years old who have uncomplicated diabetes.

Is the combined pill suitable after childbirth?
Breastfeeding mothers are generally advised not to use the combined pill. For them, the combination of the minipill *(see pp.146–7)* and the naturally contraceptive effect of breastfeeding *(see p.162)* should be sufficient. For mothers who are not breastfeeding, it is advisable to start the combined pill on day 21 after giving birth (the earliest possible date for ovulation will be around day 28).

Advantages of the combined pill
- It is highly effective when used properly.
- It does not interrupt sex.
- It makes periods lighter, less painful, and more regular, and can alleviate symptoms of premenstrual syndrome and anemia.
- It reduces the risk of PID, ectopic pregnancy *(see p.14)*, benign breast disease, and cancer of the ovary or uterus.
- It has empowered women to have greater control over their sex lives, freed from constant anxiety about unwanted pregnancy.

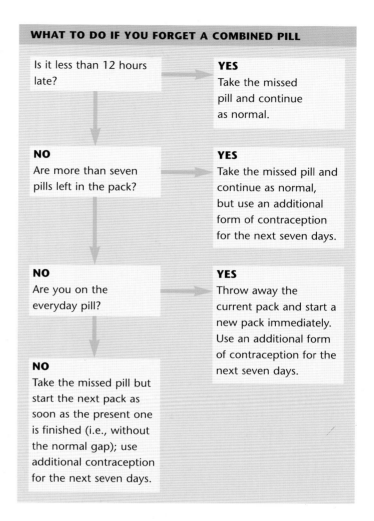

WHAT TO DO IF YOU FORGET A COMBINED PILL

Is it less than 12 hours late? → **YES** Take the missed pill and continue as normal.

NO Are more than seven pills left in the pack? → **YES** Take the missed pill and continue as normal, but use an additional form of contraception for the next seven days.

NO Are you on the everyday pill? → **YES** Throw away the current pack and start a new pack immediately. Use an additional form of contraception for the next seven days.

NO Take the missed pill but start the next pack as soon as the present one is finished (i.e., without the normal gap); use additional contraception for the next seven days.

SIDE EFFECTS: CONSULTING THE DOCTOR

Minor side effects should be mentioned to your doctor at your next appointment. But consult the doctor immediately should you have any of the following:
- severe headaches or migraines
- acute visual disturbance (e.g., blurring)
- painful swelling in the calf
- pain in the chest or stomach
- fainting attack or collapse
- numbness in an arm or leg.

Disadvantages of the combined pill
- Taking the combined pill means that the normal cycle of the woman's body is interrupted, with the very small possibility that she may develop a fatal complication (3–6 women per million pill users).

• The pill may increase blood pressure slightly, and with it the risk of developing blood clots, strokes, or heart attacks. However, these conditions are rarely caused solely by the pill, and are mainly likely to occur in women who smoke, especially if they are over 35, are overweight, and/or have high blood pressure anyway.

• It can have a number of side effects, including nausea, headaches, breakthrough bleeding (bleeding between "periods"), loss of libido (sex drive), breast tenderness, depression, or weight gain. If these occur, the doctor may prescribe a pill with a different hormonal dosage, or suggest an alternative form of contraception. Spotting (very light bleeding between "periods") and nausea are most common in the first few months and get better over time.

• There is some evidence of a link between long-term pill use and later development of certain cancers, such as cancer of the breast, cervix, and liver. This has yet to be proven conclusively.

• The pill offers no protection at all against any sexually transmitted diseases (STDs), including HIV.

DRUGS AND THE PILL

Some drugs reduce the effectiveness of the combined pill.
Anticonvulsants: barbiturates, phenytoin, Dilantin, primidone, carbamazepine
Antibiotics: rifampicin, griseofulvin, ampicillin, tetracyclines, cephalosporins
Diuretics: spironolactone
Hypnotics: dichloralphenazone
Tranquilizers: meprobromate.

The progestin-only pill or minipill

The minipill contains just one hormone—progestin (also known as progestogen), a synthetic form of the female sex hormone progesterone. It works by blocking the cervix with thick mucus to prevent sperm from entering the uterus, as well as making the uterine lining less receptive to fertilized eggs

and the fallopian tube less efficient at moving the egg from the ovary to the uterus. In some women, the minipill may also stop ovulation.

Reliability of the minipill
Used properly, the minipill has a failure rate of 0.5–2 percent; in "typical use" the failure rate can rise to about 4 percent.

Who is the minipill suitable for?
• Women who wish to use a reliable form of contraception that does not interrupt sex but does not carry the risks associated with the combined pill.
• Women who wish to use a hormonal method of contraception at a minimal dosage.
• Women prepared to commit themselves to daily pill-taking at the same time each day.
• Women over 35 who smoke but wish to use oral contraception.
• Women who wish to use oral contraception but suffer from migraines or have diabetes, high blood pressure, obesity, or a history of circulatory disorders, including a higher risk of thrombosis.
• Women who are breastfeeding but wish to use oral contraception.
• Women who experience a lot of nausea using the combined pill.

Who should not use the minipill?
• Women who are or may be pregnant.
• Women who require complete protection against the risk of pregnancy.
• Teenage girls, who require very effective contraception at the most fertile period of their lives.
• Women with a personal history of severe disease of the circulatory system.
• Women with undiagnosed vaginal bleeding.
• Women who have had an ectopic pregnancy.
• Women who have ovarian cysts, breast cancer, or severe liver disorders.

How to use the minipill
The minipill should be taken at the same time each day, 365 days a year. A woman takes the first pill—one marked with the appropriate day of the week—on the first day of her period, to protect her at once, and continues

taking a pill a day until she finishes the pack. She starts a new pack the next day. If she forgets a pill, she should take it as soon as she remembers and take the next one as normal at the correct time. If the pill is taken more than three hours late, it will give decreased protection, and another form of contraception will be needed for the next seven days.

Does the minipill affect lovemaking?

Like the combined pill, the minipill gives a woman freedom from fear of pregnancy, which may enable her to enjoy sex more. Also, it does not generally decrease libido (unlike the combined pill in some women). However, there may be irregular or breakthrough bleeding at odd times of the month.

Advantages of the minipill

• It can be taken by older women and those unable to use the combined pill because of side effects.
• It can be used by breastfeeding mothers.

Disadvantages of the minipill

• It is not as effective as the combined pill.
• It may cause irregular bleeding and periods. Some women have much lighter periods, others none at all. Breakthrough bleeding may also occur. It might help to change to a different brand of minipill.
• Like the combined pill, the minipill offers no protection against STDs, including HIV.

• It may increase the chances of having an ectopic pregnancy, although recent evidence suggests this is not in fact so.
• Some women gain weight or may feel bloated (but weight gain is less of a problem than for users of the combined pill).
• Some women experience breast tenderness.

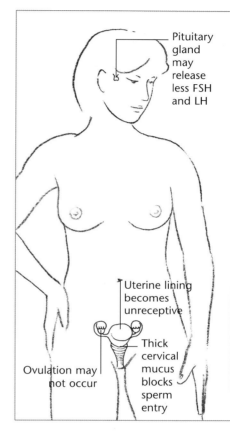

Pituitary gland may release less FSH and LH

Uterine lining becomes unreceptive

Ovulation may not occur

Thick cervical mucus blocks sperm entry

HOW THE MINIPILL WORKS

The primary effect of progestin is on the mucus produced by the cervix. Normally, this mucus becomes thinner around the time of ovulation, but in a woman taking the minipill it remains thick, forming a barrier to sperm. The progestin may also prevent pituitary-gland hormones from stimulating ovulation, and stop implantation in the uterus from happening, should fertilization occur.

QUESTIONS AND ANSWERS: CONTRACEPTIVE PILLS

Q. Does a pill user need medical checkups?
A. Yes. Her medical history, and that of her close relatives, should be considered before the pill is prescribed. She should also have a regular examination (to include a Pap smear and a check of her blood pressure and weight).

Q. With the 21-day pill, is it safe to have sex in the seven-day gap between packs?
A. Yes, it is perfectly safe.

Q. If a woman stops taking the pill, can she have a baby right away?
A. Generally, yes. But, to ensure their cycle is functioning normally, women are often advised to wait before trying to conceive until they have had

one or two periods after stopping the pill.

Q. I would like to use the pill as a contraceptive but I am really worried that I will put on weight. Is this bound to happen?
A. No. Most women who use the pill experience little or no weight gain. If you find that you are putting on weight, tell your doctor. She may prescribe another type of combined pill, or the minipill, or another form of contraception.

Q. I tend to be forgetful, but would like to use the minipill. Is this wise?
A. Probably not. To be effective, the minipill must be taken at the same time every day and, from what you have said, you might forget.

Contraceptive injections

The injectable contraceptive provides a longer-acting alternative to the pill. The main injectable contraceptive, Depo-Provera (DMPA), is currently available in more than 90 countries, including the United States, Britain, and many other European countries. The other type most commonly used is Noristerat (not available in the US). Like the progestin-only pill, the injectable contains progestin. But its primary action in injectable form is to halt ovulation. It also thickens the cervical mucus and makes the lining of the uterus less likely to receive a fertilized egg. Although it is not widely used, most women who have chosen the injectable contraceptive are very satisfied with it.

Reliability of contraceptive injections
Provided a woman returns on schedule for her injection, injectable contraceptives have a failure rate of less than 1 percent. Along with hormonal implants, they are the most reliable method of reversible contraception available.

When to have an injection
Most women who have chosen the injectable are requested to see their doctor on the first day of their period: an injection at this time means the contraceptive will be effective immediately. Given at any other time, the injection takes seven days to become effective. Women who have recently had a baby should wait until six weeks after the birth before using this method. The injection is given into a muscle, usually into the large muscle of the buttock. In the weeks following the injection, progestin is released slowly from this site into the bloodstream. How long it lasts depends on the type of injectable used. Of the two types commonly used, Depo-Provera gives protection for 12 weeks and Noristerat lasts for 8 weeks, after which more injections are required if the method is to be continued.

Does the injection affect lovemaking?
Contraceptive injections do not interrupt sex, and may enhance a woman's sex life by allowing her to relax, free from fear of pregnancy. In most cases contraceptive injections appear not to have any adverse effects on libido, but some women may notice a difference.

Who should not choose contraceptive injections?
• Women who are or suspect they may be pregnant.
• Women who want to conceive in the near future.
• Women with a personal history of severe circulatory system disease such as heart disease.
• Women with undiagnosed vaginal bleeding.
• Women with severe liver disease.
• Women who feel uncomfortable with the menstrual irregularities, including the cessation of periods, that may occur after they have been given the injection.

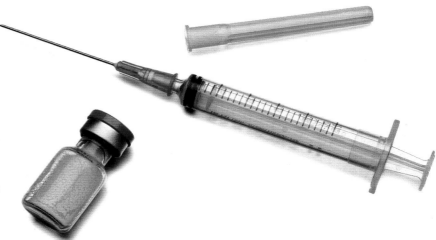

An injection of the hormone progestin provides a woman with up to three months of highly effective contraceptive protection. A major drawback of this method is that it cannot be quickly reversed if there are side effects or if the woman wants to become pregnant.

• Women with high blood pressure (unless it is treated).

• Women who show any severe side effects with the combined pill that cannot be directly linked to its estrogen component.

Advantages of contraceptive injections

• As with other long-term methods, the injectable can be taken for granted, at least until the next injection is required.

• It is highly effective, with a less than 1 percent failure rate.

• It can be used by women who are breast-feeding.

• It can be used by some women for whom the combined pill is not suitable.

Disadvantages of contraceptive injections

• It may cause weight gain.

• Once the injection has been given it cannot be reversed, so if a woman does suffer any side effects she may have to wait for at least 12 weeks—possibly as much as a year— before these subside.

• Periods may become more prolonged or irregular, or even cease.

• Some women suffer mood swings and depression.

• Fertility may take some time to return— often several months, and even a year or more —should a woman wish to conceive after using the method.

• It does not protect against any sexually transmitted diseases, including HIV.

Hormonal implants (Norplant®)

Hormonal implants provide a revolutionary new system for delivering contraceptive hormones. Inserted under a woman's skin, they release a steady stream of hormones into her bloodstream over a period of five years. Long-lasting, usually easily reversible (provided they were inserted by a specially trained doctor), extremely reliable, and with few side effects, implants have been hailed as the contraceptive of the future. Time will tell whether this is the case. Best known by the name of Norplant® (the most common formulation), contraceptive implants consist of six matchstick-sized tubes made of Silastic, a type of silicone. Each implant contains a progestin and acts as a slow-release carrier for the hormone. Once in place, the implants release the progestin into the bloodstream, which increases the impenetrability of the cervical mucus to sperm as well as reducing the chances of ovulation or of a fertilized egg implanting in the lining of the uterus.

Reliability of hormonal implants
Hormonal implants have a failure rate of less than 1 percent.

How are hormonal implants inserted?
Insertion must be carried out by a specially trained doctor, to minimize chances of complications. Women are generally asked to make an appointment for insertion on the day when

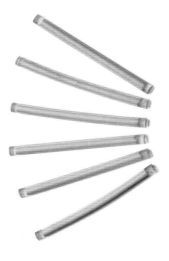

A hormonal implant consisting of six flexible tubes that, inserted under the skin, each release progestin at a steady rate for five years.

they expect their period to start. The implants are usually inserted on the inside surface of the upper arm, where they will neither migrate under the skin (as they might do at other sites in the body) nor affect the movement of the arm. After giving the patient a local anesthetic, the doctor makes a small incision in the skin—about ⅛ inch long—and inserts the six implants in a fan shape just under the skin. The whole process takes about 10 minutes, and no stitches are required. Some women may find bruising and tenderness where the implants have been inserted, but this usually subsides within a few days. Although some women are worried that the outline of the implants will be seen on the skin's surface, this is rarely the case; however, the implants can usually be felt by rubbing a finger gently over the skin's surface.

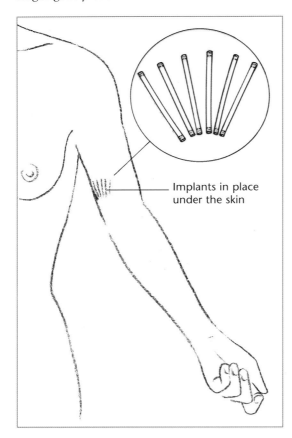

Implants in place under the skin

The six tubes in an implant are inserted by a doctor in a fan-shaped pattern under the skin. An implant is not biodegradable and remains in place until surgically removed, either because it is no longer effective or because the woman wishes to change contraception.

If inserted on the first day of a woman's period, the implants are effective immediately; inserted at any other time they take a week to become effective, and extra contraceptive protection will be needed in the meantime. The implants will provide continuous protection for five years or so. Should a woman wish to become pregnant, however, the implants can be removed by a trained doctor—this usually takes about 15 minutes. After removal, return to normal fertility is rapid.

Do implants affect lovemaking?

Like injectables, implants are reliable and do not interrupt sex. In most women they have negligible effect on libido, but in some cases there is a noticeable difference.

Who should not use hormonal implants?

- Women who are or may be pregnant.
- Women with a history of severe disease of the circulatory system.
- Women with undiagnosed abnormal bleeding from the vagina.
- Women who have breast cancer.
- Women who have severe liver disorders.

Advantages of implants

- Because of their long-term effectiveness, they can be forgotten about until the time comes for them to be renewed.
- They may be suitable for women who cannot use the combined pill.
- They can be used when breastfeeding.
- They have no long-term effect on fertility.

Disadvantages of implants

- They may cause prolonged and irregular bleeding and changes in the menstrual cycle, to the extent that 10–20 percent of women request removal during the first year of use.
- Other possible side effects include headaches, nausea, and weight gain—like other progestin-only methods.
- They do not protect against any STDs, including HIV.
- Pain may occur at the site of the implant.
- Removal of implants may be difficult, occasionally requiring two or more visits to the doctor, or even hospitalization.

Future hormonal methods

New hormonal methods are currently being researched and tested to find those that combine minimal side effects with maximum effectiveness and ease of use. Two possible future methods are described below.

The vaginal ring

Both injections and implants require a doctor to administer them and, in the case of implants, to remove them. However, a third type of long-acting hormonal contraception, which can be inserted or removed by the woman herself, may be widely used in the future. This is the vaginal ring.

Made of Silastic, the same silicone rubber that is used for implants, it is a ring about 2 inches in diameter and ¼ inch thick. The inner core of the ring contains the synthetic hormone progestin, while its outer layer consists of Silastic alone. The woman inserts it by squeezing the sides of the ring together and gently pushing it into her vagina, much as she would a diaphragm *(see p.139)*. Inside the vagina, where it moves freely, the ring releases a steady stream of progestin, which is absorbed into the woman's bloodstream through the vaginal wall. Once inserted, the ring can remain in place for three months, although it can be removed should a couple decide they wish to conceive. Fertility returns rapidly once the ring is removed.

The vaginal ring works in much the same way as the progestin-only pill: research suggests that it blocks ovulation in around 50 percent of women's menstrual cycles; increases the thickness of mucus produced by the cervix, making it impenetrable to sperm; and reduces the chances of a fertilized egg implanting in the lining of the uterus.

According to current research, the failure rate of the vaginal ring is about 3 percent, which is higher than for other hormonal contraceptives. This rate is likely to be lowered considerably when a combined ring—containing both estrogen and progestin, like the combined pill—becomes available.

In trials the ring has proven easy to use. It offers up to three months' contraceptive cover at a time, and can be controlled by the user. The main disadvantage appears to be that some users experience a vaginal discharge. The ring does not seem to interfere with sensation during sex, but should it do so, it can easily be temporarily removed for intercourse without affecting contraceptive cover. However, like other hormonal methods, it offers no protection at all against sexually transmitted diseases such as HIV or herpes.

A pill for men?

Producing a contraceptive pill for men is just one line of research directed at increasing the number of male contraceptive methods from three—the condom, withdrawal, and vasectomy. In theory, there is no reason why a male pill should not work. In practice, however, most trials of male pills have failed.

If a man is given progestin (which inhibits the release of two hormones called FSH and LH from the pituitary gland—*male hormones are described on p.21*), his testes will cease sperm production. Unfortunately, progestin also stops the release of the sex hormone testosterone, causing a loss of sex drive and thereby defeating the purpose! A combined pill containing progestin and synthetic testosterone would maintain libido, but without fully suppressing sperm production, so a high risk of pregnancy remains.

However, the results of a worldwide trial of a new type of male hormonal contraceptive, recently announced, seem more promising. This method involves weekly injections of testosterone, which evidently fools the testes into "believing" that they have already made sufficient sperm, with the result that the sperm count drops dramatically. Trials indicate that it has a failure rate of less than 2 percent, and that it does not reduce libido and may, in some men, increase it. The next step will be three-monthly injections, and the ultimate aim is to administer testosterone as an implant, a patch, or a pill. To succeed, however, male hormonal contraception needs the backing of pharmaceutical companies and, as yet, this is not forthcoming. Also, possible side-effects of a testosterone pill may include risks of prostate cancer and heart disease.

The IUD

IUD stands for intrauterine device—a small piece of plastic, placed inside a woman's uterus, which prevents conception. There are two types of IUDs currently in use. One is T-shaped with a thin strand of copper wire wound around the upright part of the T. The other type of IUD is also T-shaped, but without the copper wire; it is impregnated with the hormone progestin, which is released slowly and enhances the IUD's activity. Soft nylon threads attached to the IUD pass through the cervix and into the vagina. By inserting a finger into her vagina, a woman can feel the threads and reassure herself that the IUD is still in position.

In the United States, the only type of copper IUD available is the Copper-T 380. In Britain and the rest of Europe, various copper IUDs are available, but the Copper-T 380 is favored because of its effectiveness and lack of side effects. The progestin-releasing IUD is used in some countries: in the United States the only brand available is Progestasert, which used to be available in the UK, but was withdrawn from use because of the increased risk of ectopic pregnancy. However, a new form of hormonal IUD, the Levonorgestrel-IUD, which releases a different type of progestin (called levonorgestrel) than earlier hormonal

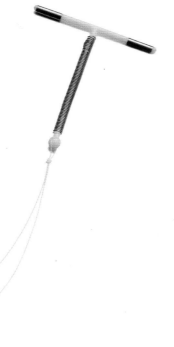

Copper IUDs (right) are coated with copper wire that improves their efficacy. A copper IUD needs to be replaced every five to eight years, depending on the exact type.

IUDs—and therefore does not have the same side effects—has recently become available in Britain and other European countries. The Levonorgestrel-IUD may be licensed for use in the United States in the future.

Reliability of IUDs

IUDs are very effective, with a failure rate of only 1–2 percent for copper IUDs and 1.5–2 percent for Progestasert. The new Levonorgestrel-IUDs have an even lower failure rate of up to 0.2 percent.

How does the IUD work?

Exactly how the IUD works as a contraceptive has always been something of a mystery, but recent research has provided some answers. The most important function of a copper IUD is to block fertilization. Under normal conditions, sperm run an obstacle course as they make their way through the unfriendly uterine environment, with few of them actually reaching the fallopian tubes. The IUD makes the uterus even more unfriendly so that no

IUDs

• That a foreign body introduced into the uterus could act as a contraceptive has been understood for many centuries. According to one ancient source, placing a pea-sized stone in the uterus of a female camel prevented pregnancy during the long journeys made by Egyptian merchants across the desert. The ancient Greek physician Hippocrates was believed to have introduced objects into women's uteri for contraceptive purposes over 2,500 years ago. And the legendary eighteenth-century Venetian sexual adventurer Giacomo Casanova was alleged to routinely place a little gold ball into his lover's cervix to avoid unwanted pregnancy.

• It is estimated that around 90 million women worldwide have an IUD inserted, of whom 66 percent live in China. Worldwide, the IUD is probably the most commonly used reversible contraception.

• Contrary to popular myth, women who have copper IUDs will not set off the alarm when they pass through metal-detecting security devices at airports.

sperm—or very few—survive the trip, making fertilization virtually impossible. Should fertilization occur, the presence of an IUD also alters the lining of the uterus, preventing implantation of the fertilized egg. The copper wire wrapped around IUDs like the Copper-T 380 makes them twice as effective as the old-fashioned "inert" IUDs (such as the Lippes loop) that were simply plastic. Because of their greater effectiveness, copper IUDs are also smaller, and therefore safer, than their inert predecessors. In addition to acting in a similar way to other IUDs, hormonal IUDs slowly release the hormone progestin, which is absorbed into the bloodstream through the uterus. Progestin causes the mucus secreted by the cervix to thicken, preventing penetration by sperm and adding an extra defense against fertilization.

Who is the IUD suitable for?

The "ideal" IUD user is a woman in her late twenties, or thirties, or forties, who is in a stable relationship and has had some or all of her children.

Who should not use the IUD?

• Women who have pelvic inflammatory disease (PID—see pp.124–5), have had it in the past, or are at high risk of getting it (i.e. are not in a monogamous relationship). Infection by PID is most common in younger women who have several sexual partners, and who are therefore more likely to contract the STDs that lead to PID. In this age group, tragically, PID can lead to sterility if it is not treated. For that reason, the IUD is not a first-choice contraceptive for young women who have not had children.
• Pregnant women, or women who may be pregnant.
• Women with uterine fibroids or uterine scars from previous surgery.
• Women who are allergic to copper (copper IUD only).
• Women who have had an ectopic pregnancy.
• Women with very heavy periods or undiagnosed abnormal vaginal bleeding—although progestin IUDs decrease menstrual blood loss and the intensity of painful periods.

THE IUD—A SAFE CONTRACEPTIVE METHOD?

Some women who have considered the IUD as a possible contraceptive choice have been put off by horror stories they may have read in the press or heard from friends about excessive bleeding, pelvic infections, and even deaths of IUD users. In fact, most women who use an IUD find it to be a virtually problem-free means of contraception, with few side effects apart from, perhaps, slightly heavier periods. It is important, however, to find a doctor who is experienced at IUD insertion and for the woman to answer questions frankly about parts of her medical history, including previous pelvic infections or sexually transmitted diseases, as these may preclude IUD use. Once the IUD is inserted, the woman should report anything unusual—possible danger signs will be described when the IUD is inserted—to her doctor immediately. But when the IUD is safely in place, there will be nothing to remember to take or put in for at least five years, and it doesn't interrupt intercourse.

THE DALKON SHIELD

In the 1970s a new type of IUD, the fish-shaped Dalkon Shield, was introduced. It caused septic late abortions, miscarriages, and even deaths. In the United States alone, the Dalkon Shield resulted in thousands of miscarriages and 33 deaths. Resulting lawsuits drove the manufacturer out of business, and many other IUD makers ceased manufacture for fear of litigation. Adverse publicity about the Dalkon Shield persuaded many women that the IUD was not for them, despite the fact that other IUDs were considered safe and effective. For a while, many American doctors stopped prescribing IUDs, although two types—the ParaGard (Copper-T 380A) and the Progestasert (a progestin-releasing IUD)— are now available.

Inserting and removing an IUD

An IUD must be inserted and removed by a specially trained doctor. The more experienced the doctor—and the better his or her track record in trouble-free IUD insertions—the less the chance of unwanted side effects in the weeks following insertion. Many doctors prefer to insert the IUD near the end of a woman's period or just after it, because it is easier to insert at this time (the cervix is a little softer) and there is little likelihood that she will be pregnant. If she has just had a baby, doctors recommend inserting the IUD around six weeks after the birth.

The IUD will have to be removed when it comes to the end of its life span (copper IUDs have a life span of five to eight years; progestin IUDs must be replaced after 12 months, and Levonorgestrel-IUDs after five years), or the woman wants it taken out. Removal must be carried out by a trained doctor: never try to remove an IUD yourself. The best time to have it removed is during menstruation. Removal is carried out using a speculum, and the device is gently pulled out by the threads. Any discomfort is likely to be short-lived.

Does the IUD affect lovemaking?
Many women like the IUD because it does not interfere with intercourse, has no effect on libido, and provides reliable protection.

Advantages of the IUD
- It is very effective and requires only that the woman check once a month that she can feel the threads.
- It is immediately reversible.
- It does not interfere with sex.
- In most women there are no side effects.
- The Progestasert can alleviate heavy periods and dysmenorrhea.

Disadvantages of the IUD
- It must be inserted and removed by a doctor.
- It can be expelled without noticing.
- A copper IUD or Progestasert may result in ectopic pregnancy *(see p.14)* if a woman gets pregnant while she is using it.
- It does not protect against any STDs.
- It can lead to increased incidence of pelvic inflammatory disease (PID—*see pp.124–5*).
- Copper IUDs can cause pains and heavy periods.
- It may perforate the uterine wall. The chances of this are about 1 in 1,000, and it usually results from faulty insertion. Initially, perforation can go unnoticed, but the woman may find she cannot feel the IUD threads, and experiences an unusual amount of pain, plus vaginal bleeding. If the uterine hole is small it will heal itself. The IUD can be removed by laparoscopy.

QUESTIONS AND ANSWERS: THE IUD

Q. Does the IUD work by causing early abortions?
A. No. Its main action is to prevent fertilization. But, in the few cases where fertilization does happen, the IUD stops the fertilized egg from attaching itself to the wall of the uterus. So the egg does not have the chance to become an embryo.

Q. I go to an aerobics class twice a week. Is there any chance my IUD will be pushed out while I'm exercising?
A. No. There is no reason to worry about this.

Q. How often should a woman check to see if her IUD is still there?
A. It is advisable for her to check whether she can feel the threads of her IUD once a month, preferably just after her period. If she can't feel the threads, or if she feels a hard object like the end of a matchstick—this could be the IUD on its way out of the uterus—she should get in touch with her doctor. In the meantime, she should use an alternative form of contraception.

Q. Does having a copper IUD alter a woman's periods?
A. Many women find that their periods become heavier when they use a copper IUD. If a woman experiences persistent pains, however, or if her period is particularly late or she has bleeding between her periods, she should consult her doctor.

Q. Does having an IUD affect a woman's chances of having a baby in the future?
A. No. Once the IUD has been removed, by a qualified doctor, a couple can expect to conceive provided they have intercourse on the days of the month when she is fertile *(for more detail, see natural methods, pp.156–62)*.

Q. Can a woman lose an IUD without noticing that it has been ejected?
A. Yes, this can happen, especially if she has a particularly heavy period that conceals its loss. This is another reason for checking the threads regularly after each period to make sure that the IUD is still there.

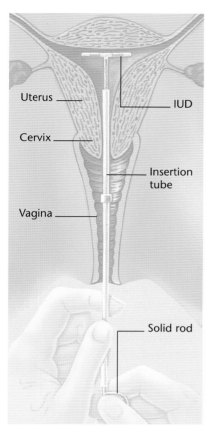

Uterus
Cervix
Vagina

IUD
Insertion tube
Solid rod

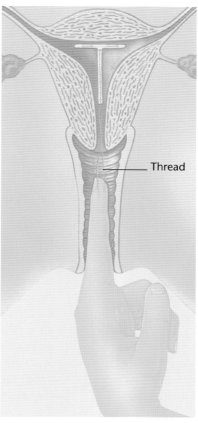

Thread

HOW AN IUD IS INSERTED

1 *Insertion is usually quick and relatively painless. Your doctor should explain what she or he is going to do beforehand and advise you to take a pain medication such as ibuprofen before insertion. You will be asked to lie with your legs apart, as you would for any gynecological examination. The doctor will then insert a speculum into your vagina in order to examine your cervix and the position of the uterus. If you feel very anxious about the insertion procedure, your doctor may give you a local anesthetic. The IUD is removed from its sterile package and squeezed into the inserter—a hollow tube—in order to flatten it. The open end of the inserter is then gently introduced into the uterus through the cervix and the IUD is deposited high up in your uterus.*

2 *When the IUD is pushed out of the open end of the inserter, it resumes its normal shape. You will probably find it useful during insertion to breathe deeply, which helps you relax. Some women feel pains, like menstrual cramps, when the inserter passes through the cervix; these may persist for some hours afterward but should disappear after that. After the inserter is removed, the threads that hang down from the IUD— which indicate that the IUD is still in position—are trimmed so they protrude into the vagina about 1 inch down from the cervix. The whole insertion procedure takes about five minutes. Once the IUD is inserted, contraceptive protection is immediate.*

THE "MIRACLE" IUD?

The Levonorgestrel–IUD is a new form of IUD that is being hailed as one of the most important innovations in reversible contraception since the introduction of the pill in the early 1960s. It is an IUD whose vertical stem contains the progestin levonorgestrel (LNG). Once the device is inserted into the uterus, it releases minute amounts of LNG—the equivalent of one to two progestin–only pills per week—at a constant rate for up to five years. This makes cervical mucus thicker and less penetrable to sperm; prevents implantation of a fertilized egg in the uterine lining; and inhibits the movement of sperm through the uterus. Because the progestin dose is so low, it reduces the risk of side effects associated with other progestin contraceptives. The LNG–IUD has a number of advantages.

- It is highly effective, with a failure rate of less than 0.2 percent.
- It is long-lasting.
- It reduces menstrual pain and makes periods lighter.
- It reduces the risk of PID.
- Fertility returns as soon as the IUD is removed.
- It does not increase the risk of ectopic pregnancy.

The main disadvantage is cost, which may be affecting use in the UK and other European countries where it has recently been introduced. It has yet to be approved in the United States. Another disadvantage is that it offers no protection against STDs, including HIV.

Natural Methods

Some forms of contraception do not require hormones, specific devices, or surgical procedures. These natural birth control methods are ideal for couples who, for whatever reason, do not wish or are unable to use "conventional" contraception. The three types of natural method are:
• natural family planning or fertility awareness, which requires a woman to monitor her monthly cycle so that she knows when she is fertile
• breastfeeding, which is—surprisingly—the most widely used contraceptive method worldwide, as well as being one of the most ancient
• coitus interruptus or withdrawal, also a very ancient method of contraception.

Natural family planning

Being aware of which days of their monthly menstrual cycle they are fertile and capable of becoming pregnant means that, in theory, women can prevent conception naturally. A woman is not fertile all the time: she ovulates (releases an egg from her ovary) only once a month, and that egg is viable—capable of being fertilized—for just 24 hours. Sperm, on the other hand, can stay alive in cervical mucus around the time of ovulation for up to three days, or occasionally longer. If a woman can predict when she will ovulate, she and her partner can deliberately avoid sexual inter-

course around the "window of fertility" that opens for about three days before ovulation and a day or two after it, thus minimizing the chance of pregnancy. This is the theory that underpins natural family planning (NFP).

How can a woman predict when she is going to ovulate?
Ovulation generally occurs 14 days (and within a range of 12 to 16 days) before the start of the next period, whatever the overall length of a woman's menstrual cycle. It is accompanied by changes in the woman's body that she can monitor. How these pieces of information are used to chart fertility, and how accurate they are, depends on the method used. There are several possibilities:
• the calendar or rhythm method
• the basal body temperature method
• the cervical mucus method
• the symptothermal method.

Reliability of natural family planning
Research indicates that failure rates can be as low as 2 percent when couples are committed to natural family planning. With less care, the failure rates can rise to 25 percent. It is clear that motivation and good teaching are vital for success. Of the various methods, the symptothermal method is the most reliable. Most couples are recommended to receive training from a trained NFP teacher, so that they feel more confident about using it.

Who is natural family planning suitable for?
• Couples who are willing to learn the techniques necessary to make NFP effective. Most programs recommend that the period of learning be from three to six months.
• Couples willing to practice periodic abstinence from intercourse.
• Women who are capable of recognizing and monitoring the signs of fertility during their menstrual cycle.
• Couples who cannot use other contraceptive methods for religious or cultural reasons.
• Couples who wish to restrict their use of barrier methods to the most fertile time of the month and use an alternative at other times.

CONTRACEPTIVE SUPERSTITIONS

Ever since the link between sex and conception was realized, there have been numerous remedies suggested for use after intercourse to prevent a woman becoming pregnant. Al Razi, a tenth-century Arabic physician, suggested that immediately after intercourse, the woman should leap up, sneeze, blow her nose several times, call out in a loud voice, and jump backward seven to nine times in order to prevent pregnancy. Interestingly, he also suggested that if she jumped forward, it would guarantee that she did get pregnant. Needless to say, we now know that such activities have absolutely no effect on the likelihood of conception.

How does natural family planning affect lovemaking?

Some couples may find that they do not want to have sex on the days when unprotected intercourse is allowed, or feel frustrated during the period of abstinence. However, others may find that periods of abstinence heighten the sexual excitement of making love on "safe" days.

Advantages of natural family planning

• There are no side effects.
• It can be used by women at any stage during their reproductive years, provided their menstrual cycle is relatively regular.
• By making women more aware of their bodies and reproductive cycle, the method can enhance their sex life—and help them achieve pregnancy should they wish it.
• It gives women control over reproduction.
• It may be the only method available to couples of certain religions and cultures.

Disadvantages of natural family planning

• Unless a couple is very committed to the method, NFP can have a high failure rate.
• Keeping daily records can be inconvenient.
• Irregular cycles—brought on by changes in daily routines, stress, or illness—can make the method unreliable.
• It requires abstinence for several days during the period of ovulation, which is when many women feel most interested in sex.
• It can be particularly unreliable after childbirth and during menopause.
• If a woman uses the BBT (basal body temperature) method and does not ovulate during a cycle, her BBT will not increase and the couple will have to abstain from intercourse throughout that month.
• It does not offer protection against any STDs, including HIV.

The calendar or rhythm method

In theory, the calendar or rhythm method looks promising as a natural contraceptive method, but in practice it is relatively crude and inaccurate, and should only be used to double-check other natural methods.

By keeping a record of her menstrual cycles, a woman will be able to calculate on which days she is fertile. Using this method, she keeps a strict record of her menstrual cycles for six consecutive months, taking the day when her period starts as the first day of each cycle. Most women find that their cycles vary in length from month to month. The timing of the fertile period can then be calculated and applied to the next month. To calculate the earliest fertile day in the cycle, subtract 20 days from the length of the shortest cycle (see example, below); the figure 20 is made up of 16 days (the maximum between ovulation and menstruation) plus 4 days (the 3 days that sperm can survive, plus 1 for safety). To calculate the last fertile day, subtract 10 from the length of the longest cycle of the previous six months; the figure 10 is made up of 12 days (the shortest time between ovulation and menstruation) minus 2 days (the maximum survival time for the egg after ovulation, plus a day's safety margin).

A TYPICAL CALCULATION OF FERTILE PERIOD

This example illustrates the method described above.

Length of shortest cycle in six months	= 27 days
Number of infertile days before ovulation	= 27–20 = 7 days
So, beginning of fertile period	**= Day 8**
Length of longest cycle	= 32 days
Probable last day of fertile period	= 32–10 = Day 22
So, end of fertile period	**= Day 23**
Intercourse should therefore be avoided on days 8–23.	

Problems with the calendar method

Unfortunately, because the method is based on evidence from earlier menstrual cycles, it cannot take account of future fluctuations in cycle length. In addition, the time at which a woman ovulates can be changed dramatically by upheavals in her daily life such as illness, stress, bereavement, or even jet lag. Also, it takes 6–24 months to know the full range of a woman's cycle. For those reasons, this method carries quite a high risk of pregnancy. It also means that a couple has to abstain from sex for an unnecessarily long time each month to allow for possible fluctuations in the cycle.

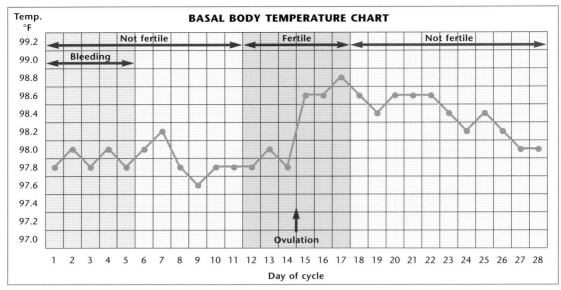

BASAL BODY TEMPERATURE CHART

Temp. °F

Not fertile   Fertile   Not fertile

Bleeding

Ovulation

Day of cycle

Basal body temperature method

Human body temperature remains relatively constant—usually at around 98.6°F, depending on the individual. However, everyone's body temperature shows a slight increase and subsequent decrease on a daily basis, reaching a peak between 3:00 and 7:00 P.M. and a minimum in the small hours of the morning between 3:00 and 6:00 A.M. This minimal temperature, attained when the body is at rest, is known as the basal body temperature (or BBT).

How can the BBT be used to calculate when a woman is fertile?

After a woman has ovulated, her basal body temperature increases by between 0.4° and 0.8°F. The chain of events happens as follows: in the ovary the ruptured follicle, from which the egg has been released, seals itself up, and starts to release the hormone progesterone, which in turn causes the temperature of the body to rise. If the egg is not fertilized, progesterone production ceases, the BBT returns to its "normal" level once more, and menstruation begins.

By monitoring changes in her BBT, a woman can determine when she has ovulated and when, accordingly, it is safe to have sex. To use this method, a temperature chart—obtainable from family planning clinics or

Each day, a woman marks her early-morning temperature on a chart. A significant rise for three days in a row, in this case days 15–17, shows she has ovulated and will not be fertile until after her next period.

doctors—and a thermometer are required. It is best to use a special fertility thermometer that shows temperature in one tenth of a degree increments to get an accurate measurement of small temperature changes. Every morning, at approximately the same time each day, the woman must record her body temperature just after waking—before getting out of bed or having anything to drink or eat. She should leave the thermometer in her mouth for 5 minutes for the temperature reading to stabilize. Alternatively, she can insert the thermometer into her vagina for 3 minutes, or, adding a dab of Vaseline first, into her rectum for the same length of time. Digital fertility thermometers give an accurate reading much more rapidly. The temperature should then be recorded by putting a dot in the center of the appropriate square on the chart *(see above)*; the dots should be joined up by straight lines to form a continuous graph.

If, for three days in a row, a woman records a BBT higher than that of all the preceding six consecutive days, this indicates that her fertile time has finished for the current cycle. She and her partner can now have unrestricted sexual intercourse until the end of her next period. After her period ends, they should not have unprotected intercourse again until she records her next significant sustained temperature rise.

Problems with the BBT method

Illness and infections can increase body temperature, while pain medications such as aspirin often lower it, masking any changes in BBT due to ovulation. Drinking alcohol the night before or getting up during the night to breastfeed a baby can also affect BBT. Charts may be hard to interpret, although interpretative skills improve with practice. But probably the greatest drawback is that the method is retrospective: it does not allow a woman to predict when ovulation is due, only when it has happened. This means a longer period of abstinence each month than with other natural methods. Furthermore, if a woman doesn't ovulate in a certain cycle, she will not be able to have intercourse at all that month.

The cervical mucus method

Secreted by the cervix, cervical mucus is a thickish liquid that changes in amount and texture during the menstrual cycle in response to changing levels of estrogen and, later in the cycle, progesterone. For certain days of the month it virtually disappears; during others it thickens to stop sperm and any bacteria in the vagina from entering the uterus; but during the most fertile time, around ovulation, it becomes thinner and sperm-friendly, with hundreds of channels through which sperm can swim into the uterus. So, the quantity and feel of cervical mucus reflects the hormonal fluctuations that precede and follow the ovulatory crescendo. By monitoring her cervical mucus, a woman should be able to predict when ovulation is about to occur and when her fertile period has finished. This is the basis of the cervical mucus method, also sometimes called the Billings method.

How does a woman examine her cervical mucus?

Most women who use the cervical mucus method do it as a matter of course after urinating. They use soft toilet tissue to blot or wipe their vulva, the area around the opening to the vagina. As moisture is absorbed, the mucus appears as a blob on the tissue. By putting a finger into the mucus and then gently pulling it away, the texture of the mucus can easily be tested (see illustration, below). Mucus texture ranges from tacky and sticky to slippery and very stretchy, depending on the stage of the monthly cycle. The color and transparency of the mucus will also change. Both texture and color of the mucus should be recorded nightly on a chart, either as a written description or by using a color code (see sample chart on p.161).

Monthly variations in a "typical" woman's cervical mucus are as follows.
- "Dry days" follow her period, when the cervical mucus forms a plug in the cervix, acting as a barrier to sperm; the vagina and vulva feel dry, and there is no visible mucus.

FERTILE MUCUS

During the fertile period, cervical mucus can be pulled out as long, stretchy threads. For that reason, fertile mucus is given the technical name *Spinnbarkeit*, the German word for spider's web.

CHANGES IN THE NATURE OF CERVICAL MUCUS DURING THE MONTHLY CYCLE

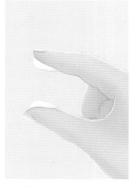

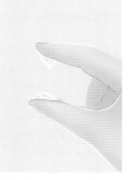

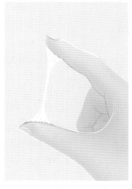

1 *Following a period, the cervix produces thick mucus that blocks the cervical canal. As mucus builds up in the cervix, sticky white or yellowish mucus appears in small amounts in the vagina.*

2 *As the egg-containing follicle develops in the ovary, the cervix produces mucus in larger amounts. At the approach of ovulation, the mucus appears watery and cloudy or transparent.*

3 *Around the time of ovulation, much more mucus is produced. This mucus is stretchy, transparent, and slippery, and indicates to a woman that she is in her most fertile phase.*

• As estrogen levels increase, mucus that is white, cloudy, and sticky to the touch appears in the vagina.

• "Wet days" precede ovulation as estrogen levels peak. Mucus is clear and slippery, like egg white, and very stretchy, and the vagina and vulva are moist. This is the fertile mucus that nurtures sperm and allows them to pass through into the cervix. The last day when this fertile mucus can be seen is called the peak day, and it coincides with maximum secretion of estrogen, which occurs just before ovulation.

• Following ovulation, a woman will find that her mucus becomes more cloudy and sticky (and thus more impenetrable to sperm). This is the result of progesterone production by the ovary, a feature mimicked by the progestin-only pill *(see pp.146–7)*. This persists until her next period begins.

How can a woman use this information?

On the "dry days" following menstruation it is considered to be safe to have intercourse on every second day—alternating because semen and the lubricants released during sexual arousal can persist overnight and may be mistaken for cervical mucus. As soon as any mucus is evident, the couple should abstain from intercourse until the evening of the fourth day after the peak day. This allows up to three days for ovulation to occur, and for the 24-hour life-span of the egg.

Problems with the cervical mucus method

One of the disadvantages of this method is that illness and vaginal conditions such as yeast infections may affect cervical mucus. Bleeding between periods may also make observations very difficult. Women who use this method need good memories, to remember when they last had intercourse, when to abstain, and so on. And mucus production may begin only two or three days before ovulation, making intercourse in the first "infertile" period that follows menstruation and precedes ovulation relatively unsafe. For these reasons, many women feel safer if they combine the cervical mucus method with other methods in the symptothermal method.

THE BENEFITS OF FERTILITY AWARENESS

By making a woman more aware of her bodily cycles, natural family planning or fertility awareness can have other benefits apart from its use as a contraceptive method.

To help conception
By being able to predict those days when the woman is most likely to be fertile, a couple can increase their chances of conceiving, especially if they have had some problem in this area. However, they should try not to turn sex into a chore by mechanically having regular intercourse during the fertile time. They should seek advice if conception has not taken place after one year of trying.

To detect pregnancy
If the BBT (basal body temperature) stays elevated for two or three weeks, this is a good indication that the woman is pregnant.

To identify low female fertility
Lack of increase in BBT repeated over several monthly cycles may indicate infrequent or non-existent ovulation.

The symptothermal (multiple index) method

The symptothermal method combines several indicators of the possible fertile period—hence the alternative name, the multiple index method—to pinpoint the fertile period accurately. In addition to basal body temperature and the appearance of cervical mucus, the woman records the following changes on her chart: the position and softness or firmness of her cervix; the pain that may occur mid-cycle when the ovary wall ruptures to release an egg *(see p.22)*; the show of blood that may occur mid-cycle; and breast tenderness, which can increase after ovulation. As with the other methods, she records her observations on a chart *(see illustration, opposite)*. The infertile period (between ovulation and menstruation) begins on the morning of the third consecutive day of high temperature, or the fourth evening after peak mucus, whichever comes last. Infertility is then confirmed by the other indicators. The calendar method can be used at

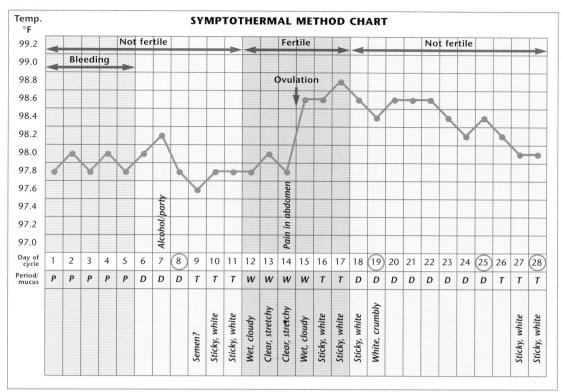

SYMPTOTHERMAL METHOD CHART

Temp. °F — Not fertile | Fertile | Not fertile — Bleeding — Ovulation — Alcohol/party — Pain in abdomen

Day of cycle	1	2	3	4	5	6	7	8	9	10	11	12	13	14	15	16	17	18	19	20	21	22	23	24	25	26	27	28
Period/mucus	P	P	P	P	P	D	D	D	T	T	T	W	W	W	W	T	T	D	D	D	D	D	D	D	D	T	T	T
Notes									Semen?	Sticky white	Sticky white	Wet, cloudy	Clear, stretchy	Clear, stretchy	Wet, cloudy	Sticky white	Sticky white	Sticky white	White, crumbly								Sticky white	Sticky white

(Intercourse days circled: 8, 19, 25, 28)

the same time to double-check and make the method more effective.

Does the method work?

The advantages and disadvantages of the symptothermal method reflect those encountered by users of any of the fertility awareness methods. The main drawbacks are that it requires time and dedication to take readings and maintain the chart, and its failure rate can reach 25 percent. Still, with careful use—providing intercourse takes place only during the part of the infertile period after ovulation but before menstruation—the failure rate should be as low as 2 percent. It also means that a couple must avoid unprotected intercourse between the end of the woman's period and the end of her fertile period. However, they do not have to abstain from all sexual activities during that time: kissing, cuddling, mutual masturbation, and oral sex are all alternatives that do not involve penetration and so can provide pleasure without risk of pregnancy.

The symptothermal method has a number of advantages, despite the frustration of abstinence. It is under a woman's personal control,

On a chart like this, a woman records her temperature and details of bleeding and mucus. She may use a code—here P = period, D = dry, T = thick mucus, and W = wet mucus—and add notes. Mucus occurring after the fertile period is disregarded. In this example, the woman has circled days when she had intercourse (once in the dry days before ovulation—although she could not at the time have been certain that she was not yet ovulating—and three times after her fertile period) to avoid confusion between semen and mucus.

and it makes both her and her partner aware of her reproductive cycles and fertility. It is acceptable to many faiths (including the Roman Catholic Church) and cultural groups that object to other methods of contraception. Being aware of her fertility also enables a woman to predict when she will be most fertile, should she wish to have a child.

New developments

In addition to digital fertility thermometers, which register body temperature within 45 seconds, there are several new techniques designed to enhance fertility awareness methods. Among these are home testing kits that detect levels of luteinizing hormone (LH) in the urine, using a dipstick that changes color. LH is the hormone released by the pituitary gland that causes ovulation to occur. By detecting the sudden increase of LH in the bloodstream, the test should show when the fertile phase is about to begin. However, it seems to be more useful for couples who wish to achieve, rather than avoid, conception.

Breastfeeding

Breastfeeding is the world's "hidden" contraceptive. It is a method that each year prevents more pregnancies than all other forms of contraception put together. Its effectiveness, however, depends on the individual woman, as well as how frequently she feeds her baby.

How does breastfeeding prevent conception?

By sucking on its mother's nipple, a baby stimulates the sudden release of a hormone called prolactin from the pituitary gland. In turn, prolactin stimulates glands in the breast to produce more milk. But prolactin also instructs the pituitary gland to stop release of the hormones that cause eggs to develop in, and be released from, the ovaries. Without ovulation, there can be no conception.

Unfortunately, the situation is not as simple as that. Prolactin levels surge to 20 times their normal levels when breastfeeding begins, but then subside rapidly when the nipple is no longer being sucked. For women who breastfeed regularly throughout the day and night, sufficient levels of prolactin are maintained to have a contraceptive effect *(see the account of the !Kung women, left)*. But in women whose babies suckle six or so times a day, prolactin levels are high only for part of the day, which means that ovulation may well not be suppressed and there is a risk of pregnancy if the couple does not use another form of contraception. Unfortunately, some women have been told—and believe—that breastfeeding will act as an effective contraceptive, and find themselves unwittingly pregnant within months of the birth of their baby.

BREASTFEEDING AS A CONTRACEPTIVE

How can a baby feeding at the breast make its mother less fertile? The answer lies in the interaction between the hormones that control the reproductive cycles. Nipple sucking causes the release of the hormone prolactin from the pituitary gland. This then halts the release of other pituitary hormones that normally cause an egg to be released from the ovary each month.

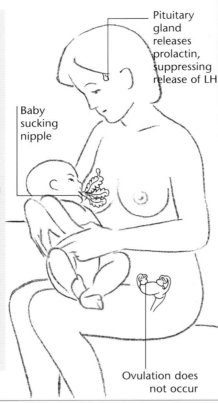

Pituitary gland releases prolactin, suppressing release of LH

Baby sucking nipple

Ovulation does not occur

THE !KUNG WOMEN OF THE KALAHARI

The !Kung bushpeople of the Kalahari desert in southern Africa are hunter-gatherers, a lifestyle they have pursued for many thousands of years. The !Kung people depend entirely on the contraceptive effect of breastfeeding to plan their families. In fact, although !Kung women have no access to other contraceptives and have sex without restrictions, they have, on average, no more than five children. The success of breastfeeding as a contraceptive lies in the fact that !Kung women keep their young children with them most of the time and breastfeed them regularly, on demand. This maintains a high level of prolactin in the blood, which suppresses the release of hormones from the pituitary gland that stimulate eggs to develop in, and be released from, the ovaries. In effect, the ovaries are switched off for long periods. Indeed, using this natural method, a !Kung woman may have only a dozen or so menstrual periods during her lifetime, with three or four years between each pregnancy.

Withdrawal (coitus interruptus)

Coitus interruptus—"interrupted intercourse" —dates from the time, tens of thousands of years ago, when humans first recognized the link between intercourse and conception. How it works is aptly described by its alternative names: "withdrawal" or "pulling out." When a man is reaching the "point of no return" and knows he is about to ejaculate, he swiftly withdraws his penis from the vagina and ejaculates on or near his partner, rather than inside her. By so doing, he reaches orgasm but stops the sperm from reaching the cervix and uterus. Or does he?

During intercourse, but without the man being aware of it, a drop of fluid called the pre-ejaculate commonly escapes from the tip of the penis. If he has recently ejaculated, that drop can contain thousands of sperm, any one of which could be well on its way to fertilizing an egg in the fallopian tubes before the man has withdrawn his penis.

The other problem with withdrawal is that it requires tremendous willpower and commitment. Young men without much sexual experience may find it particularly difficult to control the situation and withdraw in time to prevent ejaculation in their partner's vagina.

For these reasons, coitus interruptus tends to have a high failure rate, probably up to 19 percent (as against a theoretical rate of 4 percent), depending on age and experience. Couples who use the method may find that the opportunities for mutual sexual satisfaction are limited, and they may be left feeling frustrated (although if a woman has already reached orgasm she is less likely to feel unsatisfied). Certainly, withdrawal remains the most popular method of contraception in some countries, although its popularity in most Western countries has declined sharply over the past 30 years with the advent of the pill and other new and more reliable forms of contraception.

Coitus interruptus puts the pressure to make it work on the man, but leaves the possible consequence—pregnancy—to the

FAST-MOVING SPERM

At midcycle, when ovulation is most likely to take place, the chance of a younger woman getting pregnant from a single act of intercourse, if unprotected by contraception, is around 30 percent. Sperm move very rapidly: just 90 seconds after a man has ejaculated in his partner's vagina, sperm can be found swimming up through her cervix, the entrance to the uterus. This explains why douching—washing out the vagina with vinegar, lemon juice, the foam from shaken-up warm cola, water from a shower attachment, or anything else— takes place too late to be effective. It may also spread infections upward from the vagina into the uterus.

BIBLICAL CONTRACEPTION

The earliest reference to coitus interruptus appears in the *Book of Genesis*:
"Then Judah said unto Er's brother Onan, 'Go and sleep with your brother's widow. Fulfil your obligations to her as her husband's brother, so that your brother may have descendants.' But Onan knew that the children would not belong to him, so whenever he had intercourse with his brother's widow he let the semen spill on the ground, so that there would be no children for his brother." *Genesis 38:9*

woman. It puts pressure on the woman, too, because she may want the man to stay inside her longer. However, it is free, requires no equipment, and has no side effects. When no other contraceptive methods are available, withdrawal is better than no method at all, especially when the partners are young and fertile. They must remember, however, that this method offers no protection against any STDs, including HIV.

Nonpenetrative sex

Increasing numbers of couples are using nonpenetrative methods such as oral sex or mutual masturbation as an alternative to intercourse. One benefit is that nonpenetrative sex avoids risk of conception, and can be practiced, for example, during the fertile period of a woman's cycle. It would be wrong, however, to assume that this offers complete protection against STDs (see pp.117–26).

Sterilization

Sterilization is a surgical technique that blocks the pathway by which sperm or eggs travel from where they are made to their regular destination. It is highly effective, but not easily reversible. Once sterilized, a woman is most unlikely to bear any more children, or a man to father them. For this reason, careful thought and counseling are required before a couple decides to use sterilization as their contraceptive method.

The technique itself is simple. Minor surgery is used to sever the link between the ovaries or testes and the outside world. In women, this involves tubal surgery: cutting or blocking the fallopian tubes that carry ova (eggs) from ovary to uterus following ovulation. In men, the procedure is called vasectomy: literally, this means the "cutting out a portion of the vas" (deferens), the tube along which sperm travel from a testis to the penis prior to ejaculation.

Reliability of sterilization

The failure rate for female sterilization is around 0.35 percent in the first year, and 0.01 percent thereafter. The failure rate for male sterilization is 0.2 percent or less. Vasectomy does fail in a small number of cases, when the cut ends of the vas rejoin or a new passage forms for the sperm to swim along.

Who should choose sterilization?

Because of its finality, most couples who choose sterilization as a means of contraception are older, in their thirties or forties—it is certainly an increasingly popular contraceptive option in this age group—and have completed their families, or are sure that they never want to have children.

Doctors generally try to dissuade younger, childless women or men from choosing sterilization in case they change their minds later on. Most couples are advised that if there is any doubt in their minds they should not go ahead with sterilization because they may come to regret it. Reversal in both sexes can be attempted, but there is no certainty of success. (*See also dealing with infertility,*

pp.224–30: some of the techniques described can be employed to help reverse sterilization.)

Her or him? Making the decision

Once a couple has decided on sterilization, the question arises as to which of them should be sterilized. Vasectomy is quicker, simpler, and safer. No deaths have been reported following vasectomy; the death rate from female sterilization is around 3.5 per 100,000 (due to general anesthesia). Yet more women are sterilized than men. This discrepancy may be a result of motivation—the childbearing partner is more motivated to have the operation—or because, as some men argue, men retain fertility into old age and are therefore more likely to start another family if divorce or death ends their present relationship.

Can sterilization be reversed?

Sterilization should be regarded as irreversible, although occasionally—after the death of a partner, for example, or the death of children, or simply a change of mind—people request a reversal. The introduction of microsurgical techniques (the same techniques that are used for joining together the broken ends of nerves and blood vessels when re-attaching severed limbs) has increased the success of reversal operations. They are expensive, however, and their reliability cannot be guaranteed.

Female sterilization: tubal surgery

Most women's experience of tubal surgery will follow the same general procedure, although surgeons may employ a number of different techniques to effect sterilization. Tubal surgery is carried out in a hospital, normally under general anesthetic. The most common technique used today is laparoscopy. This technique is minimally invasive, leaving only tiny scars. Once the patient is anesthetized in the operating room, a surgeon makes one or two small incisions in her abdomen and inserts a laparoscope, a pencil-sized viewing tube through which she or he can see the reproductive organs. Through the same or a lower incision, the surgeon then inserts a second instrument that is used to block each fallopian tube by diathermy (heating) or with clips or rings. The instruments are then removed and the incisions are stitched up.

Most women return home within 24 hours, where they need to rest until the effects of general anesthesia wear off. An alternative method, called mini-laparotomy—once the most common method of female sterilization —involves a larger incision, and tubal ligation (tying off) of the fallopian tubes. This requires a longer stay in hospital and a protracted recovery period at home.

Are there any complications after female sterilization?

Women are likely to feel some discomfort around the incision for several days, and slight bleeding may also occur—they are generally advised to take it easy for a week or so. Major complications are rare.

Periods should remain the same following sterilization, because the ovaries, womb, and cervix are left intact. Occasionally, however, women experience heavier periods. Some doctors believe this is related to the woman's previous method of contraception—their periods may have been lighter before the operation because they were using the pill, for example—while others put it down to the operation itself—to damaged blood vessels, for instance, which could affect the flow of blood to the ovaries.

Does female sterilization affect lovemaking?

Provided there are no complications, a woman can resume sex with her partner as soon as she wishes. In general, the only effect that sterilization will have on a woman's sex life is to enhance it now that she is freed from any fear of pregnancy. The hormones controlling the menstrual cycle are released into the bloodstream by the ovaries, a process that is not affected by the blocking or sealing of the fallopian tubes. Because her hormonal levels remain unchanged, there is no hormonally induced change to her libido. However, it must be remembered, of course, that female

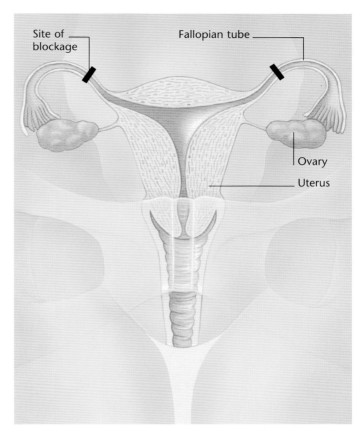

The fallopian tubes carry newly released eggs from the ovaries to the uterus. If an egg meets a sperm in the fallopian tube fertilization and pregnancy will result. Female sterilization is achieved by blocking the fallopian tubes either by tying or heating. This ensures that eggs cannot travel to the uterus, nor can sperm pass along the fallopian tube to reach the egg.

sterilization does not offer any degree of protection against sexually transmitted diseases, including HIV.

Male sterilization: vasectomy

The operation is usually carried out on an oupatient basis, either in a hospital or in a doctor's office. Most men's experience of vasectomy goes something like this: after the scrotum is shaved, the doctor gently squeezes the skin on one side to locate the vas deferens. He or she then injects a small amount of anesthetic into the scrotal skin to numb the area, and makes a small incision. The vas deferens is located and either cut or a small piece removed, and then ligated (tied off) or cauter-

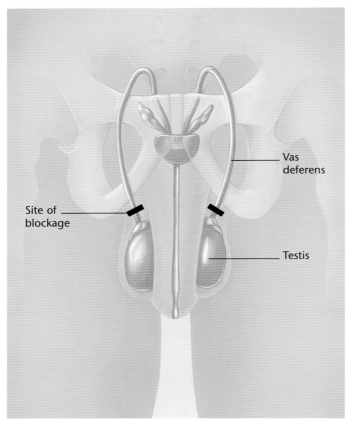

Each vas deferens is a tube that carries sperm from their production site in the testes to the penis, from which they emerge, in semen, during ejaculation. Vasectomy, or male sterilization, prevents this from happening by blocking the vasa deferentia by either cutting or heating. Although sperm continue to be produced they are not released, but reabsorbed.

Vas deferens

Site of blockage

Testis

ized (sealed by heating). After stitching up the incision in the skin using absorbable sutures, the doctor repeats the technique on the other side of the scrotum. The whole procedure should take no more than 20 minutes.

Are there any complications following a vasectomy?

Following the operation, most men are advised to take things easy for a day or so, and to avoid lifting anything heavy for 48 hours. Any aches or pains that occur as the anesthetic wears off can be treated with a mild analgesic such as aspirin; a strategically placed ice pack may also help reduce bruising and inflammation. Most men feel more comfortable if they wear tight-fitting briefs or an athletic support both day and night for a week after the operation. Stitches in the skin of the scrotum will either be absorbed or fall out within a month. However, any severe pain, swelling, bruising, or discharges should be referred to the physician without delay.

A few reports have suggested that there is a link between vasectomy and the incidence of prostate cancer. Further research is needed, but medical opinion currently believes the evidence is inconclusive. There is certainly no causal link to explain why vasectomy should increase the chances of developing prostate cancer. However, men who are worried about this should ask their doctor for advice.

QUESTIONS AND ANSWERS: STERILIZATION

Q. What happens to a man's sperm or a woman's eggs after he or she has been sterilized? Do they accumulate inside the testes or ovaries?
A. No. If sperm or ova are not released they are simply absorbed back into the body.

Q. If a man has a vasectomy, will he lose interest in sex or be unable to get an erection?
A. No. Vasectomy stops sperm from reaching the outside. It does not affect the testes, which continue to produce the hormone testosterone

—that fuels the libido—as normal. The man's desire for sex and ability to get erections should remain as they were before the operation. He will also continue to ejaculate as before, because semen production does not stop after vasectomy.

Q. Does female sterilization bring on menopause?
A. No. The operation does not affect a woman's ovaries (the organs that produce the hormones that control her menstrual cycle). Menopause will occur at the age it would have happened had she not been sterilized.

Q. Does sterilization result in a man or woman losing their interest in sex?
A. No. In general, neither male nor female sterilization has any deleterious effect on an individual's sex drive. In fact, his or her libido may be enhanced because there is no longer any need to worry about contraception or pregnancy.

Q. Is sterilization the best contraceptive option for women in their forties?
A. Not necessarily. The IUD may be an alternative for this age group.

Does male sterilization affect lovemaking?

After a vasectomy, a man can have sexual intercourse as soon as he feels comfortable. However, during the weeks following the operation, if he and his partner are having penetrative sex, they must use a condom or another form of contraception to avoid the risk of pregnancy. The reason for this is that it usually takes 20 to 30 ejaculations before all sperm are cleared out of the storage areas downstream of the point where each vas deferens is blocked; after this he starts producing sperm-free semen, or "shooting blanks." To check whether his ejaculate is sperm-free, he will probably be asked to provide semen samples 12 and 16 weeks after his vasectomy. These are then checked in a laboratory to see if they contain any sperm. Provided that both samples are sperm-free, he can have sex without any other form of contraception. However, it must be remembered that male sterilization does not offer any protection at all against sexually transmitted diseases, including HIV.

Emergency contraception

Emergency contraception refers to any method employed to prevent pregnancy after, but within a few days of, unprotected intercourse. There are two effective emergency contraception options available for women:
- the postcoital or "morning-after" pill
- the IUD.

Emergency contraception means just that: it should be used only as an emergency measure and not on a regular basis. However, it does mean that if a woman feels, in the hours and days following intercourse, that she may be at risk of becoming pregnant, she can do something about it.

The reasons why couples have unprotected sex are many and varied. They might decide to take a chance; they could get so carried away that contraception is far from their thoughts; they may drink too much alcohol to care; condoms may split, slip off, or break if

> **WHEN AND WHERE TO GET EMERGENCY CONTRACEPTION**
>
> If a woman has had intercourse without using any form of contraception, or was inadequately protected because something went wrong with the contraceptive method she was using, she may want emergency contraception. The postcoital pill and the IUD can be obtained from any clinician offering contraceptive services, family planning clinics, and some hospital accident and emergency departments.

used with an oil-based product that weakens latex; her diaphragm may not be inserted properly; a woman may forget to take her contraceptive pills correctly—or, tragically, a woman may be raped.

The postcoital or emergency pill

This is the most common form of emergency contraception. Once known as the "morning-after pill"—a name no longer used by medical professionals because it gives the erroneous impression that it works only on the morning following unprotected sex—the postcoital ("after intercourse") or emergency pill must be taken within 72 hours (3 days) of intercourse to be effective. When a woman consults her doctor she will probably be asked to take two postcoital pills immediately, and two more 12 hours later, even if that means getting up in the middle of the night (this is sometimes called the Yuzpe method, after the Canadian gynecologist who devised it in the 1970s). If lower-dose pills are used, then a woman takes four pills immediately, followed by four more pills 12 hours later.

How does the postcoital pill work?

It is not clear just how emergency contraceptive pills work. They contain the same type of synthetic sex hormones—progestin and estrogen—that are found in a standard contraceptive pill *(see pp.142–6)* but in higher doses. When absorbed into a woman's bloodstream they either stop ovulation from occurring or, if ovulation and fertilization have already taken place, the hormones prevent a fertilized egg from implanting in the wall of the uterus and developing into a fetus.

Reliability of the postcoital pill

Treatment with the postcoital pill within 72 hours of unprotected intercourse reduces the risk of pregnancy by at least 75 percent. However, couples are advised to use contraceptive protection until her next peiod in case the woman ovulates later than normal.

Are there any side effects?

Around two thirds of women experience feelings of nausea after taking the pills. If a woman vomits within three hours of the first dose, she may bring up the pills and be required to take more to ensure effective treatment. A doctor may prescribe an anti-nausea drug (or suggest an over-the-counter preparation). The woman should be made aware that her next period may be delayed, in case she interprets this to mean that she has missed a period and is pregnant. Whether she has a period or not, a woman should return to her physician three to four weeks after the initial consultation for a checkup. The postcoital pill should not be used by women who show contraindications to estrogen—such as a history of blood clots.

The IUD as a postcoital contraceptive

The alternative to using hormones to prevent pregnancy after intercourse is to insert a copper-bearing IUD (see pp.152–5). A doctor may decide to insert an IUD provided that not more than five days have elapsed since the probable date of ovulation. Because of the risk of pelvic inflammatory disease, swabs may be taken (to check for infection) prior to IUD insertion, particularly if the woman is young and is not in a regular relationship.

The woman should return for a checkup three to four weeks after the IUD is inserted. If she has had a normal period, the IUD can be removed and an alternative contraceptive method used, if she wishes.

Reliability of the IUD as a postcoital contraceptive

The IUD is virtually 100 percent effective at preventing pregnancy, and works either by inhibiting fertilization, or by stopping the fertilized egg from implanting in the wall of the uterus. Postcoital IUD insertion is more effective than postcoital pills.

RU-486: a future form of postcoital contraception?

RU-486, or mifepristone, is a drug that ends pregnancy in its first few weeks. If a woman's period is overdue, she can take RU-486, followed by another drug (prostaglandin) 36–48 hours later, and this induces an abortion. The combination is highly reliable; if used alone, RD-486 is less successful. The treatment works by nullifying the effect of progesterone, the hormone released by the woman's ovary that normally enables the early embryo to survive and develop in the uterine wall. RU-486 is also very effective as a postcoital contraceptive, but taken in this way it is expensive and rarely used.

The drug is described as postconceptional, rather than contraceptive, because it acts after implantation. This has led to controversy about the use of RU-486, with its detractors calling it the "abortion pill." Moral arguments about abortion have prevented its introduction in the United States and other countries, although it is available in France, where it was developed. Some doctors suggest that RU-486, or its successor, might be employed as a once-a-month postconceptional pill, producing short-term abortions two or three times a year—the number of times conception and implantation would occur on average in a young, fertile couple having regular unprotected intercourse.

QUESTION AND ANSWER: THE POSTCOITAL PILL

Q. Although I do not object to contraception, I do have very strong moral views about abortion and find it unacceptable. Does the postcoital pill cause an abortion?
A. No. The postcoital pill does not cause an abortion: it is not terminating a pregnancy but preventing one from starting, either by blocking ovulation or by stopping a fertilized egg from implanting in the wall of the uterus.

CONTRACEPTION CHECKLIST

CONTRACEPTIVE METHOD	FAILURE RATE‡	PROTECTION AGAINST STDS•	ADVANTAGES	DISADVANTAGES
No method (age 25)	85%	None	–	Very high risk of pregnancy
No method (age 40)	45%	None	–	High risk of pregnancy
No method (age 45)	15%	None	–	Risk of pregnancy
BARRIER METHODS				
¶Male condom	2–4% (12–15%)	Yes	Both types of condom are widely available and easy to use	Putting on, or in, the condom can interrupt sex; male condoms occasionally split; condom may slip off, or out, if used incorrectly
¶Female condom	2–4% (10–18%)	Yes		
Diaphragm with spermicide	4–8% (15–18%)	Some; not HIV* or other viruses	Cap and diaphragm can both be put in up to 3 hours before sex; no side effects; both reduce risk of cancer of the cervix	Both involve advance planning, so reducing spontaneity; can be messy; repeated sex needs addition of more spermicide
Cervical cap with spermicide	9–11% (up to 18%)	Some; not HIV* or other viruses		
HORMONAL METHODS				
Combined oral contraceptive pill	0.5% (2–4%)	No, but reduced risk of PID§	Does not interrupt sex; reduces risk of cancer of the uterus and ovaries	User must remember to take daily; may have side effects; not suitable for heavy smokers or breastfeeding women
Progestin-only pill (minipill)	0.5–2% (up to 4%)	No, but reduced risk of PID§	Does not interrupt sex; minimal side effects; can be taken by smokers and breastfeeding women	Needs to be taken at same time daily to be effective; periods may be irregular with bleeding in between
Contraceptive injection	0–1%	No, but reduced risk of PID§	As for hormonal implant; less heavy bleeding	Regular visits to doctor; periods irregular, may stop; weight gain; may have depression, loss of libido; delayed return of fertility
Hormonal implant	0–1%	No, but reduced risk of PID§	Long-lasting; does not interrupt sex; removes need to take pill daily; few side effects; can be used by breastfeeding women	Discomfort in insertion/removal, which requires a specially trained doctor; possibility of irregular, prolonged periods, mood change
Vaginal ring	3%	No, but reduced risk of PID§	Does not interrupt sex; simple to put in or remove; stays in place for 3 months	Periods may be irregular; risk of expulsion; possibility of vaginal discharge
INTRAUTERINE DEVICE				
Copper IUD	1–2%	No; may increase risk of PID§	Does not interrupt sex; can stay in place for 5–8 years (copper), depending on type (hormonal, 1 year); works as soon as inserted	Insertion/removal requires a specially trained doctor; increased risk of PID; periods may be heavier; risk of expulsion
Hormonal IUD	1.5–2%	No; may increase risk of PID§		
Levonorgestrel-IUD	0–0.2%	No; may increase risk of PID§	As implant; lasts 5 years; reduces menstrual bleeding, period pains	Insertion/removal requires trained doctor; irregular periods initially
NATURAL METHODS				
Withdrawal (coitus interruptus)	4% (up to 19%)	None	Free; no side effects; better than nothing	May be unsatisfying to both partners; not very effective
Natural family planning: sympto-thermal method	2% (up to 25%)	None	Free; no hormones or devices required; no side effects; under personal control	Requires daily record-keeping and periods of abstinence; unsuitable for women with irregular periods
STERILIZATION				
Tubal surgery (female sterilization)	0.35% in first year	None	Does not interrupt sex; effective immediately	Requires surgery, with its attendant risks
Vasectomy (male sterilization)	0.2%	None	Does not interrupt sex; involves only minor surgery	Requires surgery; not effective immediately

‡ The failure rate is the percentage of women who used that method for one year but nonetheless became pregnant. For some methods, the theoretical failure rate when correctly used differs markedly from the actual rate in "typical," less careful use. In these cases the latter rate is given in brackets below the theoretical rate. Failure rates are higher in younger, more fertile women, and lower in older (premenopausal) women.

• STDs are sexually transmitted diseases (see pp.117–26).
¶ These contraceptives can be bought in drugstores and some supermarkets. The other contraceptive techniques, apart from natural methods, require consultation with a doctor.
§ PID is pelvic inflammatory disease (see pp.124–5).
* HIV is the virus that causes AIDS (see pp.117–21); other viral STDs include herpes and genital warts (see pp.122–3).

CHAPTER 6

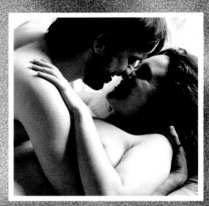

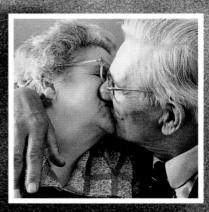

Sex and Relationships

Sex plays an important part in any intimate, loving relationship, whether the people involved have known each other for years or have met only recently. Sex is the sensual and sensory manifestation of the attraction between two people, and it can be one of the greatest pleasures in life. But sex can also cause disappointment, frustration, and unhappiness. To tackle problems such as these it helps if we are equipped with a knowledge and understanding of our sexuality and sexual behavior. Good sex is not something we know how to do instinctively—it has to be learned about and practiced.

Before looking at the area of sexual pleasure, however, it is necessary to answer a number of fundamental questions. What exactly is the human sex drive and how is it controlled? Which parts of the body respond best to stimulation? What makes one person sexually attractive to another and how do people signal that attraction? How does the human body work sexually and how can we be confident that we are sufficiently in tune with a partner's needs to give sexual satisfaction? Does fantasy have a useful role to play in our sex lives, and where does sexual variance fit in?

These are all important questions. The aim of this chapter is to look at the sexuality of women and men, as well as at some of the issues that arise from the expression of sexuality in our everyday lives.

We must always keep in mind that successful relationships have to be worked at. Too many people are surprised when their partner claims to feel unloved or unappreciated. For despite all the intimate things that people do with one another when having sex, communication between a couple is often neither good nor easy. Being able to communicate, and show enthusiasm and genuine concern for each other, is not only just as important as physical affection—it is often the first step to maintaining a deeper, long-lasting relationship.

It is not always easy to keep a relationship fresh and exciting, especially if a couple has lived together for many years, even if they have been very happy. They may find that changing their normal routine in order to spend more time together enhances their sexual feelings for each other. Relaxing and laughing together, and talking freely and openly about feelings and desires, can help boost sexual interest as well.

Above all, whatever their temporary dissatisfactions, a couple should never lose sight of the enormous benefits to be gained from a happy relationship that encompasses mutual love and respect, the enjoyment of each other's company, and a fulfilling sex life.

Sexual desire

Sexual desire is the subjective feeling that we want to have sexual pleasure, which most of us experience from time to time—ranging from many times a day to a few times a year. It is triggered by stimuli from outside the body (perhaps the sight of an attractive man or woman) and from inside the body (our natural sex drive, for example). Just because we experience sexual desire does not mean that we will necessarily engage in overt sexual behavior—if we did have sex every time we experienced sexual desire, our way of life would be very different! However, when sexual activity does take place it is generally preceded by sexual desire in both partners. That we are experiencing sexual desire is often indicated by sexual daydreams and sexual fantasies, and by genital arousal—stiffening of the penis or clitoris and lubrication of the vagina.

Sexual desire is created and controlled by the brain, but is believed not to be a single driving force: that is, sexual desire is not just a basic biological need like hunger. Instead, it is the result of a complex interaction between three different factors.

Sex drive or libido

This is a person's biological urge, their appetite, for sex. Unlike the other primary instinctive urges—such as hunger and thirst—a person's sex drive does not affect his or her ability to survive, although it obviously does affect the survival of the species. Some people seem to have a greater sex drive than others, but there is no reason to assume that men necessarily have a higher sex drive than women (see below).

Sexual motivation

A person's underlying attitude about sex—their sexual motivation—is based on their personality, expectations, sexual identity, and previous sexual experiences.

Sexual thoughts

Desire for sex may also be based on a desire for its consequences, such as a boost to self-esteem or a sense of femininity or masculinity, and by the need to be loved.

Traditionally, it was believed that men had a greater interest in sex than women. Men were thought to be driven by their libido and easily aroused, while women were more interested in sex in terms of a relationship. While it is true that male and female patterns of sexual arousal may differ, there is no evidence that male and female sexual desire does as well.

How sex drive works

While sex drive in both men and women is controlled by the brain (see box), it is triggered by hormones called androgens, the most common of which is testosterone. This particular hormone is often referred to as the "male sex hormone" because it is produced by a man's primary sex organ, the testes, and because it maintains his secondary sexual characteristics (see p.28). In fact, women also produce testosterone and other androgens. Most of their testosterone is produced in the adrenal glands, located on top of the kidneys, but some is also made by the ovaries.

Although levels of testosterone are higher in men than in women, this does not mean that men have a higher sex drive. A "suitable"

THE BRAIN AS A SEX ORGAN

Most people, if asked to list the sex organs, might include the penis, clitoris, or breasts. But few would include the brain. Yet this powerful organ, with its billions of interconnecting nerve cells, which controls and coordinates all our bodily activities, also controls our sex lives. In fact, the brain is the control center for our sexual desire and sex drive.

• The brain's limbic system controls basic emotional drives—including our sex drive.

• A specialized sexual center within part of the brain, called the hypothalamus, responds to sexual stimulation of the receptors within the genital organs, and is involved in the experience of orgasm.

• The largest, "thinking" part of the brain—the cerebrum—enables us to have the sexual thoughts, perceive the sexual stimulation, and store the various sexual memories that between them make up the pattern of sexual desire for each individual.

level of testosterone, appropriate for each sex, is essential to ensure that a man or a woman has an adequate sex drive. Lower-than-normal levels will reduce the sex drive in men and women. This may occur, for example, following illness in men or as a consequence of menopause in some women. In certain cases, a doctor may prescribe testosterone, in the form of HRT (hormone replacement therapy—*see pp.271–5*) to a male or female patient to restore their flagging libido. Similarly, naturally raised levels of testosterone typically increase sex drive. For example, many women feel more sexual around the midpoint of their menstrual cycle, about two weeks before their period is due, because their testosterone level temporarily increases when ovulation occurs.

Sex drive and age

Male sex drive is thought to reach a peak when men are in their late teens. Women, on the other hand, apparently reach the peak of their sex drive in their late thirties; thereafter it levels off and does not begin to decline until they reach their sixties. On the surface, these physiological differences would appear unfortunate: while a man's sex drive is waning, his female partner's is getting stronger. Of course, the picture is not as simple as this. Libido—as indicated by time taken to get an erection, for example—may decrease in men, but it does not mean that their sexual desire is in steep decline as well. Desire, as mentioned already, is much more complex than sex drive alone. And as a man gets older, his sexual urges often shift from being genitally focused to being more sensual and cerebral. As a result, there does not have to be an imbalance in sexual interest between partners of the same age. And a benefit of the changing nature of sexual desire is that his sexual endurance—the ability to delay and control ejaculation—will increase with age, as will her ability to achieve orgasm.

Is it love?

How to distinguish between lust, infatuation, and love is a question that faces many couples embarking on a new relationship. It is not

HOW OFTEN SHOULD WE MAKE LOVE?

It is not unusual for couples to feel that they are "strange" because they think that they are not having sex often enough. Such feelings are often triggered by magazine surveys about "how often people do it," or by friends who boast about their sex lives. But, apart from the facts that people rarely tell the truth in magazine sex surveys, and people who talk endlessly about their sex lives may often be covering up a problem, there is no reason why a couple should compare their sex lives with anyone else's. Their sexual frequency will depend on their age, the length of their relationship, their health and fitness, and their sexual desires. If both partners are happy with their sex life as it is, why worry?

LOSING THAT LOVING FEELING

There are many factors that can contribute to reducing a person's sex drive and desire for sex.
- **Alcohol** in small amounts can lower inhibition, but excessive alcohol intake frequently leads to loss of desire and arousal, as well as delayed orgasm.
- **Depression** tends to lower a person's sex drive.
- **Exhaustion**, both physical and mental, can leave little room for sex.
- **Guilt about sex**—for example, because you were brought up to believe sex is "not nice"—may reduce desire.
- **Inhibitions** may interfere with enjoyment of sex and make it hard to respond to your partner's sexual advances.
- **Stress** tends to cause a loss of sex drive.
- **Worrying** about money or business matters can diminish interest in sex.

always easy to tell the difference, particularly in the early stages of a relationship, and there is no simple test that will give an easy answer.

Sexual love is a powerful and very personal emotion. It is a state in which the happiness of a sexual partner becomes essential to that of his or her lover. Being in love can cause a number of noticeable physical symptoms, including loss of appetite, disturbed sleep, increased pulse rate, and raised blood pressure.

Only time will tell which direction a relationship will take. Love lasts; infatuation does not. And in the long term, loving has more to do with companionship than with lust.

Sexual pleasure

To have good sex, you have to work at it. Sex is not something that we instinctively know how to do well. Rather, it needs to be learned and—like most things in life—it usually improves with practice. Nor is it enough to simply understand how men and women's bodies work, because there is no universal recipe for sexual pleasure and satisfaction.

Everyone has their own individual preferences and their own unique physical likes and dislikes. Finding out about each other's sexual needs is an intrinsic part of having a sexual relationship. And that means understanding and discovering how your own body is best stimulated and sharing those discoveries with your partner.

Despite these personal differences in sexual likes and dislikes, the sexual response itself follows the same stages—arousal, leading to orgasm and finally resolution—in every individual alike.

Sexual arousal

If a couple has sexual desires, and they are attracted to each other, they may find that they want to take things further and enjoy each other sexually. The first part of sexual pleasure is arousal, when each partner becomes sexually excited. Arousal can result from the sight or smell of a partner, through thoughts about sex, or through the direct physical stimulation of foreplay. Women usually become aroused more slowly than men during foreplay; men are aroused relatively quickly, often becoming excited initially by visual stimuli such as sexy clothing or the naked body.

As arousal progresses, a plateau stage is reached, during which a high level of sexual tension is maintained. The penis and vaginal lips become engorged with blood and darken in color, and individuals tend to focus on sex and their partner, and ignore everything else that is going on around them. If sexual interest is maintained, and if sexual stimulation continues, a point is usually reached where sexual tension peaks and orgasm occurs.

Foreplay

Foreplay is the prelude to lovemaking, whether that goes on to involve sexual intercourse or other forms of sexual activity. During foreplay partners stimulate each other sensually to the point where they both become fully aroused and are ready for intercourse and/or orgasm. Foreplay can involve just about anything that both lovers find enjoyable—kissing, caressing, stroking, or licking any part of the body. It often starts with nongenital touching and culminates in direct stimulation of the most responsive erogenous zones, notably the penis, clitoris, and breasts.

Erogenous zones

The skin contains sensors that relay signals caused by touch and pressure to the brain, where they are perceived. Erogenous zones are the parts of the body's surface that evoke sexually arousing sensations when stroked, touched, or kissed. This description of erogenous areas is not intended to be prescriptive. In theory any part of the skin can be erogenous: no two people are exactly the same, and everyone likes to be touched in a different way. Still, there are certain areas that give most men and women supreme pleasure when touched, caressed, and kissed. It is important for partners to discover exactly where and how they each like to be touched.

Men and women share some common erogenous zones; areas specific to each sex—which tend to be the most responsive—are described below. In both men and women, areas that commonly contribute to arousal when stimulated include the face, lips, ear lobes, nape of the neck, arms, elbows, armpits, fingertips, buttocks, anus, backs of the knees, inside of the thighs, and feet. In fact, almost any part of the skin's surface can be erogenous, depending on the individual. In both sexes, however, there are specific areas where stimulation will generally result in intense arousal.

A woman's erogenous zones may include:
• the genitals, including the vaginal lips, just inside the vagina itself, and the clitoris—the most sensitive of all her erogenous areas, the sole function of which is sexual pleasure

• the breasts and nipples. Many, but not all, women find their breasts very responsive, and a few may achieve orgasm simply by having their nipples licked and sucked
• in some women, the perineum, the area between the vagina and the anus.

A man's erogenous zones may include:
• the genitals, including the scrotum, the shaft of the penis, and the glans of the penis, usually its most sensitive part
• the perineum, the area between the base of his penis and the anus
• in some men, the nipples.

Sexual arousal in women

As a woman becomes aroused through being sexually excited by her partner, various changes typically take place to her body.
• Her vagina becomes moist and lubricated, and the whole vulva may become moist.
• The inner part of her vagina expands.
• Her vaginal lips become thicker, separated, and turned outward.
• Her clitoris becomes larger and erect.
• Her breasts enlarge and the nipples may become erect.
• Her heart and breathing rates increase.
• Her skin may become flushed.
The clitoris plays a central role in a woman's sexual arousal. It can be stimulated by the fingers, the tongue or a vibrator, by penile thrusting, or by body pressure. When a woman is highly aroused, the tip or glans of the clitoris retracts under its hood and may no longer be seen or felt. Touching different parts of the clitoris produces different sensations: some women like the base of the clitoris to be touched; some prefer to be stimulated along the side; others get pleasure from the tip being touched. Some women like harder friction than others, although most dislike the clitoris being rubbed too hard and some find direct stimulation almost unbearable. The considerate lover will always try to find out what his partner prefers.

Sexual arousal in men

As a man becomes aroused, these changes typically take place to his body.
• His penis becomes erect.

QUESTION & ANSWER: EROGENOUS ZONES

Q. Is it true that during foreplay men only enjoy having their penis and scrotum stimulated? Or is this a myth?
A. It is true that some men do see sex as being mechanical: get an erection, have penis rubbed, put penis in vagina, and end of sex! But many men enjoy being touched, stroked, and kissed on parts of their bodies other than their genitals as part of prolonged foreplay. Of course longer foreplay benefits both partners: she will have longer to become aroused, and he will be less likely to ejaculate quickly because her stimulation of him has been less genitally focused. Try talking to your partner about what both of you want from sex.

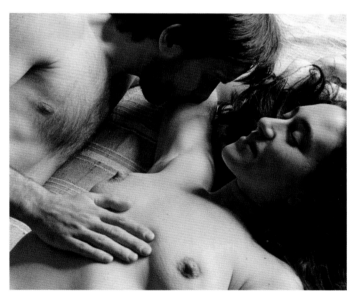

The skin is our largest erogenous zone. Stimulated by touch and stroking, skin sensors send messages that fuel arousal to the brain.

• His testes begin to elevate.
• His scrotum thickens.
• His nipples may become erect.
• His heart and breathing rates increase.
The penis, the most responsive of a man's erogenous zones, can be stimulated by fingers, mouth, or tongue, or by the vagina during intercourse. Just as a women may show her partner what she likes, a man can show his partner how he likes his penis to be stimulated so that she is neither too gentle nor too rough.

Sexual intercourse

Sexual intercourse is often, but not always, the culmination of arousal that may lead to orgasm in one or both partners. During intercourse a man, perhaps guided by his partner, introduces his erect penis into his partner's vagina. The fact that her vagina is lubricated may not necessarily mean that she is fully aroused and ready for intercourse, although he is ready: more loving, patient foreplay— without becoming mechanical or pressurizing her to hurry!—may be needed.

THE G-SPOT

The G-spot is believed to be a particularly sensitive place, located about two thirds of the way up the front wall of the vagina, just below the base of the bladder. It is named after Ernest Gräfenberg, the German gynecologist who, in the 1940s, was the first to suggest its existence. It is said to be a highly erogenous zone, which when stimulated produces an orgasm that is said to feel different from the orgasm women have as a result of clitoral stimulation. The G-spot, if it exists, is stimulated by inserting a finger in the vagina and pressing against the front wall and by rear entry positions in sexual intercourse. While some women find that such stimulation does enhance the intensity of their orgasm, women who do not experience such feelings should not worry about it. Everyone is different and whatever magazine articles say about the G-spot, its existence is still the subject of some debate.

DOES SIZE MATTER?

Some men worry about the size of their penis, just as some women worry about the size of their breasts. Surveys show, however, that women are a lot less concerned about penis size than men think they are—few women, apparently, are turned on by the sight of an enormous penis, and many may be put off by one. There is also no relationship between the size of a man's flaccid penis and its erect size, and no direct relationship between erect penis size and the degree of sexual satisfaction for either partner. Being a good lover depends on a man's understanding of his partner's needs and his ability to arouse her sexually. Women are more interested in the experience than the size!

During intercourse the man moves his penis inside the vagina or, if the woman is on top, she moves her vagina around his penis. The result is that his penis is stimulated, which may lead him to reach orgasm and ejaculate; the movement of intercourse also pulls on her labia and may move the clitoral hood over the clitoris, as well as stimulating the inside of the vagina and possibly the G-spot *(see box)*. Although a woman may reach orgasm through intercourse, it is far from a certainty, and a woman may need additional clitoral stimulation during intercourse if she wants to have an orgasm with her partner inside her.

A couple can have intercourse in many different positions—lying down, sitting, standing, kneeling—and it is up to the individual couple to discover which positions give them the most pleasure. Even when couples have found a favorite position, it is still worth having sexual intercourse in different positions because they produce different degrees of penetration and different sensations for both partners.

Orgasm

Orgasm is the culmination of arousal and the climax of sensation. But not every sexual experience results in orgasm—especially for women. While orgasm is often the high point of sex for both partners, it does not have to be. Sex should not be "orgasm-driven"; whether and how a couple achieve orgasms is a personal matter for the partners alone.

Orgasm is an intensely pleasurable sexual feeling during which the body experiences muscular contractions followed by a loss of tension before falling into a relaxed state. Any description of orgasm has to be general because it is an intensely personal feeling. And one person's experience of orgasm will vary from one sexual act to the next, depending on their mood, tiredness, relationship with their partner, and the type and amount of foreplay. Although orgasm is perceived as happening in the genitals and spreading to the rest of the body, it is orchestrated by the limbic system and hypothalamus in the brain.

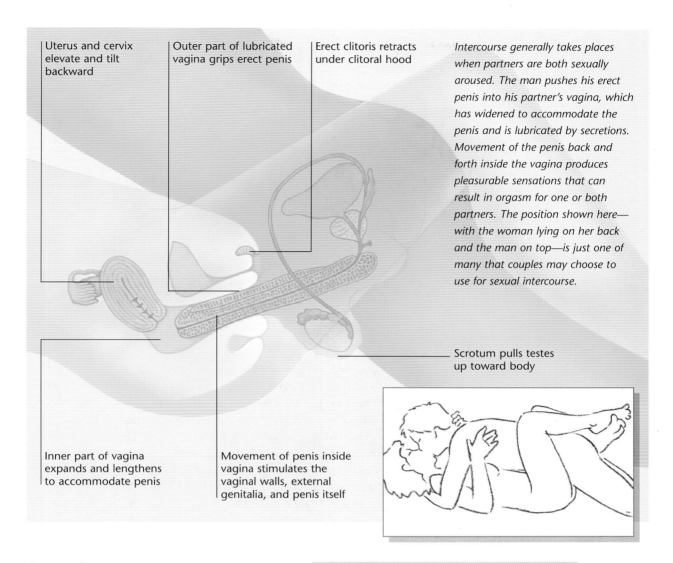

Uterus and cervix elevate and tilt backward

Outer part of lubricated vagina grips erect penis

Erect clitoris retracts under clitoral hood

Intercourse generally takes places when partners are both sexually aroused. The man pushes his erect penis into his partner's vagina, which has widened to accommodate the penis and is lubricated by secretions. Movement of the penis back and forth inside the vagina produces pleasurable sensations that can result in orgasm for one or both partners. The position shown here—with the woman lying on her back and the man on top—is just one of many that couples may choose to use for sexual intercourse.

Scrotum pulls testes up toward body

Inner part of vagina expands and lengthens to accommodate penis

Movement of penis inside vagina stimulates the vaginal walls, external genitalia, and penis itself

Orgasm in men

If a man is sexually aroused and his penis is stimulated by hand or mouth, or by the vaginal walls, he will usually reach a point of inevitability when he knows he is going to ejaculate. Within a couple of seconds, ejaculation takes place and this is normally, although not always, accompanied by orgasm *(see also pp.28–9)*. As the muscles of the urethra and penis force semen out of the penis in four or five contractions, he experiences the pleasurable sensations of orgasm. While the sensations appear to center on his penis, he may feel pleasure and a release of tension in his pelvic area and over his entire body. During orgasm he may make a sound or cry out. When the contractions cease, the man relaxes and his penis soon softens.

SIMULTANEOUS ORGASMS

In books and stories, much emphasis has been placed on the supposed value and meaning of a couple reaching orgasm together. In theory, couples who are used to each other, and who have fine-tuned their sex lives, should be able to reach a mutual climax. But this can mean that couples focus so much on climaxing together that they no longer concentrate on enjoying sex—and she (or sometimes even he) may be tempted to fake orgasms in order to achieve the "goal" together. In reality simultaneous orgasms are simply not essential for a couple to achieve sexual satisfaction in their relationship; they can be fun if they happen to occur, but they should not be the driving force behind sex.

Orgasm in women

Once a woman reaches the plateau state of arousal, stimulation of her clitoris by fingers or mouth and/or vaginal stimulation during intercourse can result in orgasm. As a woman reaches orgasm, her vagina, pubic muscles, anal sphincter, and uterus all contract rhythmically, her body may arch, and she may be thrown into spasms. Many women feel a

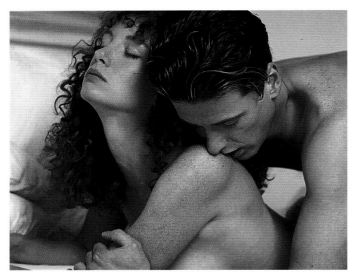

The ability to "read'"each other's bodies and understand what gives a partner pleasure is the key to sexual success. But for this to happen, both partners must communicate their needs and desires openly.

FAKING ORGASM

Some women, and a few men, find it difficult to achieve orgasm during sexual intercourse and may fake it, largely to protect their partner from feeling inadequate. According to a recent survey, as many as two out of five women fake orgasm at least sometimes, if not always. However, faking orgasm can:

• give the wrong message
• prevent you from finding mutually satisfying ways of making love
• establish a pattern of behavior that is difficult to change
• focus attention on performance rather than enjoyment.

The only way to find a solution is for both partners to talk about the problem openly and honestly and to recognize that each must take responsibility for sexual fulfillment.

wave of pleasure passing from their genitals throughout their body. She may make some kind of grimace, or cry out or even scream, depending on how intense the orgasm is for her. Once the contractions of the pelvic muscles, uterus, and vagina have ceased, she will soon begin to return to her normal state, although this process is usually much slower than in men. Unlike men, many women are capable of having several orgasms, one after the other. They remain at the plateau stage and can be stimulated to orgasm repeatedly. This is known as a multiple orgasm.

Women tend to experience a wider range of types of orgasm than men do. This appears to depend on a number of factors, including whether the clitoris is stimulated directly, or indirectly by, for example, movements of the bodies during intercourse.

While men almost always experience orgasm during sex, this may not be true for women. In men, the process of arousal and ejaculation appears to be fairly automatic, while the ability to have an orgasm appears to be, at least partially, learned in women. Some women rarely or never experience orgasm. Many of these women are believed to be potentially orgasmic, but to have never been in a suitable sexual situation. Some have been helped to experience orgasm by individual sensate focus exercises *(see pp.191–2)* and through learning about their own sexual responsiveness through masturbation.

Resolution

After orgasm, the body enters a phase of resolution: it relaxes, and heart and breathing rates return to normal. A man's penis becomes flaccid, and he may suddenly feel very sleepy. He enters a refractory period during which he cannot have a new erection; this may last for minutes in an adolescent to days in older men. In women, the period of resolution takes much longer. Her genitals can take up to 30 minutes to return to their pre-orgasmic state. Many women enjoy continued physical intimacy during this stage, and may have a sense of "afterglow" following orgasm. Unlike men, women do not experience a refractory period.

COMMON INTERCOURSE POSITIONS

This face-to-face position—known as the missionary position—is probably the most commonly used. It is comfortable and permits a couple to kiss, caress, and make eye contact during intercourse. This variation, with the woman's legs raised, allows deeper penetration.

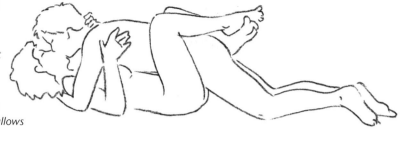

Rear-entry positions such as this allow a man to stimulate his partner's breasts and clitoris with his fingers while moving his penis inside her, a combination that can help her achieve a satisfying orgasm. This position allows deep penetration but the man must be careful not to thrust too hard and cause pain.

Woman-on-top positions enable her to control penetration. She makes the pelvic thrusts, moving her vagina around his static penis, so she can control the speed and depth of thrusting. While she does this, the man can stroke her breasts and use his fingers to stimulate her clitoris.

In this variation of the face-to-face position the man sits in a chair, and his partner lowers herself onto his penis and sits on his thighs facing him. This position enables the couple to be very close to each other, to make eye contact, and to hold and caress each other. He can also kiss and stroke her breasts.

The advantage of a side-by-side position for intercourse for many people is that it is comfortable—neither partner has to hold the other's weight. In this variation, the woman wraps her right leg over her partner's buttocks so that he lies between her legs.

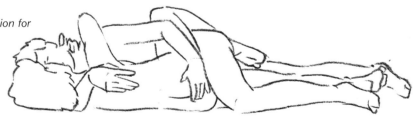

AFTERPLAY

Contact and closeness do not have to stop just because sex has finished. After one or both partners have reached orgasm, they may caress each other before sleeping. Afterplay is the postcoital equivalent of foreplay. Most couples feel very close to each other after sex; this is a good time for some gentle and relaxed cuddling. It has become a cliché that all a man wants to do after sex is to roll over and go to sleep, or get up and get a beer. It is true, however, that many women like a demonstration of tenderness and affection after making love. Compromise is probably the best solution for most couples— a kiss, a hug, or a quiet talk, and then sleep.

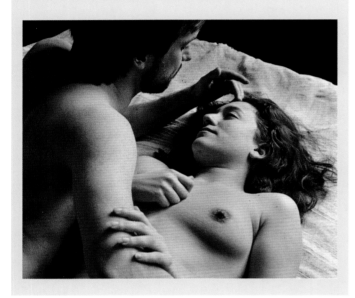

MASTURBATION IN A RELATIONSHIP

Masturbation—self-stimulation, often to orgasm —is something most of us do, with a frequency ranging from often to once or twice in a lifetime. Yet masturbation remains a taboo subject, and women in particular can be reluctant to admit that they masturbate. Masturbation is not some- thing that is always done only in private, nor something that stops as soon as a person is in a good sexual relationship. It usually gives a differ- ent type of satisfaction from that derived from sexual intercourse. Masturbation helps us learn about our own sexual needs, and watching a partner masturbate can sometimes be a useful way of learning about how he or she likes to be stimulated. Mutual masturbation can form a valuable part of a couple's sexual repertoire.

Oral sex

Using your mouth to stimulate your lover's body is one of the most loving and intimate things one person can do for another. For this reason, it can be highly satisfying to both giver and receiver. Strictly speaking, oral sex simply means mouth play on any part of the body, including the ear lobes, fingers, toes, nipples, and so on. But in practice, oral sex usually refers to oral–genital contact. Using tongue and lips to lick, kiss, and gently suck a woman's clitoris, vaginal lips, and vagina is known as cunnilingus; licking, kissing, and sucking a man's penis and scrotum, and moving his penis inside a partner's mouth is known as fellatio. While many people enjoy oral sex, some do not.

Oral sex, like other aspects of sex, is a skill to be learned. And the fastest way to find out whether it is being done properly is to ask a partner whether they are being stimulated, and how they would like to be stimulated. For example, while some women enjoy having their clitoris stimulated directly during oral sex, others find the sensation too intense.

Some people are reluctant to try oral sex because they do not quite understand what is expected of them, or because they are inhib- ited by fears. Perhaps the most common of these is the fear of smelling or tasting unpleas- ant to a partner. Provided the genitals are kept clean by daily bathing, they will generally not smell bad but will have only the normal healthy odor of sexual arousal, which should be both pleasant and exciting for a partner. A woman may worry that she will gag on her partner's penis, but how much of it she takes into her mouth is up to her. She may also be reluctant to perform fellatio for fear that her partner may ejaculate in her mouth—some- thing that he should avoid doing unless she agrees. A man, on the other hand, may be especially unsure what to do, or worry that he will find the smell or taste of the vulva over- powering. No one should be afraid to talk about what they would like to do and what they prefer not to do. However, it is advisable not to perform oral sex if a partner has a cold sore or a sexually transmitted disease.

The "69" position

The "69" position—so called because a couple lying head-to-toe resemble the figure 69—allows both partners to give and receive oral stimulation at the same time. This is a highly exciting experience for many people. However, others prefer to take turns giving each other oral sex because they find it better to concentrate on one thing—either giving or receiving sexual pleasure—at a time.

Anal sex

The anus and its surrounding region form an area that is just as erogenous, in many people, as the nipples or genitals. Touching or stroking the anal area—known as postillion-age—can be highly arousing, especially if done while stimulating the clitoris or penis or during vaginal intercourse. Some men and women enjoy having their partner's finger inserted a short distance into the anus and rectum. Lubrication in some form may be needed to make insertion painless. Some men derive great pleasure from having their partner insert a finger to stroke the prostate gland, as this can intensify feelings during his orgasm. Fingers that have been in contact with the anus or rectum should be washed before touching the genitals to avoid the risk of vaginal or urinary infection.

Some people stimulate the area around their partner's anus with their tongue, a form of stimulation known as rimming—a risky practice, as partners are putting themselves at risk of developing a gastrointestinal infection and, possibly, hepatitis.

Anal intercourse involves a man inserting his penis, from behind, just into his partner's rectum. This is made easier if lubrication, such as K-Y Jelly, is used and if the partner can relax the anal sphincter, the ring of muscle that normally keeps the anus closed.

Men tend to enjoy giving anal intercourse more than women enjoy receiving it because the penis is gripped tightly by the anus, enhancing the pleasure of intercourse. Many women simply do not find anal intercourse arousing, and may experience pain on penetration. If a couple has anal intercourse, it is wiser to do so after rather than before oral sex or vaginal intercourse, to avoid infection of the mouth or vagina. Apart from questions of hygiene, the wall of the rectum is more likely to tear during intercourse than that of the vagina because it is much thinner. This means that the passing on of sexually transmitted diseases, including HIV *(see pp.117–21)* is more likely by the anal route. For this reason, unprotected anal sex is regarded as being a particularly unsafe form of sexual contact and couples who have anal intercourse are advised to always use a condom. In some countries and states, anal intercourse is illegal.

Gay sex

Sex between homosexual couples is essentially the same as sex between heterosexual couples, but without vaginal intercourse. Kissing and caressing are the usual preambles to sexual arousal. Many homosexuals use oral sex or mutual masturbation to arouse their partner and bring him or her to orgasm. Some lesbian couples use a vibrator to stimulate the clitoris and vulva, and sometimes other sex toys to insert into the vagina or anus. Gay men may use anal intercourse to reach orgasm, although not all gay couples enjoy anal sex.

Sexual attraction and body language

Exactly what it is that makes one person feel attracted to another and find the idea of going to bed with them exciting remains, by and large, a mystery. The sexual chemistry of physical attraction is not easily explained—one person's idea of attractiveness leaves another person cold; some people seem to prefer a particular physical type, while others are attracted by a certain kind of personality. But there is actually a lot more to it than that.

If someone is widely perceived as being "attractive," that does not necessarily mean that they are conventionally good-looking. Good looks do, however, tend to be particularly important to teenagers and young adults.

This is because young people are often less secure in themselves than mature people, and the approval and envy of others is therefore very important to them. As they get older and more secure, they will probably place less importance on good looks in a partner.

It is generally accepted that far more men than women consider good looks an important element of attractiveness. So it may come as something of a surprise to learn that in a recent survey conducted by a women's magazine, men rated personal qualities more important than physical attributes as prerequisites for feeling attracted to a woman. As many as 70 percent of the men polled rated (or claimed they rated!) warmth and kindness more important than good looks. "Nice" breasts and bottom, together with shapely legs, came at the bottom of the poll, with only 30 percent of men saying that these were important to them. It may be that the emphasis on physical attributes in men's public appreciation of women is more closely connected with impressing other men than with what they really feel about women.

Women seem to place a strong emphasis on kindness—to themselves and others. Surveys reveal that they value a man who, more than being good-looking, is understanding, intelligent, and monogamous, and has a good sense of humor.

Body language

Body language is the way we communicate with each other without words, by moving and positioning our body. Touching someone's arm, making eye contact, leaning toward someone—these are all elements of body language. It is a language we all use, and in fact cannot help doing so. Most of the time we are unconscious of the messages we are conveying through our body language, but we are constantly, albeit subconsciously, monitoring the messages conveyed to us by other people's posture and gestures.

The environment we live in is bound to have a certain amount of influence on our body language. For example, people who are used to living in the country seem to need more personal space and therefore tend not to stand close to other people, while people who live in towns and cities are usually more used to the close physical presence of others.

Generally, however, body language is understandable wherever you live. Even people who speak a different language and cannot communicate with each other verbally are often able to communicate through gestures and facial expressions.

Posture and gesture in body language

The most obvious clues about what two people think of each other are to be found in their posture and gestures. Even if they are quite far apart, a couple who are mutually attracted will often sit with their bodies facing each other.

Body language is not simple, however. A single gesture does not determine whether or not one person is attracted to another. Rather, the message conveyed is a complex interplay of posture and gesture signals that may say "I find you attractive" but which are being constantly modified in response to the language shown by the other person.

Interest in another person and openness to being approached are shown in various ways (see box). These include leaning toward someone; standing in an open posture, with the arms loose or outstretched, as opposed to crossed in front of the body (a defensive pose); and exposing the wrists or turning the palms outward, an extension of this open posture.

MUSCLE TONE

Researcher Albert E. Scheflen claims that as soon as we are sexually attracted to someone, our muscle tone tightens in a form of readiness for flirtation and sexual activity:
"People in high courtship readiness are often unaware of it and, conversely, subjects who think they feel active sexually often do not evince courtship readiness at all. It is most clearly evinced by a state of high muscle tone. Sagging disappears, jowling and bagginess around the eyes decrease, the torso becomes more erect, and pot-bellied slumping disappears or decreases."

POSITIVE AND NEGATIVE BODY LANGUAGE

It may indicate that someone finds you attractive if they do any or all of the following:
- make frequent eye contact
- regularly take quick glances in your direction to check how you are reacting
- sit opposite you without arms or legs crossed
- sit next to you and lean toward you or cross their legs toward you
- lean toward you
- make encouraging hand movements
- touch your arm gently while talking.

It is very likely that someone is not attracted by you if they do any or all of the following:
- avoid making any eye contact with you
- sit opposite you and create a physical barrier between you by folding their arms across their chest
- clasp their hands in their lap, as if they were unconsciously covering their genitals
- sit next to you and lean or cross their legs away from you
- lean away from you.

When two people who are attracted to each other are standing near each other, their feet may "do the talking." In a group of men and women who are talking to each other, for example, there will probably be nothing in what they are saying to indicate who is interested in whom; but a close look at their feet can reveal unspoken messages—those who like each other might unconsciously be pointing a foot in the other's direction.

Mirroring and displacement

According to psychologists, the best clue that people are close and get along well with each other—or would like their relationship to be even closer—is if they mirror each other's actions. These behavior patterns can be observed between people who know each other well, such as close friends and family, as well as between potential sexual partners, even those who have only just met.

Mirroring means unconsciously copying the other person's posture and gestures. Thus if one person leans forward, the other does, too; if one person folds their arms, so does the other; and if one person crosses their legs, the chances are the other person will, too. In general, people tend to be unaware that they are doing this, but it is fascinating for an informed bystander to watch.

This behavior pattern not only says a lot about what people are feeling but can also be used deliberately to elicit a desired response. For this reason, some salespeople use mirroring in order to help their clients feel at ease and increase their chances of making a sale. Deliberate mirroring may also encourage a potential sexual partner.

Men and women also tend to fidget when they are attracted to one another. Experts call this "displacement behavior," and it plays a noticeable part in almost all early flirtatious exchanges between two people who are sending each other tentative signals. Displacement grooming behavior is common, too—looking in the mirror, patting the hair, or adjusting clothing. These gestures all indicate that the person is seeking reassurance that they look their best because they are particularly anxious to impress.

To touch or not to touch?

There is an almost irresistible desire to touch those to whom we are attracted. Two people who have up to this point shown each other only nontouching sex signals will probably follow these with tentative physical contact.

It's important not to assume, however, that if anyone touches you it means they want to embark on a sexual relationship—it may not have even occurred to them! Some people naturally touch much more than others. Touch may be used in various nonsexual situations and it can be embarrassing if a person jumps to the wrong conclusion. For example, people often touch someone if they are:
- offering a piece of friendly advice
- asking a favor
- extending sympathy
- expressing happiness.

Eye contact

The importance of eye contact cannot be exaggerated. Eye language between potential romantic partners is very important, although it is in some ways more subtle than the messages given out by posture and gesture.

Lovers are often happy just to gaze into each other's eyes longingly and lovingly for hours at a time, unlike people who are "just good friends." Staring into their loved one's eyes is a sure sign that a person is fascinated by what they see, almost as if they were trying to see into their minds.

More importantly, perhaps, it reveals whether someone is genuinely attracted to the other person or is merely playing some sort of flirtatious game. When someone is experiencing feelings of intense attraction, the pupils dilate with pleasure. On the other hand, when someone is experiencing strong feelings of dislike, the pupils contract with distaste. However, our pupils also react in this way in response to changes in light—expanding in dim light and contracting when the light is bright—so it is only possible to gauge intense emotion in someone when the light is constant and not too bright.

Voice

How people speak to each other, in terms of both tone and timbre of voice, is often another good indicator of how they feel. People who are sexually attracted to one another tend to talk in a lower, more intimate tone of voice than usual, and to adopt a slightly hushed, confidential way of speaking, as if they were trying to exclude the rest of the world from the conversation.

Finding a partner

Most of us have heard tales of an "ordinary" girl or boy who marries someone from a wildly different background, but partnerships like that tend to be unusual. Most people pair off with someone who comes from a similar background or lifestyle. Obviously this is likely to happen because it is easier to meet people who live close by, share the same interests, go to the same place of worship, belong to the same clubs, or work together. The similarities that bring people together tend to keep them together, and having things in common seems to increase the chances that a relationship will last.

Any great difference between a couple, be it in race, religion, wealth, or education, may

FIRST-TIME SEX

Whether it is the first time you ever have sex or the first time you have sex with a new partner, the situation needs to be handled sensitively. Either way, it may not be the magical experience that most people hope for, and it can leave you feeling surprisingly depressed. You may both be nervous or tense, or just overcome with lust, and you won't know at this stage exactly what the other person might enjoy sexually. Ways of making the first time more enjoyable include:

• taking things slowly and gently, however aroused you feel

• showing caring and loving behavior, as this is a time when both partners may feel insecure

• choosing positions that are not difficult to achieve or uncomfortable, and which allow you to maintain eye contact —or to avoid it if you feel shy. The missionary position is often the favored position when a couple first has intercourse

• asking your partner, or watching his or her reactions, to see which of your actions are pleasurable

• remembering that a woman may not have an orgasm the first time, but this does not mean that she did not enjoy having sex or that the experience was a failure

• most important of all, remembering to use a condom in order to ensure that neither an unwanted pregnancy nor a sexually transmitted disease occurs at the very beginning of a sexual relationship.

GETTING THE TIMING RIGHT

The secret of success is often nothing more complicated than getting the timing right. You might have met someone who you are sure would be just right for you, but they are already involved with someone else, or they've just split up with a long-term partner and are not ready to try another relationship, or they are about to go abroad. Meeting someone at the right time, when both of you are ready for commitment, is often all that is required for a successful relationship. If the same people were to meet at a different time, in different circumstances, their relationship might turn out quite differently.

not seem to matter at first but, as marriage counselors have frequently observed, seems to matter more as people get older. Certainly a shared interest often appears to help partners form a bond—although having separate interests and hobbies can also invigorate and refresh a relationship.

When looking for a relationship, it is unwise to have too rigid a view of an ideal partner, especially their physical attributes. If, for example, a man is only willing to consider women who are tall, with blue eyes and long blond hair, he is considerably reducing his chances of ever finding a partner, when he might have turned out to be very happy with a brunette. And even if by some chance he does manage to find his ideal partner, inflexibility may continue to be a problem in a long-term relationship: people change, and a partner will not stay just as he or she was when the relationship began.

Sex before marriage

Whether or not it is advisable for people to have sex before marriage is a question that is tied in with their moral and religious outlook. If they feel comfortable about it, having sex before marriage can be a good idea in that it may help them to establish that they are at least sexually compatible before tying the knot. In the long term, however, this offers no guarantee as to the success of the marriage.

Sexual preferences

There are no hard-and-fast rules as to who we are attracted to, or whether we should be attracted to someone of the opposite sex or the same sex. Conventional wisdom "pigeon-holes" most people as being heterosexual (having a sexual preference for members of the opposite sex) or homosexual (preferring same-sex relationships) or bisexual (enjoying both hetero- and homosexual relationships). In fact, humanity cannot be divided easily into distinct groups on the basis of sexuality. It is more realistic to see each of us at some point on a continuum of sexual preference ranging from completely heterosexual at one end to totally homosexual at the other.

QUESTION AND ANSWER: SEXUAL ATTRACTION

Q. I am a woman in my late thirties and I have recently started a sexual relationship with a man in his early twenties. My friends are skeptical and say it won't last, but so far we seem to have a very good relationship.
A. There are couples whose relationship survives as big an age gap as yours, but it is not always easy. You should consider whether your relationship is based mainly on sex, or whether you have other things in common. You should also think about the possibility of your partner wanting children when you are past childbearing age, and you should consider, too, what life is likely to be like when you are, say, 70 and he is in his fifties. Such a big age difference means that the relationship should not be entered into lightly.

Homosexuality

Men and women who are sexually attracted to people of the same sex are described as being homosexual. Homosexuality, however, is a more subtle and complex concept. Rather than simply describing same-sex attraction, homosexuality encompasses the attitudes, affections, friendships, standards, and social expectations of people whose predominant or sole sexual preference is for members of the same sex. Identifying someone as being homosexual, however, does not define a person's identity, personality, skills, or attributes: it is simply an aspect of their whole life experience.

The word "gay" is commonly used to describe homosexuals of both sexes, but is more commonly applied to homosexual men. Homosexual women usually prefer to use the term "lesbian" to describe themselves.

Many people have homosexual feelings —or even experiences—at some time in their adolescent or early adult lives. These experiences do not mean, however, that they will necessarily be gay or lesbian as adults. If a man reaching adulthood has no interest in heterosexual activity, the chances are that he will be gay. It is estimated that about 1 percent of all men are exclusively homosexual throughout their lives. Similarly, a woman who finds she enjoys sexual contact with women but not men is likely to be lesbian. In the United States, social surveys have found that approximately 0.6 percent of women have a sexual preference for members of their own sex alone. Nonetheless, many adult heterosexuals fantasize about homosexual behavior and may even have occasional homosexual experiences: this does not make them homosexual, any more than gays or lesbians who enjoy occasional heterosexual sex are heterosexual. A person's sexual orientation may, however, change during the course of their adult life.

Homosexuals, especially gay men, are commonly exposed to discrimination and prejudice, despite a more open attitude to homosexuality, on the whole, in most Western societies nowadays. It is important for gays and lesbians to be able to feel positive and free about sexual orientation and sex—a valuable aspect of adult life.

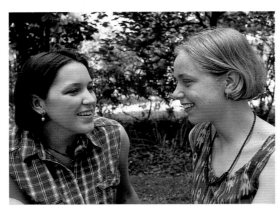

Two women can enjoy a sexual relationship which is just as close, warm, and fulfilling as a relationship between a man and a woman, or between two men.

Bisexuality

Some men and women are bisexual—they are attracted to and can enjoy sex with members of both sexes. Bisexual behavior can vary considerably. Some people may have sexual relationships with men and women at the same time, while others spend part of their life in same-sex relationships and part in relationships with the opposite sex. Some people are bisexual as young adults, while "opting" for either homosexual or heterosexual relationships as they get older. Occasional bisexual behavior, however, does not define someone as being bisexual.

Sexual fantasy and variance

A lively imagination is the best sex aid of all, and fantasies can greatly enrich a couple's sex life. Fantasies may be private or shared between partners. And if someone's fantasy world is not exciting enough for them, they may prefer to buy some "real," in the sense of tangible, sex aids. Other types of sexual variance, which don't appeal to everyone but nevertheless have a role to play in many people's sex lives, include fetishism, sado-masochism, and transvestism.

Fantasy

Many people are able to enrich their sex lives simply by using their imagination. A rich fantasy life is one of the greatest aphrodisiacs at our disposal. People are notoriously coy about their fantasies and reluctant to reveal them to their friends—and even to their lovers. Yet sharing their fantasies with each other and exploring them together can add an exciting new perspective to a couple's sex life. The most common time for people to use fantasy is while they masturbate, while the second most common time is during foreplay. Fantasy can also play an important part in intercourse, helping many people, especially women, to reach orgasm.

Sex aids

Sex aids have been around for at least 2,500 years. Some, such as alleged aphrodisiac tablets and potions, are fairly useless and not worth paying good money for. Others, such as erotic lingerie, are harmless fun and may help to spice things up a little. And still other sex aids, such as vibrators and ribbed condoms, do actually help many people, particularly women, to reach orgasm.

A vibrator, an electrically powered device that is used to give sexual pleasure, is one of the most popular sex aids. It is often used by women to give themselves sexual pleasure during masturbation, although it can also be used by couples as part of foreplay. Vibrators can have cords or be battery powered. The battery-operated ones are usually noisier. Some types have interchangeable heads, and some offer a choice of speeds. There are also special double vibrators intended to be used in both vagina and anus, while others have a special attachment for the clitoris. If the vibrator is to be used in the anus, it is important to check that it is suitable for this purpose, as otherwise it can disappear into the rectum and require medical intervention to remove it.

Another popular aid is a penis ring, which fits closely around the base of the penis, supporting it and helping to sustain an erection.

Sexual variance

Variant sexual behavior is a term used by sexologists to describe sexual behavior that is not engaged in by everyone but nevertheless provides sexual pleasure for a minority of people. It is a purely descriptive term, not implying right or wrong.

Fetishism
Fetishism is a sexual habit in which a particular object or a specific part of the body (other than the sexual organs) gives the fetishist sexual pleasure. Common fetishes include rubber, leather, fur, and feet.

Whether or not this is a problem depends largely on how dominant such feelings become. For example, there is a big difference between someone whose enjoyment of sex is enhanced if their partner wears fur, black leather, or a plastic raincoat while having sex and someone who *only* enjoys sex when their partner is wearing such garments.

It is often possible for a couple to incorporate the fetishes of one partner into their sex lives. But if a person becomes totally reliant on their fetishes in order to enjoy sexual activity, this is likely to become a problem, and they may need to see a marital and sexual counselor or therapist.

Sadomasochism
Some people enjoy playing sadomasochistic games during sex. Such games may include spanking, whipping, or bondage. These games

---

COMMON FANTASIES

The most common fantasies for women are said to include:
- sex with a complete stranger
- sex with a celebrity, or film or pop star
- sex with a friend's husband
- sex with another woman
- group sex
- being forced to have sex
- having sex in front of an audience.

The most common fantasies for men are said to include:
- being forced by a woman to have sex
- group sex
- watching two women have sex
- watching a woman masturbate
- being dominated by a woman
- oral sex
- sex with two women
- sex with a prostitute
- sex with a celebrity, or film or pop star.

---

can be fun if both partners enjoy them, but they should not be taken too far. Both partners should enter into them willingly, neither should be drunk, the object should never be to hurt anyone, and either partner should be able to call a halt to the game whenever they want to, ideally by a special "stop" signal agreed upon beforehand.

Providing you follow these rules, there is no reason why you should not include such games in your lovemaking.

Transvestism
This is the practice of dressing in clothes of the opposite sex as a means of achieving sexual excitement. It is most usually practiced by men. This is probably more common than many people realize, but because it is nearly always done in secret, there are no accurate estimates of the number of men involved.

A transvestite can spend years leading a double life—male one day, female the next, with two distinct personalities. In most countries there are support groups that will provide help and counseling for transvestites. Support groups also enable transvestites to meet other people who have the same needs and interests as themselves.

Most transvestites are heterosexual, and many of them marry and have children. Some wives are able to accept their partner's need to dress in women's clothes and will not only tolerate it but may actually encourage it, perhaps by buying them clothes. Some transvestites are homosexual and dress as a woman in order to enhance their effeminate traits. A homosexual transvestite may choose to dress as anything from an ordinary woman to an exaggerated woman—a drag queen.

Transsexuality

This is a rare gender-identity disorder characterized by a person's persistent sense of discomfort with their anatomic sex, as well as a need to change their sex organs and live as a member of the opposite sex. A transsexual will often take his or her conviction to what he believes is its natural conclusion, and have a sex reassignment operation.

Most doctors are understandably reluctant to refer transsexuals for drastic and irreversible surgery until they are absolutely sure that this is the right decision for him or her and that the patient will be able to cope with their new role in life. A therapist or counselor should be able to help someone prepare for the operation, and hormonal treatment may be prescribed to help ease the passage to being a member of the opposite sex.

In the sex reassignment operation for male transsexuals, the testes and penis are removed and a vagina is constructed from the skin of the penis and scrotum. The operation for women generally involves breast removal and the construction of a penis from other tissues. Some transsexuals find that it is difficult to come to terms with their "new self," and may

be disappointed by their reduced sexual capabilities. They may also face prejudice from other people. However, many transsexuals are happy with their sex reassignment.

Communication between sexual partners

Sexual partners do the most intimate things to each other, yet they can't always talk to each other about what they do. But good communication between partners is believed to be as essential to good sex as any particular ability to stimulate a partner or any physical attribute. Few of us would go into a restaurant and expect the waiter to know, without being told, what we want to eat. Yet many people are reluctant to convey to their partner precisely what their sexual desires actually are. And they end up with a sexual cheese sandwich instead of the orgasmic banquet of their dreams! However, a lack of communication is not surprising. Partners—both men and women—may think they know what their partner wants, or may simply feel deeply embarrassed by talking about sex, however long they have been in the relationship. But, in the long run, communicating about sex usually not only improves a couple's sex life but is sexually stimulating in itself.

Talking about sex

There are a few rare couples who never need to talk much about sex. They are so in tune with each other that they always know exactly when their partner is in the mood for sex, what their partner wants them to do in bed, and so on. However, most people cannot be expected to know instinctively what their partner enjoys—even if they know sometimes, they will not always get it right—and need to rely on communication, often verbal, to convey their feelings about what arouses them and what sexual positions they prefer. Lovers should be prepared to ask each other questions, to make requests, and to suggest different ways of making love. It is the

QUESTION AND ANSWER: TRANSSEXUALITY

Q. Is it possible for a transsexual to have children?

A. It is possible if she or he has not had a gender reassignment. If they have "changed sex," they can still have intercourse and may experience satisfaction from this, even achieving orgasm.

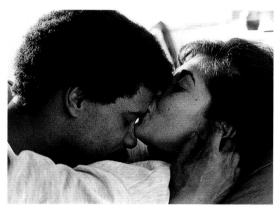

To enjoy each other sexually, and to have fulfilling sex lives, partners need to communicate their needs openly. Communication can be verbal, or nonverbal, touching or showing a partner to indicate what gives pleasure.

exchange of these confidences that helps build up a better physical relationship, and often creates greater emotional closeness as well. Never discussing sex may result in sex lives that seem boring or routine.

Nonverbal clues

Verbal communication is not the only, nor always the most appropriate, way of communicating sexual needs. It is possible, for example, to communicate by moving your partner's hand to a part of your body where the sensation is more exciting, or by making appreciative sounds when what they are doing feels good, or by shifting your position as and when the situation demands.

People should pay particular attention to what their partner does to them in the course of sex. It is usually valid to assume that if someone makes a particular sexual move, particularly if he or she does it repeatedly, this is something they themselves particularly enjoy. Nonverbal clues may therefore be a valuable way of communicating sexual preferences. So if one partner sucks their lover's nipples, or fondles their genitals, or stimulates their anus, the chances are usually high that reciprocation would be appreciated.

A question of timing

Some people find it easiest to talk about sex when they are in bed, while others feel less threatened when they are both relaxed and on neutral ground, such as over a meal or a drink. This may well be true of people who are not in the habit of talking about sex, even if they are involved in a longstanding relationship. In these circumstances it is important to broach the subject gently, even casually, perhaps by first talking about the experiences of a friend or acquaintance. It is essential, too, to respect each other's feelings and never say anything accusatory or angry, or make cruel personal remarks. Negative comments or views about your partner's sexual behavior are both inappropriate and self-defeating.

Assertiveness

Sexual relationships may be one-sided, with one partner taking the lead and dictating the pace and direction of the relationship, and the other unquestioningly following that lead. Learning to be more assertive can often be a good way of making a relationship more equal. Being assertive is not the same thing as being aggressive; rather, it means making decisions and saying yes or no firmly in response to another person's actions or wishes. And a

MEN TALKING ABOUT THEIR FEELINGS

Many men find it difficult—if not impossible—to talk about their feelings. Often the reasons for this are linked to the way in which they were brought up. From a very early age, men are discouraged from expressing their emotions. Tears are considered unmanly in many cultures. Feelings such as fear, anxiety, or love are often hidden away, unexpressed. The fact that "I love you" are three words that some men find particularly difficult to say can cause a lot of frustration and unhappiness in a relationship.

Unfortunately, by repressing their feelings many men allow their frustrations to fester away below the surface. It is often claimed that the only emotion that men don't mind admitting to is anger, so that if a man is unhappy about something, this may reveal itself as aggression—a state of affairs that certainly does not make for a successful relationship.

The man who is able to say "I love you" will do wonders for his relationship.

person should learn to be just as assertive in their sexual relationships as in other areas of their daily lives.

Men often see themselves as the dominant partner in a sexual relationship, and it is often men who take the lead in making love. There is no better way, however, for a woman to show her sexual enjoyment than by occasionally taking the lead and making the first move. Her partner may be surprised by this change in the pattern of their relationship, and his initial reaction may even be one of alarm, but not only will this variation take the pressure off him but he may well get a great deal of pleasure from it.

Any couple's sex life can, all too easily, become stuck in the same old routine. Nothing kills pleasure in sex more effectively than the feeling that it has become predictable. So if the same person always initiates sex and dictates the pace, it is often an excellent idea to change the usual pattern. Moreover, if the relationship is still a fairly new one, it's a good idea to introduce this kind of varied approach now, before sex has a chance to get stuck in a routine.

Sexual difficulties

Sex is not always as straightforward as it might be. It is rare, in fact, for a couple in a long-term relationship never to experience any kind of problem with their sex life.

There are both physical things that can go wrong with people's sexual organs and psychological problems that can compromise a sexual relationship. Both can damage the relationship, because they call into question the most intimate aspect of a couple's partnership.

If these difficulties are transitory, a couple can usually weather them if their relationship is reasonably strong. But more serious, longer-lasting problems can adversely affect their sex life to such an extent that even the closest relationship is threatened. This is another reason why it is so important for a couple to communicate openly and honestly throughout their relationship. If it is not discussed, a minor problem can be exaggerated, and a serious one cannot be solved.

Lack of desire

One of the most common sexual problems is lack of desire. Among the many reasons why a person may feel a lack of desire are
- stress
- tiredness
- feelings of tension or anxiety
- a disturbing sexual encounter in childhood
- feelings of guilt associated with sex.

Lack of desire may respond well to treatment, and in particular to sensate focus exercises (see opposite). These are widely used by many sex therapists as a way of combating one or other partner's inability to respond sexually. Sensate focus exercises are particularly

---

QUESTIONS AND ANSWERS: SEXUAL BEHAVIOR

Q. Sometimes I am not in the mood for sex, particularly if I have had a very tiring day, but I am afraid to say no for fear of upsetting my partner and making her feel rejected.
A. You're right insomuch as a sexual rebuff can make a person feel very hurt and rejected; however, it is as important sometimes to say no as it is to say yes. You must learn to reject the invitation without rejecting the person. Try explaining how tired you are and gently declining the invitation to have sex, suggesting a talk or holding instead.

Q. There are things that I would really like my girlfriend to do for me in bed, but I'm scared to tell her for fear that she'll think I'm too demanding. What should I do?
A. If you find it difficult to talk about sex with your girlfriend, you might be able to convey what you want either by doing something similar to her, which—with a bit of luck—will give her the right idea, or you might try moving her hand to the right position and hope she gets the message. Your best bet, though, and the only way of avoiding any misunderstanding, is to say openly and honestly what you want. She is unlikely to object, provided you're tactful and appreciative, and it might work wonders for your sex life.

Q. I would like to masturbate in front of my husband and for him to watch me, but I can't gather the courage to tell him. Am I crazy to want to do this, and will he think less of me for it?
A. No, far from it. Watching someone masturbate is often the best way of learning exactly how and where they like to be touched, and the surest way of bringing them to orgasm. A lot of men fantasize about watching a woman masturbate, so watching you may really excite him!

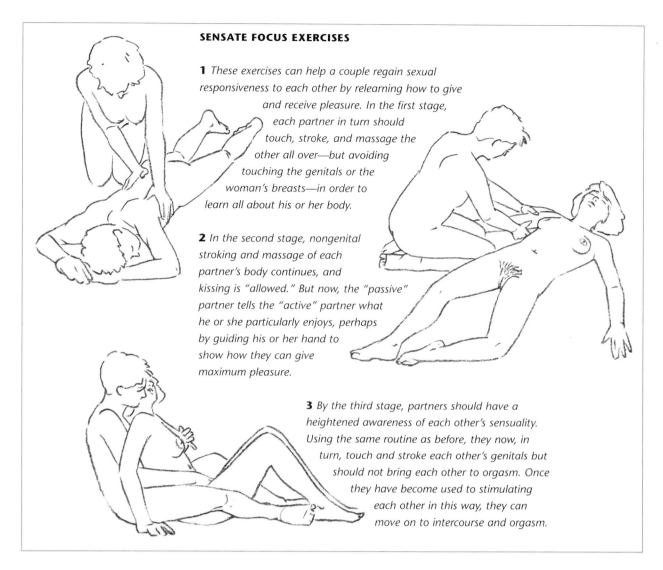

SENSATE FOCUS EXERCISES

1 *These exercises can help a couple regain sexual responsiveness to each other by relearning how to give and receive pleasure. In the first stage, each partner in turn should touch, stroke, and massage the other all over—but avoiding touching the genitals or the woman's breasts—in order to learn all about his or her body.*

2 *In the second stage, nongenital stroking and massage of each partner's body continues, and kissing is "allowed." But now, the "passive" partner tells the "active" partner what he or she particularly enjoys, perhaps by guiding his or her hand to show how they can give maximum pleasure.*

3 *By the third stage, partners should have a heightened awareness of each other's sensuality. Using the same routine as before, they now, in turn, touch and stroke each other's genitals but should not bring each other to orgasm. Once they have become used to stimulating each other in this way, they can move on to intercourse and orgasm.*

beneficial when they are conducted under the guidance of an experienced therapist. But if lack of desire is the result of sexual trauma, ingrained socio-cultural attitudes, or a mental disorder, treatment will be more complicated and, perhaps, less likely to succeed. And if lack of desire is caused by a couple disliking each other, there is probably no solution.

Sensate focus exercises

Sensate focus exercises are of particular benefit to couples who are experiencing sexual difficulties brought on by lack of desire in one or other partner, or perhaps both.

The exercises are intended to focus a couple's minds on the sensations produced by exploring each other's bodies. Each partner follows a series of progressive exercises in which he or she touches, strokes, fondles, massages, kisses, and generally gets to know and appreciate every part of their partner's body. The exercises always stop short of intercourse.

Stage 1 of the program is to learn pleasure in giving. This stage should be practiced at least three times a week for at least two weeks. Both partners should be naked and should feel as relaxed as possible. Partners should take turns being the active or the passive partner, also alternating their roles so that the person who was the first to give pleasure at one session becomes the first to receive it at the next. In the instructions that follow, the active partner in the first stage is the woman and the passive partner is the man, but this will obviously vary according to who chooses to adopt which role.

• The active partner should lubricate her hands with body lotion or oil. The passive partner should lie down, face down, and the active partner can either kneel beside him or sit astride him.

• The woman should now gently stroke and massage the man's entire body, working from head to toe. She can do anything she likes at this stage, using either her hands or mouth. If she does anything that he does not like, he can show this by pushing her hand away. This part of the exercise should continue for at least 10 minutes.

• The partners should now change places. It's the woman's turn now to relax and simply enjoy the feelings evoked by her partner's caresses. She should allow herself to let go as much as possible and to feel each touch as fully as she can. This stage should last for at least 10 minutes.

• The partners should now change places again, and change position so that the man is lying on his back while she massages his body and face. She should not touch his genitals. Do this for at least 10 minutes.

• The partners should now change places again, so that she is lying on her back while her partner strokes her face and body. He should not touch her breasts or genitals. Continue for at least 10 minutes.

When Stage 1 has been practiced for a minimum of two weeks, the couple can progress to Stage 2, which is pleasure in receiving. This stage should be practiced at least three times a week for at least two weeks. The exercises are the same but the passive partner should give his partner positive feedback on what he finds particularly pleasurable. He can do this either by telling her or by guiding her hand. He should let her know not only where he likes to be touched but also how firm or how gentle he likes that touch to be. She may also kiss him wherever she wishes (but not on his genitals) and he should let her know what he finds most pleasurable. There is still a ban on intercourse and on touching the genitals.

At the end of Stage 2, the couple should talk to each other about what they liked best.

If they feel happy with Stages 1 and 2 after practicing them for at least a month or so, they are ready to move on to Stage 3. This involves taking turns to arouse each other by touching the genitals. Once again, the couple should not have intercourse, and they should not bring each other to orgasm. This stage should be practiced at least three times a week for at least two weeks.

By the end of Stage 3, a couple should be ready to move on to full intercourse. The exercises should have done much to improve what they now know not only about their own sexuality but also about each other's. Even if there weren't sexual difficulties within the relationship, the couple should be able to enjoy sex even more now.

SEXUAL BOREDOM

Boredom can eventually become a problem in any sexual relationship. This is often because a couple's sex life has become fixed in a predictable routine and has lost much of its thrill and excitement. Spontaneity and passion, however prominent in the early days of the relationship, seem to have faded into the background.

There are perhaps two main reasons for this. The first is that, while sex is often very important in the early part of a relationship—often referred to as the honeymoon period—initial excitement often lessens as the couple get to know each other and the relationship becomes more relaxed.

The other reason is that, once a relationship has become permanent and more secure, one of the unfortunate paradoxes of sexuality is that sex automatically seems to become less exciting. This doesn't need to be as depressing as it sounds: ultimately sex can become even better. The lesson to be learned is that monogamy does not have to mean monotony, but good sex does not just happen—you have to work at it. You need to talk to each other about what kind of sexual activity gives you the most pleasure; you should be prepared to try new things; and both of you have to put sex high on your list of priorities.

Abstinence

A period of temporary sexual abstinence can be useful for recharging the batteries when the thrill has gone out of a sexual relationship—and can actually do a lot to heighten sexual enjoyment when a couple return to having sexual relations.

If a couple's sex life has lost its edge, it is often best to abstain from sex for a while. Partners should try behaving like new lovers and learn to be friends again, enjoying each other's company in ways other than sex. By taking the focus off a sexual relationship, the problem may resolve itself.

Inhibitions

Most people are, to a greater or lesser extent, inhibited. Inhibitions are generally the result of childhood influences that have instilled feelings of anxiety or guilt about sex. Unfortunately, inhibitions about sex can permanently damage a person's sex life. They interfere with their natural sexual response and prevent a person from enjoying sex, or even from becoming aroused in the first place. We therefore should try to "unlearn" our sexual inhibitions as quickly as possible. We can do this by:
• learning to like our bodies, preferably through masturbation
• realizing how many inhibitions come from the way we were brought up
• giving ourselves permission both to receive and to enjoy pleasure
• allowing ourselves to fantasize.

Women's sexual problems

Painful intercourse

A woman should not find intercourse painful. There are several reasons, however, why penetration may cause persistent pain, all of which —apart from insufficient vaginal lubrication (see box)—should be investigated by a doctor. Among the possible causes of painful intercourse are:
• insufficient vaginal lubrication
• a vaginal or pelvic infection

INSUFFICIENT LUBRICATION

If a woman's vagina is very dry, this may cause friction during intercourse, which can be uncomfortable. Insufficient lubrication is generally caused by inadequate stimulation before intercourse, in which case the problem is easily solved. A woman's vagina is more likely to be dry at certain times of her menstrual cycle than at others. It can also be a particular problem during or after menopause (see pp.267–8). At such times, some additional form of lubrication may become necessary. If the problem is not serious, sufficient lubrication may be provided by saliva. If this is inadequate, it may become necessary to use a lubricating gel, such as K-Y Jelly.

REDUCING VAGINAL TENSION

If a woman feels tense about intercourse, this exercise may help reduce her feelings of anxiety. Try to stay completely relaxed while you do it.
• Use a hand mirror to look closely at your genitals, and part the lips of your vulva gently, so that you can see better.
• Touch the entrance to your vagina with the tip of your finger.
• Lubricate your finger, either with saliva or with lubricant gel, and put the tip of the finger into your vagina; bear down a little as you do this, as if you were trying to push something out of your vagina, to loosen your vaginal muscles.
• Leave your finger there for a few minutes until you are used to the feeling, then move it in a little farther. Tighten your vaginal muscles around your finger and then relax them. Repeat this several times, inserting your finger a little farther each time.
• If you feel less anxious about having something in your vagina after the previous exercises, try inserting two fingers.
• Try doing this exercise with a partner; he should lubricate his fingers well and insert them only as far as you want him to.
• Try intercourse when you feel ready, choosing a woman-on-top position; your partner should not move at first and should allow you to control the depth of penetration.

- recent childbirth
- involuntary tightening of the vaginal muscles
- endometriosis *(see p.106)*.

Vaginismus and fear of intercourse

This is a muscle spasm of the vagina, which causes the muscles around the entrance to close so tightly that intercourse becomes impossible. Many women who experience this problem, although sexually responsive in other ways, have a deep fear of intercourse. The more a couple attempts intercourse, the more painful it becomes and the tighter the vaginal muscles squeeze. This reluctance to have sex may be because the woman:

- has been brought up to believe that sex—even with her husband—is wrong
- is scared of becoming pregnant
- had an earlier unhappy experience of sex
- has been sexually molested or raped.

Fortunately, vaginismus can be treated in almost all cases. Treatment involves muscle relaxation; pelvic floor or Kegel exercises (learning to control the muscles that are in spasm); using fingers or a vaginal dilator to open the vagina; and counseling to help the woman, and her partner, overcome the feelings that caused the problem in the first place.

Men's sexual problems

Problems of erection

A form of sexual dysfunction experienced by some men is the inability to achieve an erection, or to sustain an erection once it has been achieved. This may happen only occasionally, in which case it is unlikely to be a serious problem, or it may happen on a longer-term basis and require professional help.

Problems of erection (which used, misleadingly, to be called impotence) can be caused by overindulgence in alcohol or by extreme fatigue. This can happen to any man from time to time, and there are few men who have never experienced this problem.

Most occasional erection problems have a psychological cause. Men suffering from problems with erection should ask themselves:

- Do I feel guilty about sex?
- Am I bored with my relationship?
- Am I no longer attracted to my partner?
- Do I feel anxious?
- Do I feel guilty about any aspect of my relationship?
- Am I worried about my sexual performance?

A man who answers "Yes" to any of these questions may well have found the cause of his problem and be halfway to solving it.

There are ways in which a man can help himself deal with this situation. The chances are that he is trying to have sex with the wrong person, at the wrong time, or in some other respect under the wrong conditions. The self-help measures below are designed to help ensure that erection failure occurs as rarely as possible. He should:

- have sex only when he really feels like it
- avoid casual encounters—at least until he has regained his sexual confidence
- try not to become overanxious, but make light of the situation as much as possible
- remember that he is a human being, not a machine, and can't expect everything to work like clockwork every time he has sex.

If the problem of lack of erection persists or if the man has never had an erection, he should see a doctor to have tests for medical causes such as diabetes, hormone problems, and diseases of the nerves or blood vessels. Some drugs, especially some of those given to treat high blood pressure, can occasionally cause loss of erection.

Self-help for erection problems

If the problem is a long-term one, masturbating is one way of reassuring yourself that you can indeed achieve an erection, and that even if your erection subsides it can usually be brought back by gentle stimulation. Take this program slowly, one step at a time. Within a few weeks or months your confidence should return. Do this exercise when you are feeling completely relaxed.

- Stimulate your penis with your hand. Use whatever fantasy most turns you on. If you have trouble achieving an erection in this way, try again every day until you get an erection.
- Once you have an erection, stop stimulating yourself and let it subside completely.
- Once your penis is soft, start to stimulate it

again, using fantasies as before, until it is fully erect. If you find this difficult, using a lubricant may help. Then let the erection subside again.

• Now stimulate your penis for a third time and, this time, continue until you ejaculate.

• Do this exercise several times, until you feel confident that you are in charge of your erections and can control them at will.

• Having regained your confidence, you should be ready to move on to the next stage, which you need to do with a partner. Follow a program of sensate focus exercises (see pp. 191–2), while avoiding full sexual intercourse.

• When you have done these exercises several times a week for three or four weeks, you are ready to progress to the next stage, full sexual intercourse. It is probably best to start with one of the woman-on-top positions. If all goes well, you can then progress to one of the man-on-top positions.

If erectile dysfunction has a medical, rather than a psychological, cause—as it does in many elderly men, and in some younger men with specific medical problems—the condition can often be successfully treated. Medical treatments currently in use include the following:

• A vacuum device may be placed over the penis. This produces a partial vacuum that draws blood into the penis, creating an erection that is maintained by putting a ring around the base of the penis. However, not all users are happy with this device as the erection is not very firm.

• Easy-to-use injection systems involve a man injecting a drug directly into the spongy part of his penis, which increases the volume of blood flowing into it and produces a firm erection. The erection will then last for an hour or so. While some men find this satisfactory, others find self-injection unacceptable. A few users experience priapism (see p.114), a condition in which the penis stays erect for a prolonged period. Priapism requires urgent medical attention to prevent damage to the blood vessels inside the penis.

• Penile implants are surgically inserted hydraulic devices. The implant consists of two hollow cylinders inside the penis, which are connected to a fluid reservoir in the abdomen

and a pump, often in the scrotum. By pumping fluid in the cylinders, the man achieves an erection; by opening a valve, fluid drains out of the cylinders and the erection subsides. While not suitable for all men with erectile difficulties, especially if they have reduced penile sensitivity or sex drive, penile implants have enhanced the sex lives of many men.

Premature ejaculation

Premature ejaculation—meaning that a man ejaculates sooner than he wants to—is not only a problem experienced by many men but may also be a cause of marital conflict. It is

QUESTIONS AND ANSWERS: SEXUAL PROBLEMS

Q. My partner has had trouble achieving an orgasm for the last couple of years. He's too embarrassed to go to the doctor and says we should be able to deal with this problem ourselves. I feel really sorry for him and want to help. Is there anything I can do?

A. You sound very sympathetic and understanding, which is important if you are to help him. There are a number of things that may help you deal with the problem.

• Watch him masturbate.
• Make it clear that you do not think of his semen as dirty.
• Masturbate him.
• Give him testicular or anal stimulation.
• Straddle him when he is near orgasm.

If none of these things helps after several weeks, your husband should see a marital and sexual therapist. He should not feel embarrassed by this—any therapist has heard about virtually every sexual problem many times before and will deal with his concerns sensitively.

Q. My husband has recently developed problems in achieving an erection. This never used to happen and I'm afraid that it means he doesn't find me attractive anymore.

A. Most men experience difficulties with their erections from time to time, and it does not mean that your husband has lost interest in you. The more trouble he has with his erections, the more he will worry about it and the more likely it is to happen again. Be reassuring and understanding, without making too much of the situation. Try to help him by stimulating his penis gently, either with your hand or your mouth, but do not be too insistent as this may only make him feel worse if he doesn't respond quickly. Above all, do not behave as if you are feeling rejected, as this will only make matters worse. If the problem persists he should see his doctor and discuss the possibility of being referred to a specialist.

very common in young men in the early years of their sex life, when they are still learning how to control their ejaculation. There is no way to predict exactly when premature ejaculation may happen. A man may ejaculate before the penis becomes erect, it may be at the moment of penetration, or it may be immediately afterward.

There are many possible causes for premature ejaculation. These may be psychological (such as problems in a relationship), although in the vast majority of cases premature ejaculation is simply caused by a lack of sexual sensory awareness. Exercises that deal with this sensory deficit (such as the squeeze technique—*see right*) can usually cure premature ejaculation. Although rare, there can also be physical reasons, including:
• an infection of the genitals
• an injury to the spinal column
• a disease of the nervous system, such as multiple sclerosis.

The good news is that most cases of premature ejaculation can be treated successfully. If the condition is mild, the couple can usually treat it themselves, without seeing a doctor.

First of all, the woman needs to make it clear that she loves her partner, is sympathetic to his problem, and will do everything she can to help. When they make love, he should give her a signal that he is about to come and she should lie still, not making any movements, including vaginal ones. She can also use the squeeze technique, which means that she holds her partner's penis in a special grip that will inhibit ejaculation.

In the rare cases where a patient suffering from premature ejaculation does not respond to behavioral treatment, he will almost always respond to medication prescribed by a doctor.

The squeeze technique

This is a technique that a couple can use to treat premature ejaculation. When the woman applies this method, it will inhibit her partner's urge to ejaculate. To apply this method, follow these steps.
• Stimulate your partner's penis manually or orally until he is about to ejaculate.
• Squeeze his penis by holding it just below the glans. Grip it firmly, with your thumb on the frenulum—the part of the underside of the penis where the head and shaft meet—and your first finger opposite the thumb and the other fingers around the shaft (*see illustration*). Apply firm pressure for 15–20 seconds without moving your fingers—even the slightest movement may arouse him, which is not what is required at this stage.
• Release your grip. This should have stopped him from ejaculating for now (but if he does ejaculate, put it down to experience and try again another time). Repeat the stimulation/squeeze procedure several times before going on to have intercourse.
• Repeat the process each time you have sex.
• As his control improves, start having intercourse without using the squeeze technique, but get him to withdraw when he is about to ejaculate, and repeat the squeezing process.
• Finally, move on to sex without squeezing. With his newfound confidence, he should gain greater control over his ejaculation.

Retarded ejaculation

Some men find it difficult—even impossible—to reach orgasm in the vagina. They become aroused and maintain an erection but, despite prolonged stimulation during intercourse, orgasm does not happen. Retarded ejaculation may be caused by a number of factors, psychological or physical. Physical causes can include consumption of too much alcohol, spinal injuries, hormonal imbalances, and the effect of certain drugs, including anti-depressants and drugs for high blood pressure.

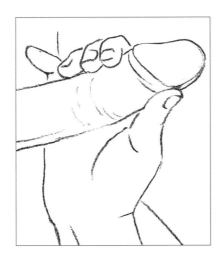

One way of stopping premature ejaculation—coming too quickly—is the squeeze technique. During sex play, the woman squeezes the man's penis as shown each time he thinks he is about to ejaculate. This usually stops ejaculation from happening yet and, in time, gives a man a greater sense of control.

Psychological causes can include a belief that sex is "dirty," fear of losing control, fear of a partner becoming pregnant, anxiety about sex, or feeling that the woman is hostile. In these cases, retarded ejaculation can often be treated by therapy. The man's partner is encouraged to masturbate him to orgasm, so that he ejaculates in an unthreatening environment. From this they progress to a combination of masturbation and intercourse, until he reaches orgasm inside her.

Maintaining a long-term relationship

Although it is never easy to maintain a long-term relationship with a partner, some couples become even closer and more "in love" after a number of years together. But it would be wrong to assume that that particular couple are unusual or just lucky. Like many other couples, these two people may have fallen deeply in love earlier in their lives, convinced that they were right for each other and would live happily ever after. However, they will then almost certainly have found that living out their romantic dream requires a great deal of understanding and hard work. They will also have discovered that there is no magic formula and that maintaining a successful relationship depends on keeping in touch with each other's feelings, being able to adapt to changes, both in themselves and in their circumstances, and on continuing to respect each other and enjoy each other's company.

Inevitably, any couple will find that the excitement of living together wears off in time and that eventually they will have to confront any underlying problems in their relationship.

Changing lifestyles can also mean that partners move in different directions or at a different pace; sometimes one or both partners become so bored with the pattern of their lives that they may think about having an affair. But whatever their dissatisfactions, a couple should never lose sight of the enormous benefits to be gained from a long-term relationship, including mutual love and

RULES IN A LONG-TERM RELATIONSHIP

It is impossible to conduct a relationship strictly according to a set of rules, but there are a few points worth remembering if the relationship is to continue to work.

- Never take each other for granted.
- Be sure to talk to each other—openly, honestly, and often.
- Listen to the other's point of view, trying not to interrupt.
- Treat each other with respect.
- Try never to end the day angry.
- Show your appreciation of each other.
- Make time for each other and enjoy some shared activities.
- Don't be too serious—it's important to laugh together sometimes.
- Make joint plans or discuss your joint goals.

respect, the enjoyment of each other's company, and the time to develop an increasingly fulfilling sex life.

Adapting to change

All people's lives change as they get older. Their work patterns may get busier, a new job may mean having to move house, a worsening financial situation may drive them into taking on more work, layoffs or retirement may force them into a completely different way of life, or a child may put varying demands on them as he or she goes through adolescence or decides to leave home.

Ideally, both partners in a relationship will change at roughly the same pace, with the result that their relationship will absorb—and be strengthened by—those changes. What is usually more difficult for a couple to deal with is when one partner moves at a different pace and direction from the other. This can lead to a situation in which a couple, despite having been together for years, suddenly feel as if they no longer know each other.

Most of us will have heard statements like: "He's not the same man I married," "I don't understand her these days," or "We don't have anything in common any more." Remarks like these usually mean that the couple are going through difficulties in their relationship. The most misleading aspect of these statements is the implication that the relationship has only recently changed or that the partner at fault has suddenly become a different person. In fact, it usually takes years for a person to change their behavior, and it is more than likely that the person making the remark just hasn't noticed that their partner was changing. Perhaps if they had been more in tune with the partner and if communication between them had been better, the "changes" might not have come as such a shock. More importantly, they might have been able to adjust to the new situation.

Finding time for each other

Most people are prepared to spend a lot of time on all sorts of work and leisure activities. But how much time do we devote to our close relationships?

If the honest answer is "not a lot," then it would obviously be a good idea for a couple to move their relationship higher on their list of priorities and not wait until there's a problem before spending more time on it. They should remember to sometimes fuss over each other; to go out to dinner and treat it like a first date, or to cook a special meal at home with all the trimmings—wine, flowers, soft lights, and music.

Sexual relationships, too, deserve to be treated as a special part of a couple's life together. Sex is one of life's greatest pleasures and shouldn't just be something a couple does on automatic pilot or for 10 minutes last thing at night. A rewarding sexual relationship requires both time and concentration.

Showing appreciation

Whispering endearments or calling each other by a pet name isn't silly. It can make someone feel loved and special, as well as creating a private bond between two people. It is also important that both partners sometimes make an effort to look their best; and equally important that the other person be appreciative. A positive effort deserves a positive reaction.

Everyday affectionate gestures are never a waste of time. They help maintain a positive

SPICING UP YOUR SEX LIFE

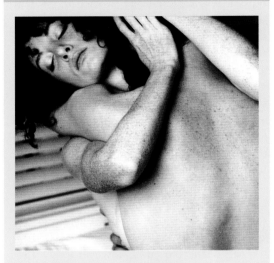

A lot of people's sex lives become boring for no reason other than laziness. Anyone who feels bored with sex should ask themselves the question, "When was the last time you tried something new in the bedroom?" If they can't even remember, chances are they could do with something to spice up their sex lives. Here are some suggestions.

- Regularly set aside time for sex.
- Talk to each other about your fantasies.
- Talk as openly as you can about what you want and expect from your sex lives together.
- Buy some sexy underwear for yourself or your partner.
- Look at erotic literature or videos together.
- Buy a sex manual to get some new ideas.
- Go away for a rest-and-recreation vacation.
- Try something new, providing your partner enjoys it and you both want to do it.

attitude toward a relationship and create a strong foundation for the inevitable highs and lows of living together.

Keeping sex exciting

Good sex doesn't necessarily always remain good; bad sex, equally, can get better. But whatever the state of a couple's sex life, this part of their life together will always need both time and consideration.

It is normal for the nature of our sex lives together to change as a relationship matures.

Sex might become more satisfying, or it might become less exciting; one partner might want sex more often than the other, or a couple's sexual preferences might not be as much in tune as they were earlier in the relationship.

Changes in people's sex lives are usually brought on by the other things happening to them. When their day-to-day lives are happy and relaxed, their sex life is likely to be good, too; when they are under stress at work, tired, or simply not getting along well, sex is likely to be one of the first things to suffer.

It is virtually impossible to keep sex exciting for both partners unless they are prepared to talk about their sexual relationship. There are surprisingly few couples who manage to set aside time to do this, however long they have been together—yet it makes no sense for partners to restrict themselves to guesswork. There is no place for embarrassment here. It is important for partners to be as frank and open as they can with each other—and that includes being honest with themselves. They should tell each other which part of their body they like to be touched, and how and what they like and, of course, don't like. They need to talk about what pleases them most about each other's bodies, what position gives them the most pleasure, what time of day they find sex most exciting—about anything, in fact, that makes sex good (or bad) for them.

Sex and illness

To enjoy sex fully, people need to be healthy, in both body and mind. When anything goes wrong with our bodies, our sex lives may suffer, although in what way and how much depends on the exact nature of the illness.

Sex may be a major concern for anyone who is seriously unwell, or recovering from illness. They may lose interest in sex temporarily, and if not, they may want to know for how long their sex life is likely to be disrupted. Poor health may also cause someone to feel less attractive and therefore less confident, and severe disability or surgery may give rise to a major change in their body image. Solutions to these problems are never easy.

Above all, the ill person will need the help of an understanding and sympathetic partner. Some of the most common illnesses that can affect a person's sex life are described below.

Arthritis

This is the inflammation of a joint, characterized by swelling, stiffness, and pain, which can be severe. It may affect the joints of the hands, knees, or hips and, although mild arthritis generally has little noticeable effect on a person's sex life, severe arthritis can cause serious problems, at least initially.

Any deformity of the limbs can cause someone to lose confidence in his or her attractiveness, while severe pain can cause loss of interest in sex. In addition, arthritis in the hips can make it difficult to find a comfortable position for intercourse, and arthritic hands can make it difficult both to caress a partner and to masturbate. Arthritis may also cause a decrease in vaginal lubrication.

However, anti-inflammatory drugs and pain medications taken before sex may help relieve pain. A hot bath before sex will help mobilize the joints. The sufferer also needs to find a suitable position in which sex is comfortable. Physical therapy and exercise may help alleviate pain and enhance sex.

USING ILLNESS AS AN EXCUSE

It is not uncommon for an ill person who was never very interested in sex to use their poor health as an excuse for not having sex. Although understandable, this reaction can cause antagonistic feelings in a partner and can pose a very real threat to the relationship if the situation continues for too long.

Diabetes

Diabetes mellitus is a disorder caused by insufficient production of the hormone insulin by the pancreas. Insulin helps control levels of glucose in the blood. In a diabetic, glucose levels can be controlled by diet and/or insulin injections. For older men, the side effects of diabetes may lead to erectile problems, although sex drive and ability to ejaculate remain unimpaired. Careful control of diabetes makes sexual problems a lot less likely, but on rare occasions some drugs used to treat diabetes may cause erectile problems, and this should be checked with a doctor. If a man finds it impossible to achieve an erection he may require medical treatment *(see p.195)*.

Diabetes in women can result in a dry, itchy vulva, difficulty in achieving orgasm, and an increase in vaginal infections, especially yeast infections. However, the problems can generally be eased by medication.

Epilepsy

This is a tendency to recurrent seizures. Some male epileptics may have trouble maintaining an erection, while some female epileptics may find it difficult to become aroused, and epileptics of either sex may lose interest in sex. Some of these problems may stem from a decrease in self-confidence, and if this is restored through counseling, sexual function may soon return to normal.

Multiple sclerosis (MS)

Multiple sclerosis is an unpredictable disease and can vary widely in both symptoms and severity. Sexual problems are common, with men reporting difficulty in achieving an erection and ejaculatory disturbances, and women reporting loss of vaginal lubrication and difficulty in achieving an orgasm.

One common feature in MS is that symptoms often come and go, with periods of exacerbation followed by periods of remission. Sexual difficulties may follow a similar pattern. It is important that patients continue sexual activity if they want, even if they are not always able to reach orgasm. Patients who still have an interest in sex should experiment to see which positions are best for them.

Stroke

How much effect a stroke has on a patient's sexuality will depend on how much disability remains afterward and on how permanent this disability is. Some patients may lose interest in sex for a time, while others may remain interested in sex but experience difficulties because they are paralyzed in one or more limbs. There is no reason why a stroke victim should not continue to have sex if he or she wishes, and stroke patients should be reassured that sex is most unlikely to induce another stroke. There may be problems finding a suitable position for intercourse because of impaired strength and problems with coordination or paralysis, but if they experiment they should find a position that suits them.

Surgery

Colostomy

A colostomy is an operation in which part of the colon is brought through an opening in the abdomen and formed into an artificial outlet so that body wastes can be removed to a special bag attached to the skin. It is often

---

SEX LIFE AFTER A HEART ATTACK

Having a heart attack need not end a person's sex life. Doctors usually advise patients who have had a heart attack to lead as normal a life as possible, and that includes sexual intercourse, provided the patient can cope with moderate exertion. Sex should be gentle at first, with the patient playing a passive role, and can gradually become more strenuous as the patient recovers. If the patient experiences any of the following symptoms during intercourse, stop intercourse. If the symptoms last longer than 15 minutes, they should be regarded as a warning sign and reported to the doctor. Symptoms include:
- breathlessness
- palpitations
- chest pain (angina).

DEPRESSION

A person's sex life is one of the first casualties of depression, and lack of interest in sex may in fact be one of the first symptoms of the condition. Depression has an effect on many other areas of a depressed person's life as well as sex, and can wreak havoc with a couple's overall relationship. If the relationship was not strong in the first place, this can cause a person to become depressed, which may then reduce the desire for sex. A vicious cycle may build up, which may easily get out of control. In such a situation therapy with a sexual and marital counselor may be a great help.

used in treating cancer of the rectum or an obstruction in the large intestine. There is no need for a colostomy to affect sex. Any problems tend to be ones of attitudes and emotions rather than physical difficulties. (However, surgery for cancer of the rectum can cause erectile problems due to nerve damage.)

Loss of a limb

This can have a major effect on a person's sex life, not least because it may have reduced his or her self-esteem and confidence and created worry that no one will find them attractive again. To lose any limb can make dexterity and positions difficult, but this can be overcome through sensitive counseling and persistent practice of new sexual positions.

Hysterectomy

This is the removal of the uterus, usually performed because of gynecological problems. There is no medical evidence to support the view that removal of the womb has any effect on sex, but some women do report that sex afterward is different. For some this may be because their orgasms feel less intense, while for others sex may be better because there are no longer any worries about the possibility of pregnancy and because symptoms such as pain or heavy bleeding are relieved. A woman should wait for six weeks after the operation before resuming sexual intercourse, to allow time for the wound to heal *(see pp.108–9)*.

Mastectomy

The removal of a woman's breast has strong sexual associations and a woman may feel she has lost an essential part of her femininity. Counseling before and after the operation should help a woman deal with this. A couple that has enjoyed a strong relationship before the operation can usually come to terms with the disability and resume normal sexual activity *(see also pp.103–4)*.

Prostatectomy

The removal of a man's prostate gland *(see pp.112-13)* when it has become abnormally large may in a few cases cause impotence. More often, it can cause retrograde ejacula-

tion, whereby the semen is ejaculated into the bladder rather than out through the penis—but this should not cause sexual problems.

Although the operation can have a major effect on a couple's sex life, problems are often psychological, and the couple should have fewer concerns if everything is explained to them carefully beforehand so that they know what to expect. A man's partner should be patient and understanding following surgery, until as near normal sexual function as possible returns. There is no reason why, in most cases, a man's sex life should not continue as normal after a prostatectomy.

DISABILITY

Those who suffer from physical disabilities often say that other people don't regard them as sexual beings and assume that they never make love. But this is not so. Those who cannot make love in a conventional sense will often obtain fulfillment from touching and cuddling. Some people say that other parts of their body have become more sensitive than they were before their disability, to compensate for any loss of sensation in the places conventionally associated with arousal. Others find that they experience arousal and orgasm just like able-bodied people. The partner of someone with a disability must be patient and supportive, but with preparation and open communication, there is usually no reason why couples cannot use their imaginations to find sexual positions that work for them.

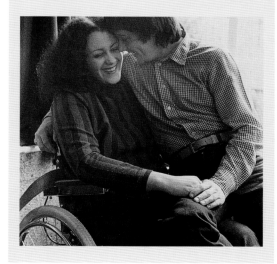

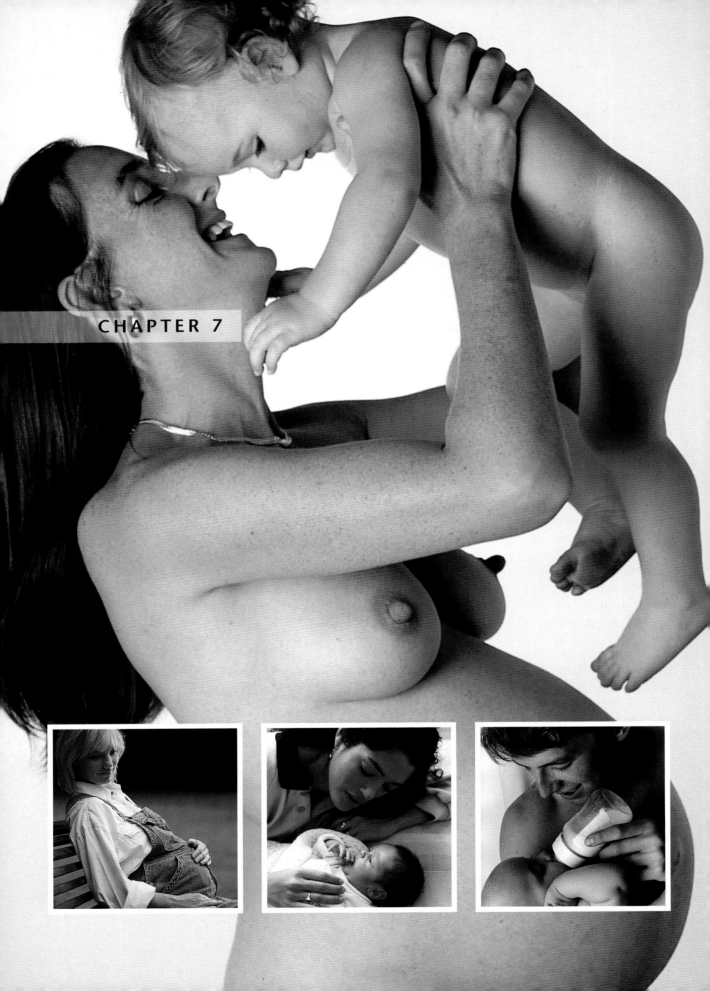

CHAPTER 7

Pregnancy and Parenthood

From the moment of conception—when sperm and egg unite and the fertilized egg embeds itself in the lining of the uterus—until a baby has grown and developed sufficiently to be born some nine months later, a pregnant woman carries and cares for another human being inside her body. Once pregnancy is completed, and the mother has given birth, she and her partner can expect to invest at least 20 years in parenting each child they produce. During this time they will forge a relationship with him or her and nurture the child to the best of their ability.

For many couples, confirmation of the pregnancy will be the culmination of months or even years of planning to have—or putting off having—a baby. The question of when to start a family has become far more of an issue in recent generations, as safer and more reliable methods of contraception such as the pill and the greater degree of control that many women have gained over their lives have led to women having children later and later. But despite their greater independence, women are still under pressure from their "biological clock"—the knowledge that as they get older their fertility levels decline until they reach the deadline imposed by menopause.

But even allowing for the pressure of the age factor, it is still advisable for a woman to wait until she feels the time is right for both her and her partner to have a child. A couple also needs to evaluate the state of their relationship, their career goals, and their financial security. If any of these three considerations seem likely to overshadow what should be a time of optimism and joy, then it may be wiser for them to postpone making such a momentous decision.

Yet although there are many couples who carefully plan parenthood, it is often the case that the most excited and happy prospective parents include many to whom the advent of a new baby has come as a complete surprise.

Once a pregnancy is confirmed, the prospect and reality of parenthood can bring with it feelings of both great joy and trepidation, as well as placing the expectant parents in new roles. Previously, the couple has been involved with and focused on each other. Now their relationship will change and grow in other directions.

Couples who expect that their lives will continue as before throughout the woman's pregnancy and after the birth are in for a shock. Talking about their feelings, explaining how they feel sexually, and saying why they feel their relationship may have changed or be changing can help couples not only to go through the upheaval of having children but also to emerge from the challenges with better and stronger relationships.

Not all relationships can survive the pressure of having children, or that of facing the prospect of remaining childless. Infertility is a distressing problem and, although improvements in infertility medicine have provided solutions for some couples, others still have to face the fact that they will never have children and will have to make adjustments to their relationships on that basis. Relationships that have suffered from these problems can be helped by active communication between the partners and, in some cases, by counseling.

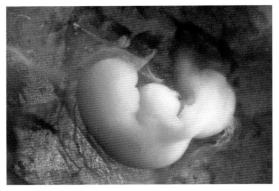

An embryo four weeks after conception is no longer than the width of a pencil. Although barely recognizable as human, the tiny embryo has a beating heart and developing nervous and respiratory systems.

Physical aspects of pregnancy

The process of growth and development from conception *(see pp.30–1)* to birth takes approximately 266 days (38 weeks). But, by convention, the length of a pregnancy is calculated from the date of the first day of the last period before conception. This is often 14 days before ovulation, making a "standard" pregnancy 280 days (40 weeks) long. This calculation is also used to estimate the likely date of birth, although such estimates are not always accurate. Normal pregnancies range in duration from 38 weeks to over 42 weeks.

For the first eight weeks of its life, a developing baby is referred to as an embryo. Thereafter, until birth, she or he, by now a recognizable human, is called a fetus. At birth the fetus becomes an infant. For reasons of convenience, pregnancy is often divided into three phases, called trimesters, of roughly 13 weeks each. The major events occurring during these three trimesters are described below. The dates denote the number of weeks into the pregnancy (measured conventionally, as described above).

First trimester
During this first phase the main organs and body systems grow and develop.
Implantation
The process called implantation is described in the conception section of Chapter 1 *(see pp.30–1)*.

EARLY SIGNS OF PREGNANCY

Some women know instinctively that they are pregnant because their body "feels" different, possibly because of changes in the levels of hormones in their bloodstream. Although not all women experience the same early signs of pregnancy, most women realize they may be pregnant when they notice particular signs and symptoms, the most common of which include:

• a missed period, although it is possible to have light bleeding around the time of a normal period as the embryo implants in the lining of the uterus. However, this sign of a possible pregnancy may be missed by those women who naturally have irregular or infrequent periods

• breast changes, which can include a feeling of heaviness and tenderness, a tingling feeling, an increase in breast size, and a darkening of the nipples and areolae

• a feeling of extreme tiredness

• nausea and perhaps vomiting, commonly known as "morning sickness" even though it does not necessarily always occur in the mornings. More than 70 percent of women experience morning sickness to some degree

• change in the sense of taste, and possibly a metallic taste in the mouth; a changed sense of smell

• cravings and/or a newfound dislike for certain foods, drinks, or smells

• feeling emotional, becoming upset easily, or bursting into tears for no apparent reason

• a need to urinate more frequently.

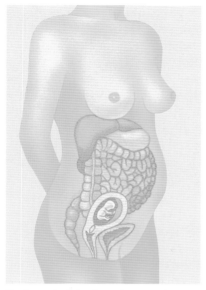

By the end of the first trimester, the fetus is 3 inches long; the woman will have gained just over 2 pounds and her shape will have changed little.

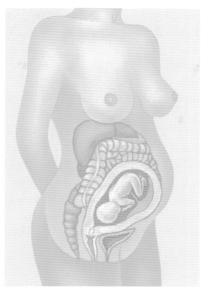

At the end of the second trimester, the fetus is 13 inches long; the mother has gained over 13 pounds and her "bump" is growing rapidly.

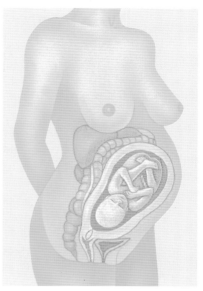

As the fetus reaches full size, the expanding uterus presses on the mother's internal organs, causing breathlessness and frequent urges to urinate.

6 weeks—size ¼ inch

A month or so after conception, the embryo's nervous, blood, and digestive systems are developing; rudimentary brain, ears, eyes, and mouth appear; its heart is beating; and four limb buds representing future arms and legs have appeared. The embryo floats in its fluid-filled protective sac, attached by the umbilical cord lifeline to the placenta. This disklike structure connects the embryo to its mother, and inside it the maternal and embryonic bloodstreams come into close enough contact to enable food and oxygen to pass into and for waste materials to be removed from the embryo's blood. There is no direct connection between the two bloodstreams, however. The placenta releases the hormone human chorionic gonadotrophin (hCG) that is detected by pregnancy-testing kits to confirm that a pregnancy has begun.

8 weeks—size 1¼ inches

The embryo's major internal organs are now formed, although they will continue to grow and mature throughout pregnancy. Fingers and toes are forming at the tips of the well-defined arms and legs, which now have elbows and knees. Facial features such as the external ears and mouth are developing.

12 weeks—size 3 inches

The fetus is now recognizably human, although its head is large in proportion to the rest of the body. The external ears and eyelids have formed; the mouth opens, closes, and can suck. The fingers and toes are fully formed, the limbs move, the external genitals are formed, and the fetus passes urine. If the mother experienced problems such as morning sickness in early pregnancy, these are probably starting to disappear. At around this time, when she visits her doctor or midwife, the mother will be able to hear the baby's heartbeat through a special amplifier.

Second trimester

By the beginning of the second trimester, the fetus is fully formed, and it now begins to grow rapidly and mature.

16 weeks—size 6 inches

The sex of the fetus can often be determined at this age during a sonogram, or ultrasound scan. The bones of the skeleton are starting to develop and the muscles are getting stronger. The mother may start to look pregnant now.

20 weeks—size 10 inches

The arms and legs have started to grow in proportion with the rest of the body. Hair grows on the head, and a fine downy hair called lanugo appears on the body. Pregnant women commonly have a feeling of well-being at this stage, and find the condition of their hair and skin improves noticeably. The mother will feel the fetus moving as it turns and kicks inside the uterus.

24 weeks—size 13 inches
The fetus grows rapidly at this stage.

Third trimester
During the final phase of pregnancy, the fetus continues to grow in preparation for its emergence into the outside world.

28 weeks—size 14½ inches
Considerable brain development takes place around this time, and the baby has a good chance of survival if it is born prematurely. The woman starts to look noticeably larger and to feel "more" pregnant.

32 weeks—size 16 inches
By now the fetus is starting to store fat under the skin. Usually around this time the fetus moves so that it lies head downward in preparation for the birth. Because of its size, the fetus presses on the mother's internal organs, which may cause her to feel breathless and to urinate more frequently.

36 weeks—size 18 inches
The body of the fetus becomes more rounded as it stores more fat, and the head may move lower into the pelvis in preparation for birth.

40 weeks—size 20 inches
At 40 weeks, the fetus is fully developed, the pregnancy is complete, and the baby is ready to be born.

Confirming a pregnancy

Although missing two consecutive periods is a strong indicator of pregnancy for most women, nowadays women are usually advised to get the pregnancy confirmed sooner than this so that they can start caring for themselves and their growing baby during the vital early weeks of its development.

Pregnancy can be confirmed as early as the first day of a missed period by carrying out a pregnancy test. This involves the detection of

---

PREGNANCY AND THE OLDER WOMAN

The biologically "ideal" time for a woman to have children is in her mid to late twenties. But many women are choosing to delay starting their family until they have reached their thirties or later, when they have established a career and financial stability. Waiting to start a family does have its risks, but the odds are still in favor of an older couple having healthy children.

• A woman's fertility decreases from her thirties onward, so she may have problems conceiving.

• The risks of having a difficult pregnancy increase over the age of 35, although they are reduced if a woman is in good shape and healthy and if she has regular checkups.

• The chances of having a baby with Down's syndrome increase after 35, and sharply after 40. In many countries, pregnant women over 35 are given amniocentesis to test whether the fetus has this chromosomal abnormality.

• Older women are more likely to encounter birth hazards including fetal death, low birthweight, and premature birth.

TESTS DURING PREGNANCY

The health of both mother and fetus is monitored throughout pregnancy. A woman visits her doctor or midwife once a month between 12 and 28 weeks; every two weeks up to 36 weeks; and every week thereafter. These tests are carried out routinely:

• urine sample, to check that her kidneys are working properly, and that she is not diabetic

• measurement of weight gain to make sure it is neither too great nor too little

• a check that blood pressure is not too high

• listening to the baby's heartbeat

• checking the mother's legs/ankles for swelling

• feeling the abdomen to check the uterus.

Other common prenatal tests include:

• ultrasound around week 16 to check that the baby is growing normally

• alpha fetoprotein (AFP) as part of a screening test for genetic abnormalities, before week 18

• amniocentesis (week 14–18) and chorionic villus sampling (week 6–8)—neither routine—to check for inherited disorders.

the hormone human chorionic gonadotrophin (hCG), released by the embryo into its mother's bloodstream and excreted in her urine. Home pregnancy testing kits are available from drugstores and many grocery stores. The test should be performed on the first urine sample of the day and, depending on the type of test, a positive result will be shown by the presence of a color change or the appearance of a dark ring. Follow directions carefully. If the result is positive, the woman should seek confirmation from her doctor, who may send another urine sample to a laboratory for similar but more sensitive testing. If the woman obtains a negative result with a home testing kit but still feels that she may be pregnant, she should repeat the test a week later—perhaps there was insufficient hCG in her urine—or go to her doctor for a urine test.

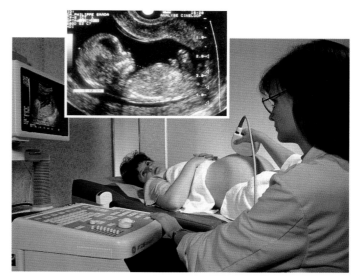

A sonogram is a safe method of monitoring the development of the fetus inside the uterus. A hand-held probe (above) sends sound waves into the uterus and uses their reflections to create an image (top).

Caring for the mother and baby

During the nine months of pregnancy, the woman plays host to the developing baby in her uterus. The way in which that baby grows and develops depends on the overall health of his or her mother. As long as the mother is in shape; eats a well-balanced diet; and avoids alcohol, nicotine from cigarettes, and other drugs—all drugs pass across the placenta to the fetus—there is a good chance that she will give birth to a healthy infant. In addition, by maintaining and possibly improving her own fitness, a mother can help alleviate some of the symptoms such as aches, pains, and tiredness that she will naturally experience during pregnancy. Continuing a fitness program after the birth will also help the mother return to her prepregnancy shape and tone.

Good health is important throughout pregnancy, but especially during the early weeks, when the baby's vital organs are formed. Of course, many babies are unplanned, but parents are commonly advised, if possible, to adopt a healthy lifestyle before conception if they do not have one already *(see box, right).*

Fitness and exercise

Regular exercise is good for health at all times, and during pregnancy is no exception.

MEDICATIONS AND PREGNANCY

All drugs, whether they are prescribed by a doctor or bought over the counter in a drugstore or supermarket, may have harmful effects on a baby. Women who intend to get pregnant or who are already pregnant should avoid taking any drugs without checking first with their doctor. And if the woman finds herself away from home and being treated by a different doctor, she should make it clear immediately that she is pregnant.

PREPARING FOR PREGNANCY

By paying special attention to health *before* they conceive, a couple can give their baby a head start in life. Potential parents are advised to take these steps three months before conception.

• Cut down on alcohol, or cut it out altogether.
• Stop smoking.
• Lose excess weight by adopting a balanced diet, rich in fresh fruit and vegetables, and by doing regular aerobic exercise.
• To help reduce the risk of spina bifida, women are advised to take folic acid supplements.
• If either partner's work involves using chemicals, X-rays, or other hazards, these may affect conception; eliminate the risk if possible.
• Wear gloves when using chemicals at home.

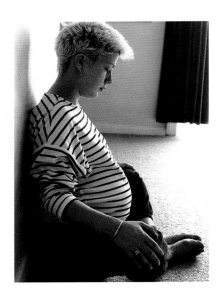

Exercise and relaxation both help counteract the demands put on your body by pregnancy. Tailor sitting (right) *encourages flexibility and suppleness while strengthening the thighs. Swimming* (below) *provides exercise without undue strain on the joints because the body is completely supported by the water.*

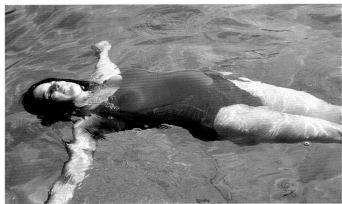

Although strenuous exercise is not advisable, especially in very early and in late pregnancy, regular exercise helps a woman prepare for labor and birth; exercise can reduce the effects of discomforts resulting from pregnancy, such as backache, and can help a woman return to her prepregnancy figure after the birth. When doing exercises, pregnant women should drink plenty of fluids, wear loose clothing, and stop immediately if they get tired. Any unusual aches or pains felt while exercising should be referred to a doctor. Useful and sensible exercises include the following:
• swimming—tones many of the body's muscles while supporting the body's weight
• walking—a good aerobic exercise that helps maintain fitness
• pelvic floor exercises—tone the muscles that form the base of the pelvis, and help improve control during childbirth *(for how to carry*

out these exercises, see opposite and p.221);
• squatting—helps strengthen the back and thigh muscles, and improve general flexibility.

Diet before and during pregnancy

During pregnancy the fetus has but one source of food—her or his mother. The better and more balanced her diet, the more likely it is that the fetus will develop normally and optimally, and the more likely (provided she also exercises) that the mother will avoid gaining excessive weight during her pregnancy.

Pregnant women are advised to:
• increase the amount of fresh, raw fruit and vegetables in their diet (many vitamins are destroyed by heating)
• reduce their intake of processed foods—these contain a range of preservatives and other chemicals that may "upset" the fetus
• reduce their intake of large amounts of sugary foods, which can lead to weight gain;
• reduce their intake of salty foods, which can cause fluid retention.

When cooking food, broiling, poaching, or microwaving reduces the amount of fat in the diet. A pregnant woman should also aim to drink plenty of fluid—especially water—each day to keep her kidneys healthy.

Contrary to popular belief, pregnant women do not need to "eat for two." However, most pregnant women find they need to slightly increase the amount of calories they consume each day because of the demands of the fetus, and weight-loss diets should be avoided during pregnancy. A well-balanced diet suitable for both mother and baby should generally contain the following:
• vitamins and fiber obtained from whole grains, fruit, and vegetables;
• proteins from lean cuts of meat, white meat such as chicken, eggs, fish, nuts, dairy products, and whole grains;
• fats from oily fish (such as sardines and herring) and vegetable oils (such as olive oil) that are rich in unsaturated fats;
• folic acid from leafy vegetables and walnuts;
• minerals, including calcium (from sardines, dairy products, whole-grain bread, green and root vegetables), iron (from lean red meat, liver, oily fish, peas and beans, nuts, whole-

PRENATAL EXERCISES

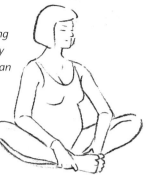

With the back straight, tailor sitting can be very comfortable, especially during later pregnancy. The feet can be pushed together or the legs crossed. Tailor sitting strengthens the back and thighs, makes pelvis and thighs more flexible, and increases blood flow to the lower body.

This exercise to strengthen the pelvic floor muscles can be done lying down as shown here, or while sitting or standing. Tighten the muscles that stop urine flowing from the bladder, hold for a few seconds, release gradually, and repeat 10 times, three or four times a day.

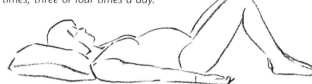

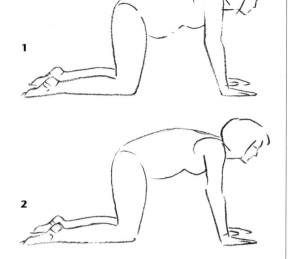

1

2

This pelvic tilt exercise helps make labor easier by making the back and pelvis more flexible and the abdominal muscles firmer. First, kneel on your hands and knees. Then tighten your abdominal and buttock muscles, rock the pelvis forward, hold for a few seconds, and release. Repeat several times.

grain bread, and dried apricots) and zinc (from meat, seafood, eggs, milk, whole grains, and wheat germ).

Smoking and pregnancy

Smoking is a risky habit not only for a mother but for the developing baby in her womb as well. Unfortunately, the addictive nature of nicotine—the active drug in tobacco—may make it difficult for her to give up. But during pregnancy one of the components of the smoke that she inhales (the gas carbon monoxide) is carried across the placenta and through the umbilical cord to the baby. Carbon monoxide decreases the capacity of the baby's blood to carry vital oxygen, thereby impeding its development. Other components of cigarette smoke, including nicotine, are also carried across the placenta into the baby's bloodstream. Women who smoke are more likely to have premature babies of low birthweight. There is also a greater likelihood that a woman will miscarry, or give birth to a stillborn or malformed baby.

FOODS TO AVOID DURING PREGNANCY

There are some foods that may make the mother ill and possibly harm the fetus, or even cause a miscarriage.
• Eggs should be cooked thoroughly to avoid the risk of salmonella poisoning. Cook chicken thoroughly for the same reason.
• All types of pâté and soft, ripened cheeses, such as brie and camembert, should be avoided because of the risk of developing *Listeria* food poisoning.
• Unpasteurized milk should not be consumed unless boiled before drinking.
• Raw meats, fish, and shellfish should be avoided.

Alcohol and pregnancy

When a pregnant woman drinks alcohol it is carried, like other drugs, across the placenta and into the fetus. Drinking alcohol during pregnancy probably increases the risk of miscarriage and stillbirth. "Safe" levels of alcohol consumption during pregnancy are not established, and women are often advised not to drink at all in the weeks before conception and during pregnancy itself. Excessive alcohol consumption during pregnancy can result in a baby being born with serious mental and physical abnormalities, known as fetal alcohol syndrome.

Miscarriage

If a fetus is lost before the 24th week of a pregnancy, this is described as a miscarriage or, in strictly medical terms, as a spontaneous abortion. About 20 percent of pregnancies end in miscarriage, although it is difficult to determine how many miscarriages actually occur each year—some women do not seek medical help, while others miscarry without realizing that they were pregnant, perhaps thinking that they have merely had an unusually heavy period.

Most miscarriages occur in the first trimester (three months) of pregnancy *(see pp.204–5)*. The most common causes of miscarriage include abnormality of the fetus and maternal illness. Symptoms of a threatened miscarriage include vaginal bleeding, cramping, and backache, although many women who show these symptoms may go

on to continue their pregnancy to term. A sudden gush of clear pinkish fluid from the vagina indicates that the amniotic sac has ruptured and that a miscarriage is now inevitable. If any of these symptoms are experienced, a woman should consult her doctor.

Losing a fetus through miscarriage is a profoundly upsetting experience for both the woman and her partner. Women commonly blame themselves for what has happened, searching for what they may have done wrong in early pregnancy. In most cases, however, a miscarriage is "nature's way" of rejecting a fetus because it is abnormal—but knowing this offers little comfort. A woman, and perhaps her partner, may find it helpful to seek advice from a counselor or support group. In most cases having a miscarriage will not prevent a woman from having more children.

Stillbirth

The loss of a baby before birth is deeply distressing at any stage of pregnancy, but probably more so when the baby is stillborn. A stillborn baby is one that dies in the uterus after the 24th week of pregnancy, or dies during birth itself. Unfortunately, this clear but cold definition fails to express the feelings experienced by a couple when they lose their baby. In addition to sadness, many feel anger, shame, and guilt. They may blame themselves unnecessarily for "causing" the stillbirth, or feel betrayed by medical staff. Their deep sense of grief often encompasses not only the actual loss of the baby before they could know and love him or her, but also the evaporation of all the hopes and expectations that had gradually been building up during the course of the pregnancy.

Stillbirth is rare, occurring in between 5 and 10 out of every 1,000 births in the developed world, but it is something that prospective parents should be aware of. Possible causes of stillbirth include severe malformation or chromosome abnormality of the fetus; a lack of oxygen passing to the fetus because of a problem with the placenta or umbilical cord; and severe infection or high blood pressure in the mother. However,

QUESTIONS AND ANSWERS: CARE DURING PREGNANCY

Q. Before I became pregnant, I went to step aerobic classes twice a week. Can I keep going?
A. Although it is probably safe to continue with your aerobic classes if you are careful and don't push your body too hard, you may wish to switch to a less strenuous form of exercise. For example, a combination of swimming, walking, and gentle yoga may prove more appropriate, giving you both cardiovascular fitness and muscle tone.

Q. I have been told to avoid cats and dogs now that I am pregnant. Is this true?
A. Not really. The advice is to avoid cat or dog feces—as might be found in a litter box or garden. These feces may contain the microorganism that causes the disease toxoplasmosis, which can seriously harm the fetus, and may cause premature birth. Toxoplasmosis may also be picked up from raw meat, so it is advisable to wash hands thoroughly after handling raw meat, and to cook meat thoroughly.

in around one third of cases, the cause of death is unknown.

In its effect on a couple's relationship, a stillbirth may draw them closer together or—especially if they both find it difficult to deal with their loss—it may push them apart. Couples who are having problems accepting their baby's death should seek help from friends and relatives and/or from support groups and counselors; medical staff or chaplains at the hospital will be able to advise them who to contact for help.

Emotional aspects of pregnancy

During pregnancy, women commonly find their emotions changing, especially during the early months. These changes are usually normal and temporary, the result of fluctuations in levels of hormones in the body.

How a woman reacts to pregnancy depends on many factors, but there are some common feelings shared by many women at this time in their lives, especially during their first pregnancy. These emotions are often conflicting, and can produce a feeling of well-being at one moment that suddenly gives way to a feeling of isolation the next. Worries and problems are best resolved by talking to partners, family, friends, and other pregnant women—it may be a great relief to discover that other people are experiencing the same or similar feelings.

Common emotional reactions of a pregnant woman may include:
• changing feelings—pleasure, elation, and satisfaction at being pregnant one day, followed by weepiness and depression the next
• concerns about the responsibilities of having a child—will she be a good mother?
• a feeling that she is trapped, that there is no going back, and that she and her partner are now committed to having a child
• anxiety about the health of the fetus and of the baby when it is born
• negative feelings about her body as it grows larger, concern that she is becoming increasingly unattractive to her partner, and self-consciousness at how she is perceived by other people
• worrying about the pain she may experience during the birth, and about loss of control at this time
• a dislike of being examined by the midwife or the doctor.

Looking good during pregnancy

Pregnancy can unnecessarily undermine a woman's self-esteem. She may feel that the growing "bulge" is making her less attractive, a feeling compounded by tiredness or nausea. But feeling good about oneself and being confident are very important during pregnancy. Being relaxed and happy about the way she looks helps a woman stay mentally healthy during those nine months, boosts her confidence in social situations, and enhances her relationship with her partner. Pregnancy itself contributes toward looking good in many women, especially during the second trimester, because the hormonal changes going on inside their body improve the condition of their hair and make their skin smooth and healthy-looking. Exercise, as described already, is great for relaxing the body, improving circulation, and toning the muscles. But there are many other ways of looking good.

Hair
A woman's hair tends to improve naturally during pregnancy, becoming brighter, softer and more shiny. Frequent appointments at the hairdresser keep the hair looking good and give the mother time to relax.

Skin care and makeup
Skin may change during pregnancy—it may become softer and moister, or drier, or oilier—and skin care should be adjusted accordingly. A rich moisturizer, used on skin that tended to be dry before pregnancy, may not be suitable for skin that has suddenly become oily. Any darkening of the facial skin—as experienced by some women during pregnancy—can be concealed by using a foundation. Makeup proves a good morale booster for many women. It may help to consult a beauty therapist about skin care and makeup during

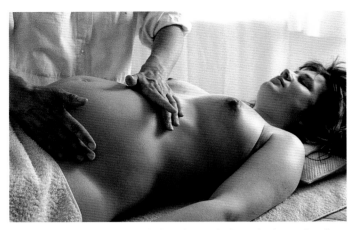

Massage can help induce a feeling of calm and well-being. Massage oils should be checked to see whether they are suitable for use during pregnancy.

pregnancy in order to get an objective view on what is most suitable for each individual.

New clothes

Clothes make an important statement about a person, and that is as true during pregnancy as at any other time. Obviously clothes should be comfortable, lightweight, and loose-fitting. Accessories such as earrings, necklaces, and scarves can help ensure that clothes look good. It is also important to consider shoes, because the feet have to bear increasing body weight during pregnancy and may swell or go up in size. Be sure shoes are the right size and comfortable, with low heels.

Underwear

Being pregnant is no reason to give up wearing pretty or sexy underwear. Buying new underwear that looks good and feels comfortable can give a woman a real boost, especially if she is feeling unattractive.

Feeling pampered

An expectant mother should let herself be spoiled during pregnancy. Choose a massage, a facial, a manicure, a pedicure and foot massage, or a complete head-to-toe treatment. (However, pregnant women may be advised to avoid certain essential oils, such as sage, basil, ho leaf, and perhaps birch, camphor, clove, fennel, and lavender. If in doubt as to which oils to avoid, check with a beauty therapist.) Equally beneficial may be a long afternoon spent relaxing by a swimming pool, punctuated by an occasional swim.

The father's emotions

Although the father-to-be is not the one who will actually give birth to the baby, he will probably share many of the emotions experienced by his partner. Initially he may feel a basic pride in his ability to produce children, but he may also have sleepless nights worrying about his new, lifelong commitment. He may have feelings of rejection and of being excluded by the pregnancy. There could be a number of reasons for this.

• Many men have little knowledge about pregnancy and may feel estranged when their partner—whom they thought they knew well —changes her behavior as well as her shape.

• Some men equate sex with love, perhaps unconsciously, and if their partner loses interest in sex, they may feel unloved and rejected.

TALKING ABOUT FEELINGS WITH A PARTNER

However strong a relationship is between partners, there is usually a need for adjustment on both sides in order to deal with the novel experience of pregnancy. If changes in the relationship are implemented by just one partner, the shift can be bewildering for the other partner. Build a framework of mutual support and understanding by talking and sharing your feelings, both good and bad. Voicing your concerns may help dispel any anxieties you are experiencing and lay a pattern of good communication for the future.

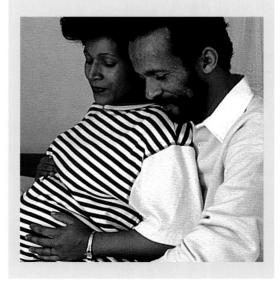

• A number of men may feel unsettled by their perception that their partner has changed her role from lover to mother.

Of course, not all men experience these feelings; many find a deeper understanding and love for their partner as a result of the pregnancy. Those men who do feel isolated and rejected may find it helps to talk through their feelings with their partner, a family member or friend who has had similar feelings, or an independent counselor.

Telling other children in the family about the new baby

The arrival of a new baby is bound to change the dynamics of a family. Many parents worry that an older child will be jealous of a new sibling, and feel concerned about whether they can provide sufficient love and attention to both children. It is probably true that in many cases the first-born child, having been the sole focus of his or her parents' attention, initially feels displaced and insecure when a "rival" appears. However, preparing the child well in advance of the birth can help alleviate such feelings. If a child, however young, is informed that he or she will have a brother or sister, and encouraged to feel involved with the new arrival—seeing the baby as someone whom they will be able to help care for now and play with in future years—and if the parents are aware that the new baby will cause a family rearrangement, and do their best to ensure that the change is a positive one, then feelings of rivalry and jealousy—although unlikely to be eliminated altogether—can be minimized.

PREPARING OLDER CHILDREN FOR THE NEW ARRIVAL

There are various strategies that can be helpful in preparing a child, or children, for the arrival of a new brother or sister. Obviously, the effectiveness of any of these suggestions will depend on the age of the child, his or her individual personality, and the relationship the child has with their parents. Whatever preparatory methods are used, the child should constantly be reassured that the new baby will not change the love that the parents feel toward the older sibling.

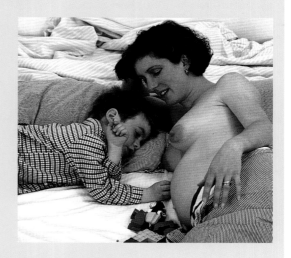

• Explain carefully and clearly to the child that a new brother or sister will soon be joining the family; it's probably best to start explaining this when the pregnancy starts to show. Remind the youngster about any friends of the same age who already have younger siblings. Repetition of the information may help it sink in.

• Show the child photographs of themselves at various stages from birth to the present day as a reminder that they were once a tiny baby, just like the new arrival.

• As pregnancy advances, let the child touch the growing "bump" and feel any movement of the fetus as it kicks or turns in the uterus.

• If he is not sharing in these activities already, make sure the father gets involved with caring for, feeding, playing with, and reading to the child. In this way, after the baby is born, it will seem completely natural for the child to spend more time with their father as the mother spends time with the baby.

• When the baby is born, give the child a present "from" the baby as an indication that the new arrival loves his or her brother or sister.

• Some children may enjoy feeling they are more "grown up" by being given small tasks or extra responsibilities after the baby arrives.

• After the birth, get the father to carry the baby when possible, so that the mother has her hands free to hug and hold the child and make sure that he or she does not feel rejected.

Pregnancy and sex

Pregnancy affects all aspects of a couple's life, including their sex life. And yet sex during pregnancy is a subject that is rarely addressed. There is nothing wrong with enjoying an active sex life during pregnancy, unless your doctor or midwife tells you that there may be a risk to the developing fetus. In many ways, a couple can feel more relaxed about sex during pregnancy. There is no worry about contraception, and women tend to become more aware of their bodies at this time—many find they have a greater capacity for sexual desire and pleasure during pregnancy. The reason for this is that blood flow to the genital and breast areas increases during pregnancy, as does the level of the hormone progesterone in the blood—both factors that are believed to encourage and increase sexual arousal. However, there is no right or wrong attitude about sex during a normal pregnancy, although whether in practice a couple continues sexual activity depends on a number of issues.

• A woman may feel too ill, exhausted, or uncomfortable to have sex, especially in the early and late months of pregnancy.
• A couple may feel—especially in the later months of the pregnancy—that the baby is there and "watching" what is going on.
• There may be worries that having sex will trigger labor or harm the baby. In a normal pregnancy these fears are unfounded.
• Some women feel unhappy about their body shape and attractiveness; some may feel "turned off" by the whole process of pregnancy—sexual arousal and response depend on having good, positive feelings about oneself. Also, the woman may feel that pregnancy and motherhood are incompatible with sensual and sexual behavior.

Many couples continue to enjoy sex during part or all of the pregnancy, with around 30 percent still having sex up to the very last weeks. Although there are no norms here, many women find that interest in sex decreases in the first months of pregnancy, increases in the middle months when initial problems of emotional upheaval and nausea have passed, and decreases once more in the later months when sex has become significantly more uncomfortable.

For some women sexual intercourse can be uncomfortable during the later part of pregnancy, but there are other ways of enjoying sex at this time. Exploration of sex during pregnancy can not only help bring a couple closer during a particularly emotional time in their lives, reducing the stress and tensions that pregnancy might bring—it can also enhance their future sex life.

When to avoid sex during pregnancy

There are certain circumstances when a couple is advised by their doctor to avoid sexual intercourse, or any sexual activity, during part or all of a pregnancy. It is important to find out from their doctor what sort of sexual activity they should avoid—for example, is it all right for the woman to reach orgasm through masturbation?—and whether the ban applies for just the first few months of pregnancy or for the full term. Reasons why a couple should avoid sex during pregnancy can include the following:
• If a woman has had a previous miscarriage, she may be advised not to have sex in the first three months of pregnancy.
• Spotting or light bleeding occurring in the first weeks of pregnancy may indicate the possibility of miscarriage and doctors may advise against having sex. In the middle part of pregnancy, bleeding may indicate a problem with the placenta, and intercourse and orgasms may need to be avoided.
• Painful cramps in the abdomen may indicate the possibility of miscarriage in early and middle pregnancy, of problems with the placenta in middle pregnancy, or of premature labor in later pregnancy. If pain does occur, it is advisable to abstain from sex until the cause has been determined.
• In late pregnancy, if a woman's water has broken (the membrane around the fetus has ruptured) it is advisable to avoid intercourse, even in order to stimulate labor (see p.216), because the fetus is no longer protected against infections reaching it via the vagina.

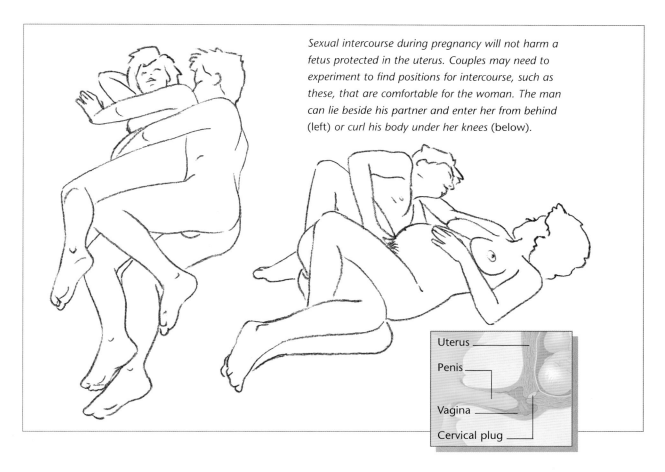

Sexual intercourse during pregnancy will not harm a fetus protected in the uterus. Couples may need to experiment to find positions for intercourse, such as these, that are comfortable for the woman. The man can lie beside his partner and enter her from behind (left) or curl his body under her knees (below).

Uterus

Penis

Vagina

Cervical plug

Sexual intercourse during pregnancy

In normal circumstances, there is no reason why a couple should not include sexual intercourse as part of their lovemaking during pregnancy. The fetus is well protected inside the amniotic sac, and the cervix is sealed with a plug of mucus. While orgasms cause the uterus to contract, this will not usually cause premature onset of labor unless there has been a previous history of miscarriage. Putting the penis into a well-lubricated vagina or gently inserting one or two (clean) fingers will not cause any harm to the baby, and neither will ejaculation. However, a couple should never put anything else, such as a vibrator, inside the woman's vagina while she is pregnant, nor blow air into it (which should never be done at any time). And during intercourse a man should move his penis gently, without powerful, deep thrusting.

The positions used for intercourse may change as the pregnancy progresses. For the first few months of the pregnancy, a woman and her partner can usually enjoy sex comfortably in all positions. But as her abdomen and breasts enlarge, and the latter become more tender, the couple will find some positions—especially the man-on-top missionary positions—increasingly uncomfortable. They may actually find that this need to try out different positions leads them to discover more exciting ways of having sex that will even enhance their sex life. Some of these positions are described below *(see also pp.176–81)*. The descriptions are intended merely to serve as examples of which positions some couples may like to try. It may be helpful during intercourse, especially in the later stages of pregnancy, to have some pillows or cushions nearby in case extra support is required. Suitable positions for intercourse could include:

Modified missionary positions
These variations of the "standard" face-to-face position *(p.179)* avoid the man resting his

weight on his partner's abdomen and breasts. He can, for example, support himself with his arms, keeping his upper body upright. Alternatively, she can lie on her back, or sit, with her legs over the edge of the bed, while he kneels on the floor between her legs.

Side-by-side positions

The couple lie on their sides facing each other, entwining their legs. A variation of this is a rear-entry position *(see right)*.

Lying down

A woman lies in a half-sitting position, propped up with pillows, and with her knees up. Her partner lies with his body curled under her knees so that he can put his penis into her vagina. This allows for very gentle penetration, and can be especially helpful if a woman is tired.

Sitting positions

These are really a variation of the woman-on-top positions described below. The man sits on a chair while his partner sits astride him, and facing him. This only allows limited movement, but it enables the couple to be very close and intimate.

The next three positions, and all their variations, can be enjoyed at any time during the pregnancy. But many women find them to be the most comfortable after the fourth or fifth month, when lying in certain positions, and pressure from the man being on top, becomes increasingly uncomfortable.

Rear entry

In rear-entry positions, the couple are facing in the same direction, with the man pushing his penis into her vagina from behind. One way of achieving this is by the couple lying side by side—slotted together like spoons, with him lying against her back. While having intercourse in this position, he can caress his partner's breasts and clitoris. In later pregnancy, however, it is often more comfortable to have rear-entry intercourse with the woman on all fours and the man kneeling behind her, or with both partners kneeling and upright; both these positions remove pressure from the belly, but allow the man to stroke the woman's clitoris and/or her breasts.

Woman-on-top positions

This could be either with the woman kneeling astride the man, controlling the pace of intercourse and the depth of penetration by moving her body up and down on his penis, or with her lying with her legs between or outside his. These last two positions will be less comfortable in later pregnancy.

Alternatives to sexual intercourse

During pregnancy, as at any other time in a relationship, there are other ways that a couple may choose to give each sexual and sensual pleasure other than through having sexual intercourse.

USING SEX TO ENCOURAGE LABOR WHEN BIRTH IS DUE

When the baby is due, or overdue, some couples choose to use lovemaking to help start labor naturally, although if the birth is long overdue, the hospital may induce labor by using drugs. Of course, many couples may not feel like sex so late in the pregnancy, and these methods are not guaranteed to work. But in a normal pregnancy, there is no risk that making love will cause labor to begin prematurely. Here is how sex can help with starting labor:

• Any form of sex—be it intercourse or oral sex—that results in a woman having an orgasm will cause her uterus to contract, and if the woman has multiple orgasms the uterus will contract even more. Each orgasm should produce between five and 10 uterine contractions.

• Sexual intercourse involves the ejaculation of semen into the vagina. Semen contains substances called prostaglandins that cause the uterus to contract. Some women are apparently more sensitive to the action of these prostaglandins than others. It may be better to choose a position for intercourse that will cause the maximal deposit of semen on the cervix—such as the woman lying on her back with her legs raised—although such positions may be impractical or uncomfortable at this stage of the pregnancy!

• Stimulation of the nipples causes the release of the hormone oxytocin from the pituitary gland, and oxytocin will cause the uterus to contract. A partner can kiss and suck the nipples, or the nipples can be massaged with warm oil and then stroked and gently pinched.

● Kissing, cuddling, and caressing brings a couple close to each other.

● Massage is especially helpful in relaxing a pregnant woman and providing relief for aches and pains.

● Masturbation, either of one partner or mutually, can provide sexual relief and satisfaction when other forms of sex are not possible or desired.

● Oral sex (provided care is taken not to force air into the vagina and thereby into the mother's bloodstream) can be ideal.

● Sucking and licking a woman's nipples during lovemaking may be highly pleasurable and may also help prepare the nipples for breastfeeding.

New baby, new relationships

The arrival of a new baby means reassessing relationships within the family, and both parents and siblings establishing a relationship with the new arrival.

Bonding

As soon as a baby is born, the process of forming a relationship with his or her parents begins, a process known as bonding. This formation of a deep attachment between parents and their newborn infant is an important factor in determining a child's normal emotional development.

The initial—and perhaps the strongest—bond is usually established between the baby and its mother. If a mother has her newborn baby with her following the birth, the baby will focus on the mother within hours of being born. She reciprocates by establishing close eye contact; by holding, touching, and stroking the baby; and by talking soothingly. In this way, a bond is gradually built between mother and baby.

The bonding process is enhanced by breastfeeding when the baby is not only in close contact with the mother's skin, but can also taste and smell her. The baby soon

BONDING BEFORE BIRTH

Modern technology has meant that the bond between parents and baby can start to develop before the baby is even born. The use of sonograms (ultrasound)—which use sound waves to produce an image of the baby inside the uterus—enables parents to see the developing fetus from the early months of pregnancy, and even to discover its sex. Such images can evoke a deep feeling of recognition for "their" baby. Some parents may carry sonograms of the baby around with them to show to their friends and relatives.

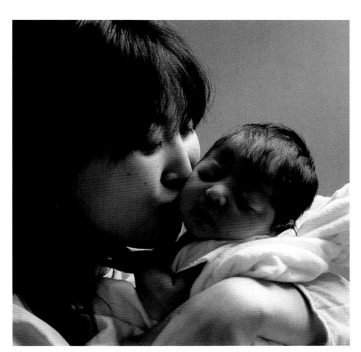

The all-important bonding process between a mother and her baby starts soon after birth. Sight, touch, and smell establish the bond between mother and infant.

responds to the mother's appearance and attention by smiling and other facial expressions, and this increases the attachment between them. As the bond develops, mothers become more attuned to their infant's needs.

The importance of bonding in a child's development, and the need for a mother, and father, to be close to their infant during the period after birth highlight the inadequacy of the policy in some hospitals where infants are separated from their parents after birth and access to the baby is restricted. Fortunately, this is becoming less common. Obviously, seriously ill babies, or those born prematurely and kept in an incubator, cannot remain close to their mothers, but they can still be touched, stroked, and talked to until they are healthy enough to be held.

Fathers should also be encouraged to bond with their newborn child. There is evidence to show that fathers who are present at the birth are likely to be closer to their baby than fathers who do not attend. And although fathers cannot achieve the same level of closeness that the mother and baby experience during breastfeeding, they can hold and talk to their baby so that the infant comes to recognize and respond to their face, voice, and smell. Bonding will also take place with other people such as grandparents or older siblings if the attention shown by the person toward the baby is consistent, caring, and long-term.

Although the bonding process sounds natural and miraculous, some mothers feel indifferent to their new baby and unable to show any maternal feelings. This should not be a cause of worry, because in the majority of cases a feeling of love and attachment develops toward the baby sooner or later. If there are lasting bonding problems between parent and baby, however, counseling may help mothers interact successfully with their baby. Similarly, being taught how to bond may be necessary for couples who adopt an infant, although usually they will find that the bonding process comes naturally.

Breastfeeding

Milk is manufactured by mammary glands in the breasts during the later stages of pregnancy, and continues to be produced for as long as the mother breastfeeds her infant. Breastfeeding serves not only to feed the growing baby but also to strengthen the bond between mother and infant. But if the mother finds she is unable or unwilling to breastfeed, she should not feel guilty. She can still show as much love, care, and attention to her baby while she is feeding him or her with a bottle.

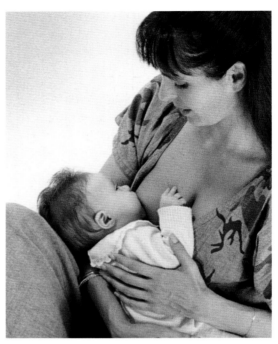

Many women find breastfeeding to be a rewarding and satisfying part of baby care. If a mother wants to breastfeed but has difficulties, she should seek help.

If the mother has decided to breastfeed her infant, she should put the baby to her breast as soon as possible after birth. Most babies have a strong instinct to suck when they are born, although they may need some guidance to find the nipple. Some mothers may need to be patient for a few days while the baby gets the hang of concentrating on sucking. A lactation consultant can help.

For the first few days after birth a yellowish liquid called colostrum is released through the nipples. Colostrum is rich in proteins and antibodies that help defend the newborn against infection, especially infections of the digestive system—such as gastroenteritis—which can be particularly serious if they occur in babies at this stage.

Two or three days after the birth, colostrum is replaced by breast milk itself—a thinner, bluish white liquid that also contains some antibodies, as well as a balance of nutrients required by the infant. Some mothers may feel concerned, initially, that their breast milk is too "thin" when compared with the more familiar cow's milk. This is perfectly natural: cow's milk is, quite simply, richer.

Initially, providing small feedings frequently will help to establish milk flow. Thereafter, the baby should be fed on demand to maintain the milk supply.

Breastfeeding is the natural way of feeding babies between the time they are born and the time they are weaned. Nowadays it is usually seen as a normal part of family life, and not something to be hidden away from children or other adults. In general, mothers today tend to favor breastfeeding their infants rather than bottle-feeding, in contrast to mothers of the previous generation. There are several reasons why breastfeeding is advantageous for both mother and infant.

• Breastfeeding helps establish a close bond between mother and baby, as well as giving both of them emotional and physical pleasure.

• The thick colostrum that is released in the first two or three days after birth helps to protect the baby against infection, as does breast milk itself.

• Breast milk is sterile and provides all the nutrients that a baby requires in balanced amounts.

• Breast milk aids the baby's digestion, helps avoid indigestion or constipation, and makes the baby's stools and regurgitated food relatively odorless.

• Breastfeeding helps avoid obesity in babies because the flow of milk gradually slows during each feeding, enabling the baby to satisfy itself without overeating.

• The release of the hormone oxytocin caused by suckling in the days after birth also causes the muscles in the wall of the uterus to contract (these contractions are called afterpains), which helps the uterus to return to its normal size more rapidly.

• Breastfeeding mothers tend to return to their original weight and figure more rapidly. Breast size inevitably increases markedly during pregnancy in preparation for breastfeeding, both as a result of hormonal action increasing the size of the milk-producing glands and because the blood supply to the breasts is increased. Some women fear that if they breastfeed, their breasts will lose their shape and sag. In fact, the opposite is generally true: breastfeeding can enhance the shape

BREASTFEEDING AND SENSUALITY

Many societies regard breasts, outside the context of pregnancy and parenthood, as part of a woman's sexual being. For this reason, some women find it difficult to come to terms with regarding their breasts as the source of their baby's food, or to expose their breasts to feed the baby, however discreetly, in public. Some women who have chosen to breastfeed may be taken by surprise by the sensual or sexual feelings they experience as the baby suckles. Such feelings are natural. Having experienced these sensations, some women may find increased enjoyment in having their breasts sucked and stimulated during sex with their partner, thus adding to that relationship. Breastfeeding should be a natural, pleasurable experience for both baby and mother.

of the breasts. What can adversely affect their shape, however, is lack of good support during pregnancy itself, when they become fuller and heavier.

Body changes after birth

Within six weeks of the birth—the post-partum period—a woman's body has started to get back to normal. Despite the inevitability of some aches and pains for a few weeks after the birth, rest (including as much sleep as is possible with a newborn baby), a good diet, and avoiding straining the body will all help the body return to normal.

In the first week it is important to get as much rest and sleep as possible, to allow the body to recover from the stresses and strains of birth. Thereafter, normal activity can gradually be increased each day, and the woman should feel better and stronger as each week passes. A woman who has just given birth should expect a number of changes to occur to her body. These include:

• Once her baby has been born, a woman will notice an immediate weight loss, but when she looks in the mirror, her body may look quite swollen and puffy, especially in the arms, legs and abdomen. Much of this puffiness is due to accumulated water, most of which disappears naturally in the first week. Exercises will help the woman to strengthen muscles, such as the abdominal muscles, that were stretched during pregnancy and birth *(see postpartum exercises, opposite)*. Attempting to lose weight by following a reduced-calorie diet is not advised at this stage, especially if a woman is breastfeeding. It is important that she follows a healthy, balanced diet *(see p.208)*, whether breastfeeding or bottle-feeding, to aid in the

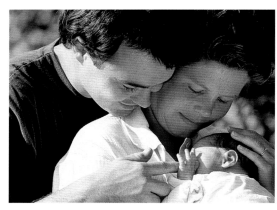

While the bond may be naturally stronger between mother and baby, fathers have an important part to play in the processes of bonding and baby care.

MAKING TIME FOR A PARTNER

The days and weeks following the birth of a baby are likely to be hard work for both parents, especially, perhaps, the mother, who is bound to find herself spending almost all her time looking after her baby's needs. And because of her disturbed sleep patterns, she may well take advantage of the time her baby is asleep to take a nap. This combination of tiredness and preoccupation may mean that she has little time to spend with her partner. When they are together, they may be dealing with the baby together rather than focusing on each other. But however tired, upset, depressed, or out of shape a mother may feel, it is important that she and her partner make sure they spend some quality time together. A new father, however involved he is with the baby, may feel pushed out by the new arrival, ignored by his partner, and isolated from the pair of them. So now is the time to make a date with each other to reestablish communications and talk about changing circumstances. Making time for each other now, however short the period, will help set a good pattern for your future relationship.

recovery of muscle tone and keep her body functioning properly.

• Two to three days after the birth, the uterus starts to shrink, returning to its prepregnancy size within six weeks. This process is usually accompanied by contractions (afterpains), which may be severe but can be alleviated by acetaminophen or other pain medications, and which subside in a few days. Medications should be avoided or kept to a minimum if breastfeeding. Shrinkage of the uterus can be assisted by breastfeeding *(see above)*.

• Vaginal bleeding, called lochia, occurs for two or three weeks after birth, as the uterine wall where the placenta was attached bleeds until it is healed. The vaginal discharge is initially red and then becomes brownish, and may increase when breastfeeding. If, after turning brownish, it becomes heavy and red again, a woman should consult her doctor.

• There may be pain in the perineum, the area between the anus and vagina, for a few weeks. This is especially likely if the woman has had stitches, either because she had an episiotomy —a cut in the perineum to make delivery of the baby easier and prevent the perineum from tearing—or because the perineum tore and was stitched up. Until the area heals, sitting may be uncomfortable without a cushion. Perineal soreness may be relieved by using an ice pack or taking a warm bath. Gentle pelvic floor muscle exercises *(see p.209)* may also help. If the area remains sensitive, it may be inflamed or be sewn too tightly, and the woman should see her doctor or midwife.

• The mother may become constipated for a few days after the birth. The best ways to counteract this are to take gentle walks, drink plenty of water, and eat food high in fiber such as raw fruit and vegetables.

• The mother may urinate more frequently in the days following the birth, as the body eliminates excess fluid.

Becoming a father

Although their involvement with the newborn baby can never be quite as close and intense as that of the mother, fathers can and should involve themselves with the processes of

POSTPARTUM EXERCISES

1

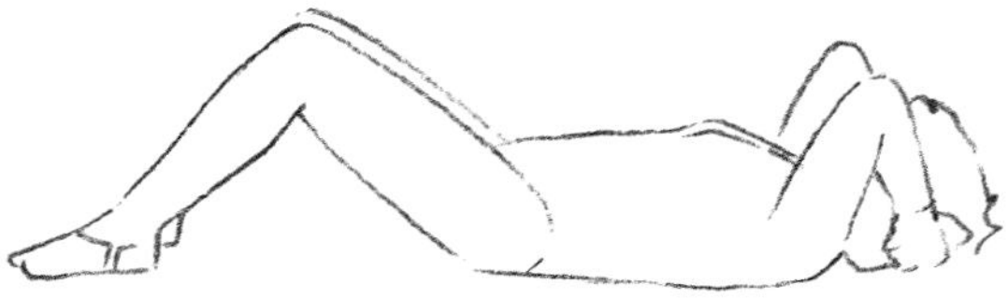

2

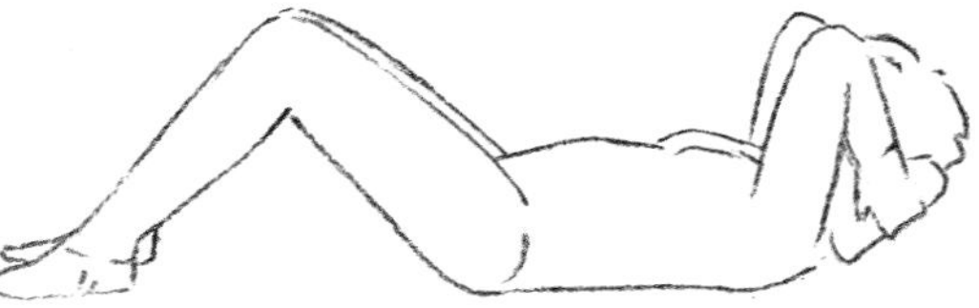

TONING THE ABDOMEN
Holding a small cushion behind your head, lift your head upward, feel your abdominal muscles tighten, then relax. Repeat this twice initially, increasing the number of repeats as you get stronger.

1

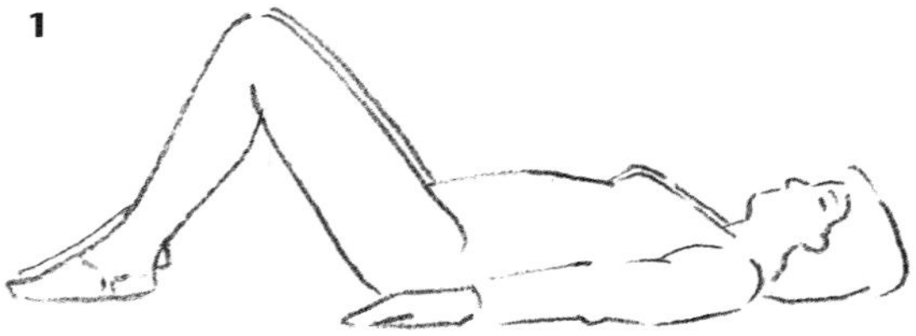

2

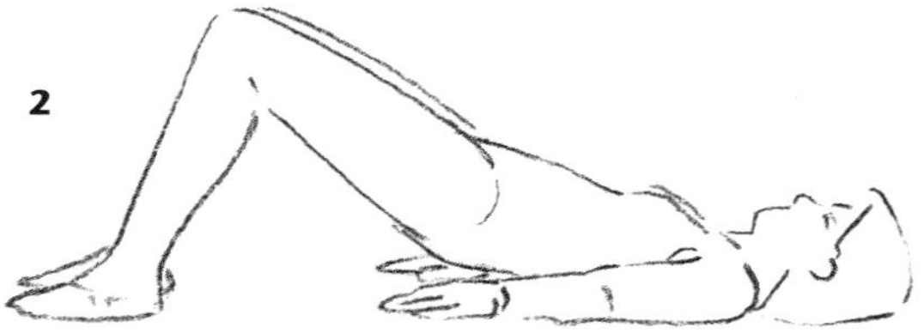

PELVIC LIFT
This strengthens the buttocks, thighs, and lower back and relaxes the head and neck. Lie with your arms by your side. Lift your buttocks off the ground, hold the position for a few seconds, relax, and repeat.

bonding and child care. And even though the mother may feel totally absorbed by her new baby, she should find the opportunity for "quality time" with her partner so that he does not feel excluded.

In the past, fathers often missed out on the early months of a child's life because it was not part of their perceived role. If they did play a part in a child's upbringing it was to play with him or her at the toddler stage or later. Today, fathers take a much greater part in their child's development. Many are not only present at the birth but also assist with it as a birthing partner. The father can then help his partner look after the newborn baby, so that she has more rest and sleep, especially if she is getting up during the night to breast-feed. If the baby is being bottle-fed, the couple can take turns with the feeding.

Fatherhood is often perceived as being more peripheral than motherhood, but fathers have an important role in the family, both as supporter of their partner and in helping to care for the baby.

Postpartum exercises

These exercises can help the new mother restore muscle tone and body shape by strengthening those muscles—such as the abdominal and pelvic floor muscles—most affected by pregnancy and birth. If the woman has exercised regularly during pregnancy, she will find that other body muscles are still firm. It is important to remember, however, that the postpartum exercises illustrated above should only be attempted progressively—starting very gently, and then building up—to avoid physical damage. If there is any pain, stop exercising immediately. (A woman who has had a cesarean should wait until the third week after the birth and take things even more gently.) Other exercises that will make the woman feel better and healthier, when she has recovered from the birth and when she has the time or opportunity, include jogging and swimming. With regular exercise a woman's figure can return to normal within three or four months after the birth.

Sex and contraception after birth

The return to an active sex life after the birth of a baby may take weeks or months, depending on each individual couple. As with other aspects of sex during pregnancy and parenthood, there is no right or wrong way, although if a couple who previously had an active sex life has difficulty in resuming their sexual relationship, they may need outside counseling to help solve any problems.

The best time for a couple to resume their sex life is when they both feel ready and able.

POSTPARTUM DEPRESSION

Often known as "baby blues," postpartum depression is experienced by almost two thirds of mothers after giving birth. Most commonly they suffer mild depression, which may begin soon after the birth but usually develops four or five days later. Women typically feel confused, tired, miserable, and discouraged, and cry easily. The most likely causes are sudden fluctuations in hormone levels, a feeling of anticlimax after the stress of childbirth and, perhaps, fear of the new responsibility of looking after a baby. With loving care and emotional support from partner and family, the depression should pass after a few days. Occasionally, however, it continues for months or even years; this seems to be caused not by hormones but by difficulty adjusting to a new identity as a mother, and by feelings triggered by the experience.

In about one in 1,000 mothers, a more serious condition, postpartum psychosis, develops. Here the mother becomes severely confused and can be a danger to herself and her baby. She needs to be admitted to hospital to receive treatment in the form of drugs and counseling, which should also involve her partner, to effect a full recovery.

QUESTION & ANSWER: RESUMING SEX AFTER CHILDBIRTH

Q. Will my vagina be too stretched after birth to make sexual intercourse enjoyable?
A. The vagina is highly elastic and will return to around its original size after birth. In addition, if you did pelvic floor exercises during pregnancy and continue to do them, you should have an increased ability to control the muscles around your vagina and so hold and squeeze your partner's penis during intercourse.

At the end of the four- or six-week postpartum period, the woman will return to the doctor's office or midwife for her postpartum checkup, and the couple may want to wait until after this before they start having sex again. Although there is no reason why they should not resume their sex life sooner than the postpartum checkup, there are a number of reasons why this may in fact not happen.

• The soreness felt by many women around the vagina and perineum in the first weeks after the birth may make them uninterested in sex, especially if they had stitches.

• Hormonal imbalance after the birth may make a woman lose her sex drive. This may also be affected by breastfeeding; some breastfeeding women find that their desire for sex decreases or becomes nonexistent.

• Tiredness after the birth, exacerbated by lack of sleep caused by getting up during the night to feed the baby, may leave no energy for sex or even sexual thoughts.

• A mother's relationship with the baby may be so intense and absorbing that she temporarily loses interest in the physical relationship she had with her partner. She may also find it hard at first to reconcile her new role as a mother with her sexuality.

Lack of sex may cause problems between the couple if she lacks desire while his libido is bubbling over. Failure to discuss their sexual relationship at this stage can create strain, and may lead to continuing sexual problems in later years. It is far better for a couple to talk about their feelings, and if necessary try to find alternative ways of giving each other comfort and pleasure.

If a couple has decided they want to resume their sex life after the birth of a baby, they should take it slowly at first—for example, sex could take the form of mutual exploration in order to rediscover each other's bodies. If the area around the woman's vagina is still sore, it may be better to avoid full intercourse at first, or to use positions that put little pressure on the vagina, or on the breasts if they are full and swollen (see pp.218–19). The vagina may be drier than usual at this time and extra lubrication, such as K-Y Jelly, may be useful.

Fertility after birth

During pregnancy, a woman is effectively infertile because her normal ovarian and menstrual cycles are suspended: she does not release any eggs from her ovaries, and she does not have any periods. After giving birth most women return to normal fertility quite quickly, with periods resuming within four to seven weeks after the birth if they are not breastfeeding. Even before she has a period, a woman's fertility may return—that is, she may ovulate. In women who are breastfeeding, the resumption of ovulation and menstruation may be delayed until she stops breastfeeding altogether, but breastfeeding is no guarantee of infertility. Whether a woman breastfeeds or bottle-feeds, therefore, she and her partner should use contraception.

Contraception after birth

The choice of contraception available to a couple depends on their preferences, the suitability of particular methods as advised by their doctor, and whether the woman plans to breastfeed or not. It may be better to discuss plans for contraception before the birth, rather than having to think about it, along with everything else, after the baby is born. In any case, it is better to be prepared and not to delay starting contraception until the first menstruation or the first postpartum visit. There are various options for contraception.

Condoms
Male and female condoms are easy-to-use forms of barrier contraception that can be used at any time after the birth. If combined with the natural contraceptive effect of breastfeeding, there is very little chance of pregnancy *(see also p.162)*.

Diaphragm and cervical cap
The diaphragm and cap fit inside the vagina and in most cases prevent sperm from reaching the cervix and entering the uterus. Both are suitable for use by women after birth, and neither has any effect on breastfeeding. The old, prepregnancy diaphragm or cap will no longer be suitable, and a new one will have to be fitted in order to compensate for changes in the shape and size of internal organs. Fitting or refitting should be delayed until four to six weeks after birth, when the uterus and cervix have settled down. Couples should bear in mind, however, that the internal organs may have changed shape to such an extent that these methods may no longer be suitable once a woman has given birth *(see also p.139)*.

Hormonal methods
The main actions of hormonal contraceptives are either to prevent ovulation or to thicken the mucus at the entrance to the cervix so that sperm cannot enter the uterus.

Combined oral contraceptive (the pill)
The pill is not recommended for breastfeeding women as it may decrease the volume of breast milk or alter its composition. It can be prescribed for women who are not breastfeeding, although it should not be started until at least two weeks after the birth because of the increased risk of side effects in the immediate postpartum period.

Progestin-only contraception—the minipill, implants, and injectables
In general, these are suitable for all women after they have given birth. If combined with breastfeeding, the contraceptive cover will be all the more reliable. The progestin-only pill, or minipill, can be started about three weeks after delivery. The hormonal implant and injectable contraceptives can be given to a woman within a few days of the birth *(see also pp.148–50)*.

BREASTFEEDING AS A FORM OF CONTRACEPTION

Q. I have been told that breastfeeding is an effective contraceptive. Is this true, or do I need to use another contraceptive method as well when we have sexual intercourse?

A. Breastfeeding, if done frequently and regularly, will generally prevent ovulation, and may therefore act as a contraceptive method after the birth. However, to be sure that they are well protected, breastfeeding women are usually advised to use another method of contraception, especially if the frequency of breastfeeding is reduced or when the baby has reached six months of age.

IUD

The IUD (an intrauterine device that fits inside the uterus) is suitable, especially for women who are not planning to have any more children. It has no effect on breast-feeding and is generally inserted some four to six weeks after birth, although some doctors may decide to fit an IUD immediately *(see also pp.152-5).*

Natural family planning

Natural methods involve monitoring various changes in a woman's body to determine when she will ovulate or has ovulated. These methods are difficult to use in the weeks following birth because ovulation and menstruation have not yet started again, or are still erratic, and the signs by which the fertile times of the month are normally determined are not clear-cut. If no other contraceptive method can be used, it may be better to avoid actual intercourse, practice abstinence, or use withdrawal until the menstrual cycle returns to normal *(see also pp.156–62). (Contraceptive methods are described in detail in Chapter 5.)*

Infertility

Infertility is the inability to conceive. It is not a disease, it shows no outward signs, and yet it causes great pain and upset to those men and women that it affects. Fortunately, more is known nowadays about infertility than in previous years, and there are a greater number of possible treatments available.

If a couple decides to have a child, it might appear that the only prerequisite for conception is for them to have sexual intercourse without using contraception. For many couples this is certainly the case provided that

---

MYTHS ABOUT INFERTILITY

There are many myths and misunderstandings about infertility, including the following.
- **Infertility is always the woman's fault.**
No. Only half of all cases of infertility are caused by a women's fertility problems.
- **A woman must have an orgasm in order to conceive.**
No. Although having an orgasm may help with sperm transport, conception can take place whether or not she has an orgasm.
- **If infertile couples just relaxed a little, and stopped trying so hard, the woman would soon become pregnant.**
No. This advice, so often forthcoming from friends and relatives, is not true and is of little help. The frustrations of being infertile can certainly create stress, but this stress does not of itself cause infertility.
- **Infertile men are less masculine because they have low levels of the male sex hormone testosterone.**
No. First, infertility is in no way related to a man's sexuality or any other aspect of his masculinity. Second, few infertile men have lower-than-normal testosterone levels.
- **If a woman has sex, even just once, at the right time—around ovulation—she is sure to get pregnant.**
No. Only around 15 percent of women get pregnant during the first menstrual cycle when they have regular unprotected sex.
- **If you want to get pregnant it is better for the man not to ejaculate more than once a week so that all the sperm are not used up.**
No. Ejaculating more than once a week will not deplete sperm supplies. And having sex two or three times a week should ensure that sperm are present in the woman when she ovulates.
- **Timing is all-important. A couple with fertility problems must have sex 12 hours before the woman is due to ovulate in order for her to get pregnant.**
No. First, it is quite difficult to time precisely when ovulation is going to take place. Second, sperm will survive inside a woman for 48 hours or longer. And third, strict timing turns sex into a chore, and puts pressure on a couple which may turn them off sex and each other altogether.
- **If a woman has periods, she must be releasing eggs from her ovaries as well.**
Not necessarily. Even women with very regular periods may not always ovulate.

they satisfy the requirements for conception to take place *(see box, below)*. On average, 15 percent of fertile couples conceive within a month of starting to have unprotected sex, while 95 percent of women in a relationship where both partners are fertile will be pregnant within one year.

But for a significant minority of couples pregnancy simply does not happen. Their inability to conceive may be caused by a number of different factors, some of which can be treated. By strict definition, a couple is deemed to be infertile if they have not conceived despite having unprotected intercourse for 12 months. Statistically, 70 percent of these couples show primary infertility—they have never previously had a child; the remaining 30 percent have secondary infertility—the couple already has a child or children but find themselves unable to conceive another child. However, it is important to remember that even if couples are described as infertile because they do not conceive within the 12 months, they may well conceive after this time without requiring any treatment.

The incidence of infertility has increased over the past 25 years. There are a number of possible explanations for this.
• There is a much greater awareness of infertility problems so that more couples are approaching doctors and clinics in search of advice and treatment.
• There has been an increase in the incidence of sexually transmitted diseases (STDs—*see pp.117–26*); some STDs, especially if they are untreated, can lead to decreased fertility, or infertility.
• More couples are delaying having children until they are in their thirties, by which time a woman's fertility may be decreasing. Recent figures indicate that in the developed world 1 couple in 10 in their twenties is infertile, rising to 1 in 7 aged 30–34, and 1 in 5 for the 35–39 age group.

Infertility affects men and women in different ways. The initial disappointment that pregnancy is not under way can lead to a range of emotions, including guilt, anger, and a sense of bereavement, which can put stress on a relationship. It is important that, if a couple thinks they have a problem, they seek help as soon as possible, as their problem may be fairly easy to solve. In recent years there have been major breakthroughs in the treatment and diagnosis of infertility. However, it should also be remembered that there are no magic solutions. Even the much publicized modern "test-tube" techniques are suitable only in a small number of cases, and are not always successful. Some infertile couples will never be able to have children, and they need to make the emotional adjustments to come to terms with this.

Research into the diagnosis and treatment of infertility is an active and expanding field. This part of the chapter gives a brief overview of some of the common causes of, and treatments for, infertility.

Causes of infertility

There are many possible reasons why a couple may be infertile. However, modern diagnostic techniques mean that a specific cause can now be identified in 85–90 percent of couples who consult their doctor about the problem. Contrary to popular belief, infertility is not

---

REQUIREMENTS FOR CONCEPTION TO OCCUR

That there are not more infertile couples is quite surprising when all the factors required for conception to take place are considered. These are the main "fertility factors."

In both sexes
• A normal, functioning reproductive system.
• Adequate sex drive, and full, frequent sexual intercourse.

In women
• A regular ovulatory cycle *(see pp.20–3)*.
• Fully functioning fallopian tubes *(see p.14)*.
• The production, around the time of ovulation, of watery mucus by the cervix that permits ejaculated sperms to pass into the uterus from the vagina.
• A uterus that permits implantation of the embryo and that can support and sustain the fetus for the full term of the pregnancy.

In men
• Producing semen *(see pp.27–9)* that contains sufficient numbers of healthy, motile (spontaneously mobile) sperm.
• Being able to achieve an erection *(see pp.28–9)*.
• Being able to ejaculate semen into the vagina *(see p.29)*.

just a female problem. Although in about 50 percent of infertile couples, it is the woman who has the fertility problem, in 30 percent of couples it is the man, and in the remaining 20 percent both partners have fertility problems. The reason why the figure is higher in women is simply because there are more things that can go wrong. However, in order for a doctor to attempt to ascertain what exactly is causing the infertility, it is essential that both partners be examined.

One further factor that should be taken into consideration is that the sexually transmitted diseases (STDs) that give rise to pelvic inflammatory disease (PID—*see pp.124–5*) in women, and other reproductive disorders in men, are the leading preventable cause of infertility. The probability of developing STDs increases with the number of sexual partners the person has, but decreases if he or she has consistently practiced safe sex *(see p.119)*.

Improving the chances of conception

Infertility may not be the result of an anatomical or physiological problem. Some lifestyle factors can affect fertility as well. If both partners are fertile, or if one of them has lower-than-normal fertility, changing one or more of these factors may result in conception, removing the need for any medical treatment.
• Infertility can be the result of not understanding how reproductive biology works. If a couple only has sexual intercourse just after and/or just before a woman's period, there is little chance that she will conceive. To optimize the chance of conception, they should try to have sex around the time she is likely to ovulate. Although sperm will stay alive in the fallopian tubes for over 48 hours, the egg is only viable for between 12 and 24 hours after ovulation; the "window" for fertilization is not that long. If the woman has a regular menstrual cycle, ovulation will be around 14 days before her next period begins. If menstrual cycles are not regular, there are other ways of trying to narrow down when ovulation will take place—the same techniques that are used for determining the fertile time of the month in natural contraception methods *(see pp.156–62)*.

• Working long hours and having a stressful lifestyle may cause a couple to have reduced sex drive and, possibly, lower fertility. A stress-management program may solve their infertility problems.
• Low body weight in women—a drop of 10–15 percent below recommended weight for height—may inhibit ovulation. This often happens in women who exercise excessively, and in those suffering from anorexia nervosa or bulimia *(see p.83)*. Restoring a woman's weight to relatively normal levels often results in the return of her fertility.
• Overconsumption of cigarettes and/or alcohol can reduce a man's sperm count and make him less fertile.
• Recreational drugs, such as marijuana, if used in excess, can suppress sperm production and depress testosterone levels in men, and upset the normal balance of the menstrual cycle in women.
• Wearing tight underpants, spending too long in hot tubs or saunas, undertaking strenuous cycling or other strenuous sports activities are all believed to reduce fertility in men, especially if their sperm count is already low.

Female infertility

The two major physical causes of female infertility are failure to ovulate and blockage of the fallopian tubes.

Failure to ovulate

Normally, during the reproductive years between puberty and the menopause, an egg is released from one of the ovaries each month. In some women ovulation does not happen or occurs on an irregular basis. There are three reasons why this may happen.
• There is something wrong with the balance in the bloodstream of the hormones that cause ovulation. For example, there may be too little follicle stimulating hormone (FSH) or luteinizing hormone (LH), or there may be excessive amounts of a hormone called prolactin that inhibits ovulation.
• The ovaries may be affected by a disorder, such as polycystic ovarian syndrome, or they may be abnormal or absent.

• The ovaries may be affected by a major life event that causes the woman extreme stress and inhibits ovulation.

Diagnosis

A number of procedures for attempting to identify the time of ovulation may be used to diagnose failure to ovulate.

• Basal body temperature (BBT) can be measured through the month, and recorded daily on a chart, to see if ovulation has taken place. BBT usually drops just before ovulation and rises just after it. Measuring BBT is done at home by the woman. The BBT must be taken every morning before the woman has risen from bed, and before she has eaten or drunk anything. It must be continued over at least three months before any pattern can be observed. It may be helpful to do this before the initial consultation so that the chart can be shown to the doctor. The method is not infallible, but it may be a useful initial guide to what is going on (see pp.158–9).

• A "dipstick" test can be used at home to measure levels of luteinizing hormone (LH) in urine. LH levels rise just before ovulation, so that if the kit detects a rise in levels, ovulation is probably about to occur. These kits are expensive and, some doctors argue, not much more accurate than the BBT method.

• Levels of hormones such as progesterone and FSH in the blood can be measured to determine whether they are normal and likely to cause ovulation, or to determine whether

or not ovulation has taken place.

• Endometrial biopsy involves taking a small sample from the lining of the uterus a few days before a period is due, to determine whether the lining has thickened as a consequence of an egg being released from one of the ovaries.

Treatment

If ovulatory problems are diagnosed, they are usually treated with drug therapy. There is now about a 90 percent chance that drug treatment will restore ovulation. The main drug treatments are as follows.

• Clomiphene is the drug most commonly used. It appears to stimulate the pituitary gland to produce more FSH and LH, and these hormones stimulate ovulation.

• Human menopausal gonadotrophin (HMG) contains the pituitary hormones FSH and LH. Injections of HMG stimulate the ovarian follicles to develop and, hopefully, thereby cause ovulation to occur.

• Injections of FSH work to stimulate the ovary directly.

• Bromocriptine prevents the pituitary gland from producing too much of the hormone prolactin. This hormone, which normally controls milk production, inhibits ovulation if levels in the blood are too high—this explains why regular breastfeeding is a natural method of contraception.

Blockage of the fallopian tubes

The fallopian tubes are responsible for transporting sperm in one direction to meet the egg, and the egg in the other direction on its journey to reach the uterus. Damage to, or scarring of, one or both tubes can prevent them from carrying out these vital functions. Fallopian tubes may be defective from birth, or they may be damaged by surgery or disease. A common cause of blockage is pelvic inflammatory disease (PID) resulting from infection with chlamydia (see pp.121–2). The risk of tubal blockage increases with each episode of PID.

Diagnosis

Blockage of the fallopian tubes is usually diagnosed by one of the following.

• Hysterosalpinography—an X-ray picture of

the fallopian tubes is taken after a special dye has been introduced into them so that any blockages or deformities can be pinpointed.

• Laparoscopy—a viewing tube is inserted into the abdominal cavity to inspect the fallopian tubes for damage.

Treatment

If blockage of, or damage to, the fallopian tubes is diagnosed, it may be possible to treat it in one of the following ways. However, because of the delicacy of these tubes, and the ease with which their normal functioning can be disrupted, the success rate of these procedures is not high.

• Tubal surgery often involves removing a damaged part of the tube, and then joining together the cut ends. However, it is a very delicate procedure—because the inner part of the fallopian tube is so narrow—and the overall success rate averages 35–40 percent.

• In a procedure known as tuboplasty, surgeons insert a fine tube into the fallopian tube through the uterus. Part of this tube, or catheter, can be expanded like a balloon to attempt to widen the fallopian tube where it is constricted. Success rates of up to 40 percent have been reported for this technique.

Other causes of female infertility

Other causes of infertility include endometriosis; abnormal vaginal or cervical secretions that do not allow sperm to swim through into the uterus during the fertile time of the month; and abnormalities of the uterus, such as fibroids (see p.106).

Male infertility

The reason for most cases of male infertility, or reduced fertility, is a low sperm count—producing too few sperm—and/or a high proportion of defective sperm.

Sperm count

The number of sperm in 1 milliliter (about one fifth of a teaspoon) of a man's semen varies from day to day, but the optimal average is probably between 60 and 100 million sperm per milliliter. If the number of sperm in a man's semen drops to 20 million per ml, the couple may have problems in conceiving, especially if the sperm sample also shows a high level of abnormalities.

Functional capacity

This is a measure of the percentage of defective sperm in a semen sample. Sperm are produced by the millions every day, and every man's semen contains some abnormal sperm. However, if a large number of sperm lack the normal motility (spontaneous mobility), or are incapable of penetrating an egg, fertility will be much reduced or nonexistent.

Possible causes of low sperm count include varicocele (varicose veins in the scrotum), hormonal disorders, injury to or disease of the testes, infection with mumps in adult life, and excessive use of alcohol, nicotine, or other drugs.

Other causes of male infertility include hormonal abnormalities and sexual dysfunction such as problems with erection (see pp.194–5), inability to ejaculate, and retrograde ejaculation (when semen is ejaculated into the bladder instead of out of the penis).

Diagnosing and treating male infertility

The initial examination will probably involve a physical examination of the testes and scrotum to make sure that both testes have descended, and that there is no varicocele (varicose vein) present. But the main diagnostic procedure is the examination of a sample of semen. The patient is normally given instructions about how to collect a semen sample by masturbating or during sexual intercourse. The sample is then examined to assess its volume, the number of sperm per milliliter (the sperm count), the motility of the sperm, and whether or not there are large numbers of abnormal sperm in the sample.

Sperm counts vary from day to day, and a single low count may not mean that a man has low fertility or is infertile. But if semen analysis consistently indicates a low sperm count and/or sperm abnormality, it may mean that the man is infertile. If the sperm count is low, blood samples are usually taken to measure the levels of the hormones that control (or inhibit) sperm production. Further tests include taking a small sample of tissue from the testes, and testing sperm to see if they are capable of penetrating an egg in order to allow fertilization to take place.

If a hormonal problem is indicated, drug treatment may be effective in restoring a fertile sperm count. Surgery to remove a varicocele, or microsurgery to remove a blockage in the vas deferens (the tube carrying the sperm from the testes to the outside), may also be successful in restoring fertility.

Test-tube babies—in vitro fertilization

There are cases of female infertility where the treatments described above are unsuccessful, or where treatment is impossible. In this situation, a couple may decide to try in vitro fertilization (IVF). This involves removing eggs from a woman's body, fertilizing them with sperm provided by her partner, and replacing a fertilized egg back in her body. This sounds very simple, but in fact requires great commitment on the part of the couple. And, despite considerable publicity about the "test-tube babies" conceived by this method, the chances of success are relatively low.

Women who may be suitable for IVF include those who have not responded to hormonal treatment; those whose fallopian tubes are too damaged to be repaired; and those whose infertility remains unexplained even after comprehensive testing. Of course, to be considered for IVF, a woman must have ovaries that are capable of producing eggs, usually when stimulated by drugs; she must also have a normally functioning uterus in which the embryo can implant and develop.

The IVF technique

After assessment to decide whether a couple is suitable for IVF, and whether they will have the commitment to put up with the difficult timetable, repeated hospital visits, possible side effects, and strains on their relationship, the decision may be taken to go ahead with IVF. The woman is treated with hormone injections that stimulate her ovaries to produce eggs. As egg-containing follicles grow inside the ovary (see pp.20–3), their progress

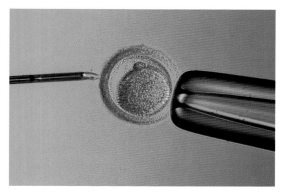

In vitro fertilization helps ensure penetration of the egg by a sperm. A pipette (right) holds the egg (center) in position while a needle (left) is inserted to make an entry point for penetrating sperm.

QUESTIONS & ANSWERS: INSEMINATION

Q. What does artificial insemination involve? How is it used to help with infertility problems?
A. Artificial insemination involves taking a sample of a man's sperm and introducing it by syringe into his partner's uterus. This may be done because his sperm count is low, or if her cervical mucus is consistently too thick to allow sperm to travel from her vagina into the uterus. Another type of artificial insemination called AID (artificial insemination by donor) may be used when a man's sperm count is very low and fertilization is impossible. It involves artificial insemination using sperm from a donor whose identity is unknown to the couple, but whose physical characteristics as nearly as possible match those of the male partner. The use of AID requires much thought and discussion, as well as proper counseling, however, before a couple goes through with it.

Q. My wife and I have been trying to conceive for two years, but without success. It now appears that I have a very low sperm count and in practical terms am infertile. Can IVF do anything to help in our situation?
A. Recent advances in IVF techniques mean that nowadays infertile men may be helped as well. At some clinics, it is now possible to inject a single sperm—from a sperm sample collected from a man with a low count—directly into an isolated egg, and place the fertilized egg back inside the woman's uterus.

can be tracked using ultrasound and hormone tests. Just when follicles are due to burst and release mature eggs, a hollow needle is introduced into the ovary—usually through the vagina—under local anesthetic and some of the ripe follicles are removed.

The delicate eggs are examined under the microscope and are kept in a special culture fluid. After the male partner has provided a semen sample, his sperm are "washed" and mixed with individual eggs. After 48 hours, if any of the eggs have been fertilized, and look normal, one or two of the microscopic embryos are introduced along a tube into the uterus through the cervix in the hope that one of them will implant in the uterine lining and develop into a baby.

IVF has a success rate of 15–30 percent, and is most likely to succeed in younger women. IVF can also help in some cases of male infertility because it brings sperm and eggs into immediate contact, thereby maximizing the possibility of fertilization.

Ending a pregnancy

Pregnancy usually brings great joy and happiness to both a woman and her partner, whether the pregnancy is planned or not. However, there may be circumstances when a doctor or the woman herself decide that the pregnancy should be brought to an end prematurely by means of a therapeutic termination, or abortion. There are three main reasons why this difficult option may have to be considered.

• The physical health of the woman may be endangered by the pregnancy, so that she risks dying if she goes to full term.

• The fetus may be suffering from severe abnormalities that may kill it, or prevent it from having any sort of sustainable and normal existence.

• The pregnancy may be unplanned and unwanted. For example, a woman may be at a stage of her life where, because of her age (she may consider herself too young or too old) or because of other commitments, she does not want to be pregnant. She may have

become pregnant because her contraceptives did not work. Or, tragically, she may have become pregnant from rape or incest. Whatever the reason for pregnancy, she may ask her doctor for an abortion because she considers that continuing with the pregnancy will affect her mental health and, perhaps, the mental health of her existing children.

Therapeutic abortion means ending a pregnancy before its 24th week. Laws regarding abortion vary from country to country and even state to state. In the United States, the decision to have an abortion is made by the woman in consultation with her doctor.

Because of its emotive nature, the decision to have an abortion is often very difficult to make. This is not helped by the fact that abortion has become a highly politicized issue in the United States. A woman who wants to be pregnant but has been advised by her doctor to have a termination may feel that she is destroying a life that she should preserve. A woman whose pregnancy is unwanted may, paradoxically, have exactly the same feelings. Partners can help in either situation by providing support, although ultimately the decision to go ahead with an abortion (except in genuinely life-threatening situations) is the woman's. However, many hospitals and family-planning clinics provide counseling services for women in order to help them come to the decision that is right for them, and, should the woman decide to go ahead with a termination, to come to terms with her loss after the abortion has taken place.

After a termination, whether it is early or late, a woman must watch for signs of any complications—such as high temperature, excessive bleeding, or painful abdominal cramps—and consult her doctor if they appear. She will also need to return to the clinic or hospital for a checkup to make sure that everything is all right. From an emotional standpoint, a woman's reaction may depend on why she had the abortion. If the pregnancy was wanted, she may have feelings of guilt and anger, similar to those experienced by women who have had a stillbirth. She may have to tell friends and family that she has had an abortion only weeks after the joyful announcement that she is pregnant. Talking through her feelings with her partner, a counselor, and possibly a support group should help a woman come to terms with her loss. If the pregnancy was unwanted, a woman may feel relieved that she can get on with her life, but such feelings are often mixed up with sadness, anger, and grief, which, again, should be talked through with her partner, friends, and/or counselors.

Having an abortion

Once a woman and her doctor have decided that her pregnancy should be terminated, the method used for the termination will depend on the length of the pregnancy. The earlier an abortion is performed, the safer it is.

• If the pregnancy is to be terminated within seven weeks of the last period, a doctor may opt to use a nonsurgical abortion technique (although this is not available in the United States). On the first visit to the clinic, a woman takes an antiprogesterone drug (RU-486) by mouth, which brings the pregnancy to an end. Two days later, she returns to have a prostaglandin suppository inserted into her vagina, which will cause the uterus to contract and its lining to be shed. After both drug administrations, the woman is observed to see if the drugs are having the desired effect, and to ensure there are no side-effects. A final visit is then required within one or two weeks to check that there are no problems.

• The most common method of termination, which is used in the vast majority of cases, is the suction abortion or vacuum aspiration. This technique can be used in "early" abortions, up to the 12th week of pregnancy. Carried out under local or general anesthetic, the operation involves inserting a flexible tube through the dilated cervix through which the contents of the uterine cavity are sucked out. In some cases, the doctor may also use dilation and curettage (D and C—see p.106), to ensure that all fetal and placental tissues have been removed. After the procedure the woman will be required to remain in the recovery room for about an hour to ensure that she has recovered before leaving the hospital or clinic. During this time she may feel

COMPLICATIONS AND RISKS

The legalization of abortion has removed the curse of the back-street abortionists who caused the unnecessary deaths of so many women. But, as with many medical procedures, there are possible risks and complications associated with terminations carried out under standard conditions, and the later the abortion, the greater the risk of a complication.

• Having an abortion should not affect a woman's future ability to have children, but any procedure may introduce infection into the uterus, which could result in infertility.

• Excessive bleeding after an abortion may be an indication of tissue retained in the uterus, or of a perforated uterus. If she bleeds heavily, a woman should contact her doctor immediately.

• Retained tissue in the uterus after an abortion may also be indicated by painful cramps, prolonged bleeding, sore breasts, or the emergence of large blood clots via the vagina. If a woman notices any of these symptoms she should report it to her doctor promptly so that any retained tissue can be removed quickly.

• A high temperature (over 100.5°F) may indicate infection, a common complication of abortion. A woman suspecting infection should seek antibiotic treatment from her doctor to prevent the spread of infection.

strong contractions of the uterus as it returns to its original size. She may also feel tired and shaky, and perhaps nauseous. These feelings should soon pass.

• In later abortions, between 12 and 22 weeks of pregnancy, the preferred method is dilation and evacuation (D and E). This involves dilating the cervix (as with D and C) and using a curette, forceps, and suction to remove the uterine contents and lining.

• Another method after 16 weeks is induction abortion. This involves the use of prostaglandins to cause the uterus to contract and expel the fetus and placenta. This technique may be more distressing for women than suction abortion or D and E because it may involve many hours of waiting until labor begins and the small fetus is expelled.

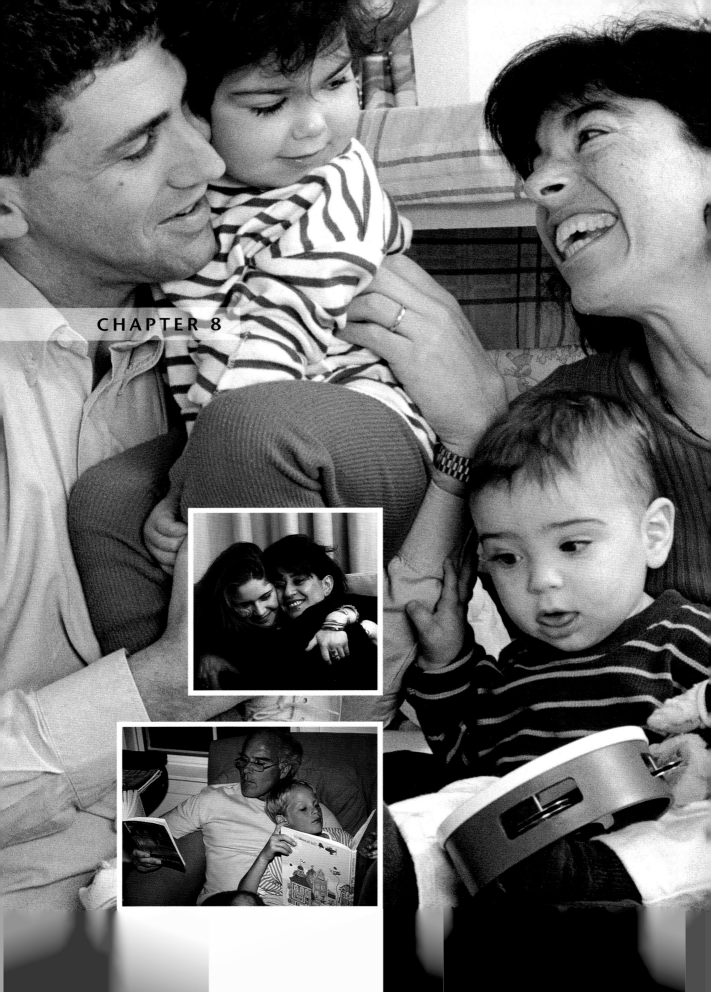

CHAPTER 8

The Family and Sexuality

What determines the nature of our adult sexuality? What controls the way in which we form relationships? And why do some people achieve longer-lasting and happier relationships than others? The answers to these questions are complex. But most significant of all the factors that mold how we relate to other people sexually and emotionally is the influence of those individuals who are closest to us during our early years—our family.

Yet what exactly is the family? In common mythology, much favored by advertising executives, a typical family consists of mom, dad, and two point four children. In reality, however, the family is not a standard-sized and readily quantifiable unit. In fact, the term "family" describes not only the members of the unit but also the complex interactions that take place between adults and children. True, this interactive unit may consist of two adults —a mom and dad—and their children. But a modern family is just as likely to consist of a single parent with one or more children, or be extended, by virtue of including stepchildren.

Despite this range of family structures, it is possible to tease out common factors that affect the way we will behave sexually as adults. The children of parents who adopt an encouraging, caring, and loving attitude, and who have a positive and open view of sex, are more likely to grow up with a well-adjusted attitude toward sexual matters. Similarly, if parents nurture and care for each other, their children are more likely to achieve a similar warmth and stability in their own relationships. Conversely, negative parental influences in the matter of sex and relationships may have a detrimental effect on their children's future relationships. The tensions, emotions, and interactions that exist between parents, between siblings, and between parents and siblings all serve to shape the family and influence a child's developing sexuality.

Another dimension of the family is its dynamism. The family is constantly changing, and parents need to note and cope with these alterations because any change in one part of the family will have an effect on the other part. Such adjustments may be positive and planned—a child starting school, for example, or a new baby. Or they may be devastating and unexpected, divorce or bereavement being the greatest changes that can affect a family. While it is true that divorce rates are increasing, it would be unreasonable to state that all children of divorced parents are unable to forge successful long-term relationships of their own. Even when parents do divorce, if they can show that as individual adults they still love and care for their children, they may be able to limit the emotional fallout resulting from their separation.

Family dynamics

Whatever the shape and size of a family, the nature of any relationships within it is of vital importance, both in terms of the happiness and stability of its individual members and as a learning environment, where children can develop an understanding of how people relate to each other.

It is important, therefore, that parents (and grandparents) monitor the way they treat their children. Although this may be obvious to most parents, maintaining a positive, affirmative attitude toward their children, especially when they are still young, will go a long way to ensuring the development of a

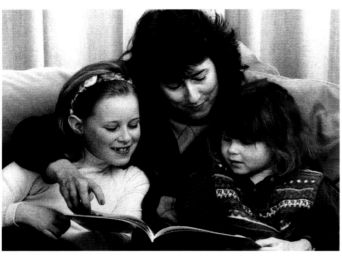

Reading together is one way for parents and children to spend quality time—a time when they focus on one another without being disturbed or distracted.

happy, well-balanced young adult. On the other hand, constantly criticizing and denigrating a young child will often have a negative effect, producing a child who is cautious and lacking in confidence. This can all too easily lead to a lack of self-esteem that can have a damaging effect on the development of personality during adolescence and young adulthood, and on future relationships.

Family relationships, and the overall shape of the family, do not remain static. From the first moment of interrelationship—be it the first meeting of two lovers, or the birth of a child to a single mother—the family ship begins its long voyage through uncharted waters. And while major family events, such as the arrival of a new child, may cause major changes in the relationships within the family, those complex relationships are also affected by events, however minor, that occur every day. Change and development within the family are ongoing processes. Parents need to monitor the dynamics of their family to ensure that the environment in which their children are growing up is appropriate, and that the family is developing in a positive and not a destructive way.

Bonding

The relationship between a baby and his or her parents is initiated very soon after birth. Visual, verbal, and physical interaction between parent and infant bring the two (or three) closer together, allowing mutual discovery and understanding to take place in a process known as bonding.

Although bonding is mostly referred to in the context of a newborn baby and his or her parents, it remains an important aspect of the relationship with both parents throughout childhood and into adolescence. In order to encourage bonding, it is important that parents make opportunities to spend "quality" time with their child regularly. Quality time can include talking, reading, or playing together, or perhaps watching a favorite television show together. For many parents and children, a key bonding time is when a parent reads a bedtime story to the child. Because this can be such a close and warm time, many children still enjoy this long after they are able to read themselves.

As children get older, especially during adolescence, the closeness between parents and child may apparently diminish. This may be true in physical terms—adolescents may prefer to be out with their friends rather than sitting at home with parents watching TV—but emotionally children will remain close to parents and still benefit from the bond between them. Talking about worries, stress, boyfriends, girlfriends, and all kinds of other problems and interests helps adolescents pass through this challenging part of their life less painfully. Independent though they may appear to be, adolescents are much in need of parental love and attention.

Parents as role models

The fact that, in most cases, parents and children spend many years in close proximity to one other within a family makes it inevitable that children will be influenced by the way parents relate to each other and to other adults. Generally, if parents have a warm and loving relationship with each other, this influence will rub off on the children. Conversely, if their relationship is not close, and if there are constant arguments, then children may well grow up with a negative model of family relationships. Fathers and sons often form close relationships, and the father is generally the son's main role model. Certainly, how the father behaves toward the boy's mother will set an example to his son, and he is likely—when he, in turn, is in a relationship—to treat his wife or girlfriend in the same way that he saw his father treat his mother. Since fathers and sons frequently follow this kind of behavior pattern, a father should be aware of the influence he has on his son when he is at an impressionable age. Similarly, the closeness between most mothers and their daughters means that the girl will be influenced by the way that her mother relates to her partner and to other men. Overall, parents should always be aware of the messages—both overt and hidden—that they send constantly to their children in the matter of relationships, for these will often have a considerable influence over the way that children go on to relate to their partners as adults.

Siblings

Siblings can be friends, and they can be allies (perhaps against their parents). They can teach, and learn, valuable lessons about sharing—possessions, love, and space—and about the importance of loyalty. The better the relationships between siblings, the more confident each child is likely to feel about forming relationships with other people.

Same-sex siblings have much to offer each other, whatever the age difference. Girls can

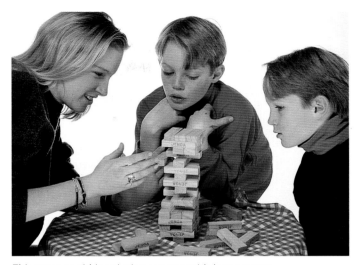

This teenage girl is enjoying a game with her younger brothers. Strong relationships can form between siblings regardless of age and sex differences.

talk to their sisters about any number of things that they might find it difficult to discuss with parents. For many girls there may be no one better to talk to than an older sister whom they can believe and trust. Boys can develop a similar kind of relationship with their brothers.

Having a sibling of the opposite sex has its value, too. For one thing, it is useful to develop an awareness from an early age of the differences between the sexes—both physical and emotional. Young people who have grown up, and had a good relationship, with an opposite-sex sibling or siblings may find it much easier to relate to the opposite sex during adolescence and adulthood than someone who has grown up either as an only child or with same-sex siblings.

In the same way that they bond with their children, parents can encourage bonding between their children. However, having a good relationship with siblings is neither universal nor compulsory. We all have personalities of our own, and just because we are closely related to someone does not mean that we have to get along well with them.

Only children

In the introduction to this chapter the myth of the "standard" family was mentioned. Just as a "normal" family may contain no children,

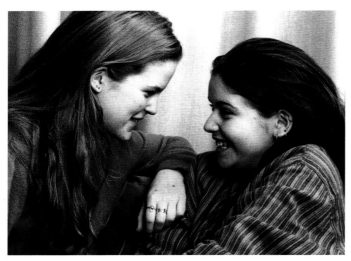

Only children do not have to be lonely children! Many children without brothers and sisters benefit from forming close friendships with other children to "fill the gap." The companionship and closeness of friends of the same age can be both reassuring and fun.

DO'S AND DON'TS FOR PARENTS OF ONLY CHILDREN

There are certain things that the parents of an only child may find helpful:

Do
• try to make sure your child has plenty of chances to meet and play with other children
• encourage him or her to share with other children
• make sure your child has interests that do not involve either parent.

Don't
• spoil the child
• be overprotective or possessive
• allow your child to grow up believing he or she is the center of the universe
• put too much pressure on the child to succeed
• lead your child to believe that his or her parents' happiness depends on the child's success.

QUESTION AND ANSWER: FAMILY RELATIONSHIPS

Q. My son is much closer to me than he is to his father. Will this mean that he is more likely to grow up gay?
A. There is no right or wrong way for children to relate to their individual parents, and your son's future sexual orientation will not be determined by his relationship with either of you. It is good that you and he are close, providing that he is not overwhelmed by you. But, unless there is great antipathy between him and his father, it may be worth finding a common interest for them to pursue together—perhaps a weekend camping and hiking—so that they can develop a closer relationship that will benefit both of them.

or five children, so it may contain just one child. While it is true that an only child misses out on some of the benefits that having brothers or sisters can bring, this does not mean that the child will grow up unable to form a close and caring sexual relationship with anyone else. Nor does it mean that she or he will become withdrawn and antisocial.

The way in which only children develop will depend on their personality, the relationship they have with parents, and the nature of their relationships with other relatives. One of the advantages of having siblings is that it may make it easier for a child to make friends. Parents can, if they wish, help an only child fill some of the gaps left by the absence of siblings by encouraging him or her to take part in activities with children of the same age, so that the child builds up a wide social network. Parents should also be aware that because an only child does not have siblings to form a relationship with, he or she may feel excluded by the closeness of the relationship between parents, or alternatively may be inclined to dominate it. While there is no need to smother the child with love or spoil him or her, parents with an only child may find it beneficial to spend more time bonding separately with the child than they would do with each child in a larger family.

There are also undoubtedly some benefits to be gained from being in a sibling-free family. Most only children get considerably more individual attention from their parents than they would if they had to share them. And, since not all brothers and sisters get along together, some children envy friends who are only children and do not have to put up with the constant bickering and teasing that seems to go on in their home.

Stereotyping roles

Parents often take on stereotypical roles in the way in which they relate to their children. For example, it is common for a mother to take her daughter to do the household shopping, while the father takes his son to watch football. But is there anything wrong with this? Probably not, because it is all part of the bonding process. While parental influences play a part in the development of gender role *(see pp.37–40),* many other factors also contribute toward a child's concept of his or her maleness or femaleness. However, it has been, and still is, traditional in many cultures to view females as the "weaker" sex and inferior to males. It is important for parents to make an effort to overcome such stereotyping by treating their children equally and providing them with equality of opportunity regardless of their gender. This will teach them valuable lessons about the equality of the sexes—both in a family context and on a wider scale.

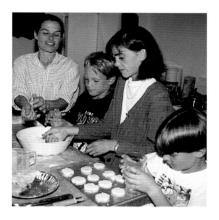

Playing together not only forges strong bonds between family members. it also allows parents to pass on—in a very subtle way—some important lessons about life and to influence their children to behave in a way they feel is appropriate.

Leisure activities

Leisure time is a great opportunity for family members to bond and strengthen ties. A family that spends time and plays together will probably also be happy together.

A way to encourage shared leisure activities might be for the family to sometimes go bowling or skating together, to share a hobby, or to go on vacation together. It is not the activity itself that matters so much as the fact that they do it together and that afterward they can talk and laugh about what happened. Anything that encourages communication is bound to improve family bonds.

Eating together is also an important event within the family. The regularity and constancy of sitting round a table and sharing food is vital in a child's development. In addition to being fed, the child learns how to behave when eating and listens to, and participates in, the conversations that take place between parents and other family members.

Outside interests

Although it is important for a family to enjoy some shared leisure activities, it is also important that individual members establish their own outside interests and friendships.

Outside interests and relationships add another stimulus to relationships within the family. They not only provide something else to talk about but also add a new focus of attention, not just for the person concerned but for the whole family.

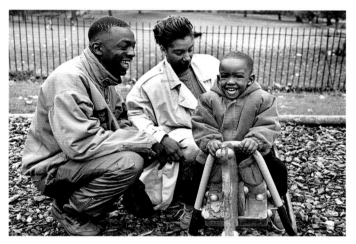

New relationships should never be seen as a threat. Far from replacing the child's attachment to his or her family, they should widen the social circle of acquaintances for both child and parents and, as a result, enrich the existing family attachments.

Learning to let go

Families are not static. Relationships develop and change as people get older. A parent's relationship with a baby is obviously not the same relationship as the one they have with a toddler, a school-age child, or a teenager, and parents must be prepared to adapt according to the changing needs of their growing child. They must accept that their offspring is gradually shedding a lot of his or her "childish" characteristics, and they must be prepared, when the time comes, for their child to become independent of her or his family. This gradual letting go may be a painful process but it should also be seen as a natural stage that most families go through *(see also pp.260–1).*

Responding to a child's development

It is not unusual for parents to feel slightly overwhelmed by the speed with which their children develop. In particular, it often comes as a shock to parents to realize that a child's sexuality develops at a relatively early age. However, this is just another stage in a child's development, and parents should simply take it in stride.

It is important for parents to discuss their feelings about their child's development, and any anxieties they may have. Parents should be careful to present a united front—if a child spots the smallest disagreement between them, he or she is almost bound to capitalize on it and to play one parent off against the other.

This is especially true when it comes to discipline. One parent may believe that children should merely have things carefully explained to them when they do something wrong; the other parent may prefer to admonish the child by raising their voice. Whatever they believe, they should agree beforehand on which line they are going to take and adopt a public policy in front of the children. Nothing is more likely to engender bad behavior in a child than any kind of contradictory message.

Sex education

Because sex is a central part of life, its importance should never be ignored. Children need to know and understand about sexual matters, although this need not be a constant topic of conversation. Parents may find it hard to broach what is traditionally seen as a difficult subject with their children. However, rather than waiting until their children are approaching their teens, it may be wiser for parents to start talking to their children about sex when they are young. At first it will probably be in response to questions such as "Where do I come from?" But if children receive sexual information—on a need-to-know basis—throughout childhood, by the time puberty arrives they will have a basic understanding of what is happening to them

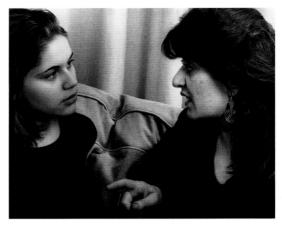

By talking to children in a positive way about sex and relationships from childhood on, parents can help ensure that they grow up to have a happy sex life.

sexually. By approaching sexual education in this way, a young person may be able to talk frankly and openly about sex with their parents at a time when it is probably taking on considerable importance in their lives. While most children have some kind of sex education at school, this tends to be fairly anatomical, and not related to the feelings and emotions of sex. Parents can play an important role in their child's future sexuality and relationships by providing them, slowly but surely, with a clear overview of sex, and by giving the message in a way that shows sex in a positive light—as something pleasurable under the right circumstances.

One specific way in which parents can help their children is to prepare them for the physical and emotional changes that will come with puberty. A girl should, by the age of nine or ten, be aware that she will over the next few years develop pubic hair and breasts, and that her periods will start. Similarly, boys should also know about body hair, penis growth, and ejaculation. While some parents regard childhood as an age of "innocence" that should remain unsullied by talk of sex, it does the child no good not to know, at an appropriate level, about sexual and emotional matters. Sex is not sinful, and ignorance about sexual matters in late childhood can allow a child to grow up with a negative and guilt-ridden attitude toward both sex and relationships.

While it is considered important for parents to be positive and open with their children about sexual matters, they may not feel the same about sexual information and images that their children see on television and in other media. Sex and sexuality portrayed on screen or in books is often dominated by a stereotypical attitude toward sex, and that attitude may not match up with the type of sexual message that parents wish to convey to their children. In movies men are commonly portrayed as sexual aggressors, and women as passive recipients. For that reason parents may find it helpful to monitor television and other portrayals of sex to which their children may be exposed.

Being a parent and a sexual partner

Once a couple has adjusted to the inevitable changes to their relationship caused by having a baby, they may be tempted to think that life will soon return to normal. In reality their life will never be quite the same as it was before the arrival of a child. A baby is very demanding and may well require attention at any time, day or night. Equally, once children are older—and capable of fending for themselves to a much greater extent—they are nonetheless bound to make demands on the time, attention, and energies of their parents. There will be school commitments, help with homework, and all the inevitable ferrying around to outside activities, not to mention simply being available for the children when they want comfort, help, advice, or just some company.

There are so many things within a relationship that vie for attention—job, housework, friends, hobbies—that a couple can end up seeming to have little time for each other. Once a couple has a child, they are likely to have less time for sex. This will be particularly noticeable if they had the kind of relationship before where it was usual for them to have sex as the mood took them. Now this part of their relationship is likely to be relegated to bedtimes and may not be as much fun as before.

New parents may also feel differently about sex because, in some subconscious way, having a child has made them identify more closely with their own parents. People rarely acknowledge that their parents had any sex life, let alone an exciting one. The fact that they, too, are now parents may lead a couple to believe that they should behave like responsible, mature adults, and this may mean that sex plays a less important part in life. There is no need for this to happen.

A couple should try to ensure that their sex life has the same importance in their life as it had earlier in their relationship. If, in spite of all their best efforts, sex has taken a backseat for a while, it is all too easy to make the mistake of ceasing even to show any physical affection, in case the more enthusiastic partner tries to take things further. But it is very important for a couple to make sure that physical affection remains an integral part of their relationship, particularly at this time, when they are both likely to need the reassurance that they are still loved and that the child hasn't ruined things between them. It is also important for partners to talk to each other during this period and tell each other what they are feeling.

Knowing that their parents have sex

It is very important for children to know that their parents are happy together. This is good for their own happiness and helps them feel secure. It is also good for their emotional well-being—and later for their own sexual development—to realize that their parents

NUDITY IN FRONT OF YOUR CHILDREN

Parents see their children naked and many parents feel there is no reason why children should not, in turn, see their parents naked. These parents consider nudity to be a natural and harmless part of life in a family. Certainly nakedness in this context allows children to develop a healthy attitude toward the differences between male and female bodies that will extend into adulthood. Other parents, however, may feel less comfortable about nudity, perhaps because of the way they were brought up. They might find such behavior acceptable while the children are very young, but feel it should cease when the children are older and more sexually aware. Whichever policy the parents decide to adopt is up to them; they should pursue the one that they feel happiest and most comfortable with.

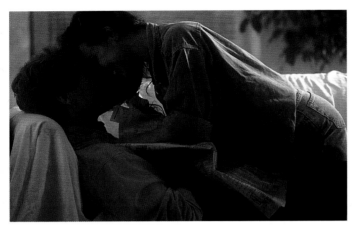

Just because they have a young family does not mean that a couple has to give up sex. Making time and opportunities for sex can spice up a couple's relationship and make sex even more enjoyable.

QUESTIONS & ANSWERS: ADJUSTING TO CHILDREN

Q. My husband has always liked to kiss and hug, and I used to think it was great. We now have a three-year-old daughter. My husband still wants to behave in much the same way but I find it oddly embarrassing in front of her. Am I being oversensitive?

A. Perhaps you are. It can only be good for your daughter to see spontaneous physical affection between you. It teaches her the value of physical closeness between two people who love each other, which is one of the first and most valuable lessons she can learn as part of her early sex education. (However, while hugging and kissing are fine, groping and fondling are too adult for a child to understand.) Don't reject your husband's warmth, welcome it.

Q. Our little girl likes to get into our bed during the night. She always manages to squeeze in between my wife and me. If we all stay in bed, none of us gets a good night's sleep, so one of us—and it's usually me—spends the rest of the night in the spare room. I feel that my bed has been taken over. My wife says it's just a phase and it'll pass, but I don't agree. What can we do?

A. There are people who express the joys of a family sleeping together in one giant bed, but the great majority of parents are like you and resent their sleep being disturbed. Other than when a child is sick (and sometimes even then), it is wise to exclude the child from the parents' bed, and you should do this now before it becomes too hard a habit to break. Some children are very good at slipping into their parents' bed and lying there unnoticed for quite a long time. If this happens, put the child back to bed right away. If the child comes back a second time, return them to bed again, but this time show that you are mildly displeased with their behavior.

enjoy a close relationship that involves them showing affection to each other both at home and in public. As children get older they will probably come to realize that an important component of their parents' closeness is their sexual relationship, although, of course, children should not in any way be overtly confronted with this fact. Making the link between sex and feelings is almost as important a part of their sex education as conversations with them about sex or their formal sex education at school. Some parents are embarrassed by the thought of their children knowing they have sex, but there is no need for this. Sex is a completely natural activity, and embarrassment or guilt should play no part in it. Anything that helps their children understand the importance of sex in a happy and loving relationship can only be a good thing.

Making time for sex

Couples who have children often complain that it is difficult to find time to have sex. This is particularly so when there is a baby, because they can demand attention at any time, day or night, but even when the children have grown it can still be a problem.

Children need to learn as they get older that there are times when their parents like to be alone and that they cannot always have their parents' undivided attention. Many parents find it helpful to teach their children to knock on their bedroom door before coming in; as children get older, a reciprocal arrangement can be established so that parents also knock on the child's door before entering their room.

If constant interruption by children, or thin walls between bedrooms, is a problem, it is essential to make time for sex (or at least for uninterrupted intimacy, if the couple are not in the mood for sex at the allotted time). It might be possible for the children to spend the night with a relative or friend or, if they can afford it, for the parents to treat themselves to a hotel for the night while a baby-sitter stays with the children.

This kind of approach may make sex seem less than spontaneous. But although

GRANDPARENTS

Grandparents have an important—yet often overlooked—role to play in the family. A grandparent is like a wise elder, more detached than a parent; this often allows a close bond to develop between grandparents and grandchildren, and grandparents may exert a valuable stabilizing influence. Because of that closeness, grandparents may be badly affected by a divorce, particularly if they are the parents of the partner who left. Separation can mean that they lose regular contact with their grandchildren, which can be a great sadness for people in their later years. They may feel frustrated that they seem to have no control over the situation. Ultimately it is not only the grandparents but also the grandchildren who lose out, as children can benefit enormously from relationships with their older relatives. Indeed, a good relationship with loving grandparents may help to offset any strained or difficult atmosphere that the child has been experiencing at home.

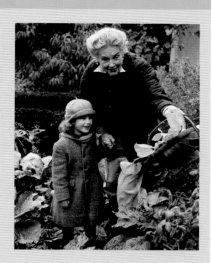

spontaneous sex can be wonderful, it is not the only way to make love. Planning a sexual enounter in advance and enjoying the anticipation of it can be just as exciting.

Separation and divorce

When any couple separates, it is likely to be a dramatic change, not only for them but also for the people around them. Separation can mean great relief or a terrible sense of loss akin to bereavement, or feelings somewhere between these two extremes, or a combination of both—it all depends on the nature of the relationship. Separation will also have an effect on the children of a relationship, although these effects may be much more subtle and less obvious.

Being the partner who moves out of the family home

When a relationship ends there is usually one partner who has to move out of the family home that he or she has shared with a partner for, perhaps, many years. Moving under any circumstances can be very stressful, but being obliged to leave because of the breakup of a relationship can be even more so. The following may help ease the pain.
• Try to take a positive approach and see finding and moving into a new home as the

beginning of the next phase of your life.
• Decorate your new home in a way that reflects your character and feelings.
• If your children are living with your partner, make space for them in a special room that they can play or sleep in when they come to visit you.
• Take your mind off your move by taking up new interests and making new friends.
• Try not to think about your old home and what may be happening to it, in the same way that you should try not to let your old relationship dominate your thoughts.
• Don't see yourself as a loser because you had to move out of the family home.

The partner who stays

Facing life alone after years of being—albeit perhaps unhappily—with a partner can be a daunting prospect. There are few people who find it an easy transition, although many experience an overwhelming sense of relief that the relationship is over and tensions have been removed. It is important to capitalize on that relief—to enjoy the fact that the house is now, for the time being anyway, yours alone:
• Move your ex-partner's things out of the way, and remove any reminders of them that you find it difficult to have around. This is your (and possibly your children's) home now, and it should feel like home.
• Rearrange your furniture as you choose.

- Enjoy your newfound freedom to do what you want, when you want.
- Invite friends over to share your new existence with you.
- Even when you're eating alone, do it properly—cook a nice meal, set the table, light some candles.

Children of separated parents

The separation of their parents can be a very sad time for most children, whatever their age. It may feel like the end of their world, and they are likely to be overcome by feelings of loss, even panic. Stability and continuity are of great importance to a child, and there are few things more worrying than an uncertain future. However, they may, at the same time, experience a feeling of relief when their parents break up, especially if they were aware of the tension between them, or if they did not get along particularly well with the parent who is moving out.

When parents separate, a child often loses daily contact with the parent who leaves. A very young child is unlikely to understand exactly what has happened, even when the circumstances are carefully explained to them—as they should be. All they know is that the parent has left them, and they may feel that it must be their fault. Perhaps they did something wrong, or perhaps they were not lovable enough for the parent to think it was worth staying around. Even an older child, who understands why his or her parents split up, may have similar feelings of guilt or rejection. Children need a lot of care at this time. They need to know that both their parents love them, that what happened was not their fault, and that their future is not as bleak as they may imagine.

A child may also worry that, if it happened once, it may well happen again and the other parent may also leave. This will obviously increase the child's feelings of insecurity and anxiety. Separation may convey the message that love can end unexpectedly and for no apparent reason, and that however strong your feelings for someone, they may still leave. Feelings such as this can affect a child's lifelong emotional development, so that when that child grows up he or she may find it difficult to trust their partner and sustain a long-term relationship.

The more acrimonious the breakup, the more difficult it will be for children to deal with. It will be even worse if they are put in the middle and encouraged to take sides. Children understand from an early age that they are made up of half mommy, half daddy. If they learn to hate one parent, they may well begin to hate part of themselves. Children need to respect both parents in order to develop healthy self-esteem. And to this end it is very helpful if a separated parent refrains, whatever his or her feelings, from denigrating his or her ex-partner in front of the children. Of course it is healthiest for children if the separation can take place quietly and calmly, with ex-partners remaining friends and the children seeing both parents regularly.

MOVING

The child who is forced to move homes very frequently—perhaps because parents have broken up or because of changing financial circumstances—may grow up feeling insecure. A child's relationship with his or her home is very close. Moving often produces concerns for a child about, for example, changing schools or having to make new friends. If everything else in a child's life is secure—the child gets along well with their siblings and parents, and there is no friction between the parents—frequent moves are unlikely to cause any serious problems. But if families move often, and there is a background of other difficulties, their parents or parent must anticipate that the child will feel even more insecure.

QUESTION AND ANSWER: MOTHER AND CHILD

Q. My relationship with my daughter has been a great comfort to me during my divorce. She has been very supportive and we have become very close. My friends say I was wrong to let this happen and that I should try not to involve her so much in my sadness. Are they right?
A. It is hard for a child to witness a parent's unhappiness. By all means take comfort in the quality of your relationship, but try not to cling or share intense feelings: this is a heavy burden to bear, demanding emotional maturity that she cannot yet possess, even if she seems to. It may later make her fear strong emotions, be they feelings of love or grief and sorrow.

Both during and after their parents' divorce, children often show their unhappiness in the following characteristic ways.
• Young children in particular may suffer from nightmares, become frightened of the dark, or have difficulty in getting to sleep.
• Older children may become withdrawn or depressed and unwilling to communicate.
• Children may become more disobedient or quarrelsome than usual; their unhappiness can also be shown by unexpected aggression to siblings, animals, or children at school.
• They may fall behind with schoolwork or make excuses for cutting school.

In any of these situations it is important that the parents stay calm. They should work to be understanding and supportive during an unsettling period in their children's lives.

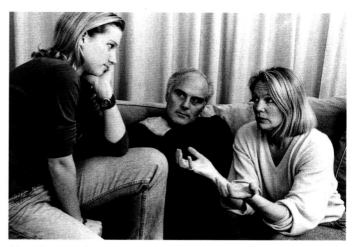

After divorce or bereavement, forming relationships within a new family can be difficult for both children and parents. Stepchildren may find great difficulty relating to a stepparent, and vice versa. Discussing matters openly can help iron out some of these problems.

New families

After separation or divorce, many people may feel that they will never commit themselves to another relationship. But after a few years —or even months—when the wounds are beginning to heal and the person is beginning to feel lonely, a new relationship may start to seem like a more attractive proposition.

Although entering a new relationship will initially be exciting and challenging, as with all major changes in life, it may also prove quite stressful. Someone who has recently escaped from a failed relationship may understandably find it difficult to contemplate the idea of committing themselves to another relationship. But unless he or she chooses to remain single for the rest of their life, there comes a time when they must be prepared to make that new commitment. Someone who has become accustomed to living on their own, sleeping on their own, and doing exactly as they please when they please may find it hard to adjust to being one half of a couple and to taking someone else into account when it comes to making decisions. They may also find that their new sexual relationship is completely different from the one they had with their ex-partner, and that they need to make adjustments sexually as well.

HELPING YOUR CHILDREN COPE WITH DIVORCE

Helping your children deal with the pain of their parents' divorce is a delicate balancing act requiring a lot of sensitivity. You must neither neglect them nor cling to them too tightly. However, there are ways you can help your children get through this difficult time.
• Let them know you love them.
• Reassure them that they are in no way to blame for the situation.
• Try not to upset their normal family routine more than is absolutely necessary.
• However unhappy and preoccupied you are, always make time for your children and never let them feel neglected.
• Do not involve them in arguments between you and your partner; try to make sure they never witness angry exchanges, especially those involving physical violence.
• Do not ask them to take sides between you.
• Do not cling too tightly to them or make them feel that they are essential to your well-being.

Stepfamilies

Forming a new relationship may involve the integration of children from previous relationships to form a stepfamily. The relationships in stepfamilies are not always easy, be they the one between stepmother and ex-wife, or stepfather and ex-husband, or stepparents and their partner's children. Stepfamilies need a particularly strong relationship between the couple for the simple reason that the parenting bond between them is based not on the fact that they had a child together but on their desire to share their life. For some people, the stepfamily works well from the beginning, and there are few problems. For the great majority of stepfamilies, however, there are bound to be tensions, which need to be resolved. Children, especially adolescents, may resent the imposition of the authority of a new father or mother, especially if they have a good relationship with the parent who has left the family home. They may not get along with any new step-siblings, or they may find that, in the short term at least, the atmosphere is not as open or relaxed as it used to be. Stepfathers or stepmothers may be angered and upset by the attitude and antipathy of their partner's children—it can be very trying to be with someone you love if their children apparently hate you. As with all family matters, it helps if members of the stepfamily can learn to communicate. This will probably take time, require a great deal of give and take, and involve restraint as family members learn not to impose their will on others. Eventually, in most cases, the stepfamily will work efficiently as a family, and the children of the stepfamily should develop "normally," perhaps enriched by the change in family structure. If things do not work out, however, it may be worth seeking family therapy so that an outsider can attempt to mediate between "warring factions" within the stepfamily.

Stepparents

Finding a new partner with whom to start again is seldom easy. Finding a new partner who is also prepared to take on a ready-made family that includes children from a previous relationship can be harder still.

The relationship between stepparent and stepchild may be difficult. Children often find the new relationship troublesome because

THE PLUS FACTORS IN COMBINING FAMILIES

There are many positive things that can be gained from combining families. For the adults concerned, the benefits include:

• companionship

• a close physical relationship

• a feeling of warmth and belonging which family life often brings

• sharing problems and responsibilities;

• another adult to talk to about day-to-day family situations.

For some children (such as an only child in a one-parent family), this may be the first time they have lived in a family group. The transition may be difficult—children can become just as set in their ways as a single adult once they've gotten used to being on their own—but the benefits include:

• companionship

• an extended social life

• the feeling of "belonging" that family life usually brings

• new sibling relationships, with all the benefits these bring

• other new relationships (stepgrandparents, aunts and uncles, and so on).

BECOMING A STEPPARENT

Taking on someone else's children by a previous relationship may seem like a good idea, but it can actually be very difficult. Even biological parents don't always bond with their own children, so it's hardly surprising that it can be difficult for a stepparent to be able to love someone else's children immediately. Advice for new or prospective stepparents should include the following.

• Don't force or rush relationships with children.

• Try to see things from the child's point of view.

• Be both patient and understanding, and don't be surprised when the child behaves badly.

• Realize that any aggressive or difficult behavior on the part of the stepchild is not so much a dislike of you as a sign of deep-seated insecurities.

• Allow the children to decide what they want to call you.

• Make sure you spend time alone with your new partner with no children around.

• Don't criticize the absent parent.

• Be prepared to act as an unbiased mediator, if necessary, between your own children and those of your new partner.

they generally find any major change unsettling. They are often reluctant to trust a new partner, and may resent the presence of someone whom they see as usurping their key position in their parent's affections. They are likely to experience a conflict of loyalty between their natural parents—and that includes the absent one—and their new stepparent. There is, on the one hand, a desire to develop a good relationship, and, on the other hand, a fear of that relationship developing too quickly. And because the stepparent and child do not share any mutual history of loving and caring, it is inevitable that tensions will sometimes erupt.

Some studies have predicted that by the turn of the century stepfamilies are likely to be the most common family unit. However, perhaps surprisingly, it is a unit that works well for many thousands of people. If things seem to be difficult at first, it is important not to become despondent, and to be patient. Time and commitment are the key factors in making new relationships work.

Being a single parent

The most common reason why people become single parents is as a result of separation or divorce. Following the trauma of separation, a single parent also has to take on the added responsibility of being in sole charge of the child, or children, of the dissolved partnership. However, despite the apparent burdens of this role, many women, and men, find it not just consoling but also inspiring. In addition to company, a child can provide an immediate focus of interest so that the parent can get over the breakup of the relationship more readily through nurturing and encouraging their offspring.

Less commonly, single parenthood is the result of being widowed. This is usually an even more difficult situation, due to the greater grief felt by both parent and children.

Another reason for single parenthood is the choice that an increasing number of women make in favor of single motherhood. A few women get pregnant with the express

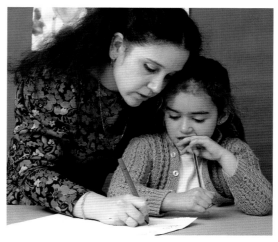

Single parenthood need not always present problems. There is no reason why children should not be brought up as happy and well-balanced individuals simply because they live with one parent rather than two.

intention of raising the baby on their own. Most single women get pregnant by accident and then decide to have the baby rather than have an abortion, even though they are not in a permanent relationship.

Facing life as a single parent

When someone first becomes a single parent it is common for them to concentrate all their efforts on their children. But although children need a lot of attention at this time, the parent should not focus every ounce of their worry and attention on the child. They must not forget their own needs; they must face their own hurt feelings and anxieties. Only by facing them can they resolve them.

The feelings of a newly single parent may include anger, loneliness, insecurity, uncertainty about the future, money worries, and a sense of panic at having to cope with everything alone. But the parent may also feel great relief at no longer being in an unpleasant and bitter relationship; or elation at finding new and unfamiliar feelings of freedom; or a positive sense of a new beginning, coupled with optimism regarding the future.

The single-parent family

If single parenthood has come about as a result of divorce or death, there is bound to be a sudden change in family dynamics.

What was once a two-parents-plus-child (or children) setup suddenly becomes a one-parent-plus-child setup. Even if the now absent parent was not at home much before, he or she was around some of the time, and members of the family were constantly reminded of them.

Departure of one parent from the family home is bound to have an effect on the relationship between the remaining parent and child. It is not unusual for the child to express sadness and anxieties at this time as anger—and the only person who is around to be angry with is the parent with whom they still live. This can be difficult for a newly single parent to cope with, but it is essential that the parent use the patience and understanding needed to make the effort now in order to avoid damaging their long-term relationship with their child. The lone parent may also be astounded—and angered—by the strong feelings held by a child toward the departed partner, particularly if that partner has behaved badly in the past. This type of behavior is common in children and should be accepted as such; a single parent should not embark on a propaganda campaign for or against an ex-partner in an attempt to bring a child around to their point of view. This will probably not work, and anyway it is better to let children make up their own mind.

The relationship between absent parent and child

Difficult as things may be, the single parent who lives with his or her children is comparatively lucky. It is much more difficult for parents to build a good relationship with children when they don't live with them.

It is not unusual for the absent parent, whose relationship with their child is often overshadowed by feelings of guilt, to try to buy their children's love by showering them with expensive presents. This is unlikely to succeed in the long term, and can only make things worse for the other parent who is living with the child and may not be able to afford to spend money on comparable gifts.

The relationship between ex-partners

However angry they are, there is no way that two people can sever all connection between them if they have a child. Contact between divorced couples may be difficult, even if they are no longer arguing about money or property. There may still be a residue of bitterness and dislike that is hard to overcome.

Children often sense these negative emotions and find them difficult to deal with. It is for this reason that it is so important to try to maintain as civil and calm a relationship as possible between ex-partners, with as little arguing and sniping as possible.

QUESTIONS AND ANSWERS: THE EFFECTS OF DIVORCE ON CHILDREN

Q. I was devastated when my parents separated when I was 10. It was as if my world had ended. I recently married but I've been postponing the decision to have children because I'm frightened of putting any kids of mine through the same situation. Am I being silly?
A. It is true that, statistically, people whose parents have split up seem to be more likely to divorce themselves. However, there is no reason why this should happen to you, and you should not allow yourself to be influenced by that part of your history. You have clearly thought about this: you know how awful it can be for a child and you know, too, how important it is to keep your marriage stable. Your self-knowledge should give you the determination to succeed.

Q. My husband thinks we should get a divorce, but I'm worried about the effect this will have on the children. I've heard that research shows that children are better off with two unhappy parents than with divorced parents. Is this true?
A. This depends to a large extent on the circumstances. Two unhappy parents are one thing, but two warring parents, constantly arguing and scoring points off each other, are another. An amicable divorce, on the other hand, may not be very damaging to the children, while an acrimonious one, with both parents doing their best to turn the children against the other parent, can cause a lot of damage. In other words, it's not so much whether or not you divorce as the circumstances along either path.

Single fathers

Although there are far fewer single fathers than there are single mothers, their numbers are increasing and the problems they face are much the same as those confronting single mothers. People are often surprised when a single father does a good job of parenting, but there is absolutely no reason why a man should not be capable of bringing up a child well and happily without the help or support of a partner.

Gay and lesbian parents

In some families, both parents are of the same sex and having a homosexual relationship. Gay families can attract considerable criticism and prejudice but there is no reason why gay parents of either sex should not have the same close and loving relationship with their children as other parents—as well as the caring, the dedication, the ups and downs, the closeness, and the fights found in all families.

Some gay parents may have had their children while they were in a heterosexual relationship, and when this relationship finished took their children with them into their new relationship. Often this happens after a custody battle in which their sexuality may have been raised as a reason why they should not be granted custody. It is more usually lesbian mothers who manage to gain custody of their children, rather than gay fathers. Social disapproval of homosexual men, together with the usual custom of awarding custody to the mother, means that there are very few openly gay fathers who have custody of their children. Many gay men even have to fight hard for access rights. It may be particularly difficult for a heterosexual partner who was left for the sake of a gay or lesbian relationship to encourage their child to have frequent contact with the homosexual parent, but for the sake of the child they need to do their best not to allow their own feelings to get in the way.

Some lesbian couples start their own families. They usually do this by selecting a man — perhaps a close friend—to provide the sperm

ROLE MODELS WHEN PARENTS ARE GAY

Does gay parenting present any problems? One possible problem when the parents are lesbian is that because both parents are women there may not be a male role model for a young boy. (The problem does not arise so much with a child living with a gay father, as there will probably be daily contact with women at the child's school so that he or she is less likely to miss out on female role models.) Some lesbians think their children see enough men—perhaps their father and adult friends—for this not to be a problem. Others think that it won't do boys any harm to be brought up in a predominantly female society, in which values such as tolerance and sensitivity are perceived to be paramount.

necessary for one of them to become a mother (conception usually takes place using artificial insemination). Alternatively, they might pay for artificial insemination by an agency that provides sperm samples with descriptive profiles of the men who supplied them.

Coming out to children

If children are brought up by a gay couple, they are sure to learn and understand the nature of their parents' relationship from the way they and their friends behave. In this way they should develop an accepting attitude toward both homosexual and heterosexual relationships but not be swayed as to the way their own sexual preferences will turn out.

Where a parent has left a heterosexual relationship to embark on a gay relationship the situation may not be so straightforward. It is rarely easy for a gay or lesbian to "come out" and reveal their sexuality to the world. It can be still more difficult for a parent to come out and reveal it to their children. This can be a major hurdle in parents' relationship with their children, partly because of the social prejudice surrounding gay and lesbian relationships and partly because many people find it difficult to discuss their sexuality with anyone, let alone their own children. However, the more open a parent can be with children, the easier it will be for those children to appreciate and understand the situation, and the less likely it is that their own relationships will be adversely affected in later life.

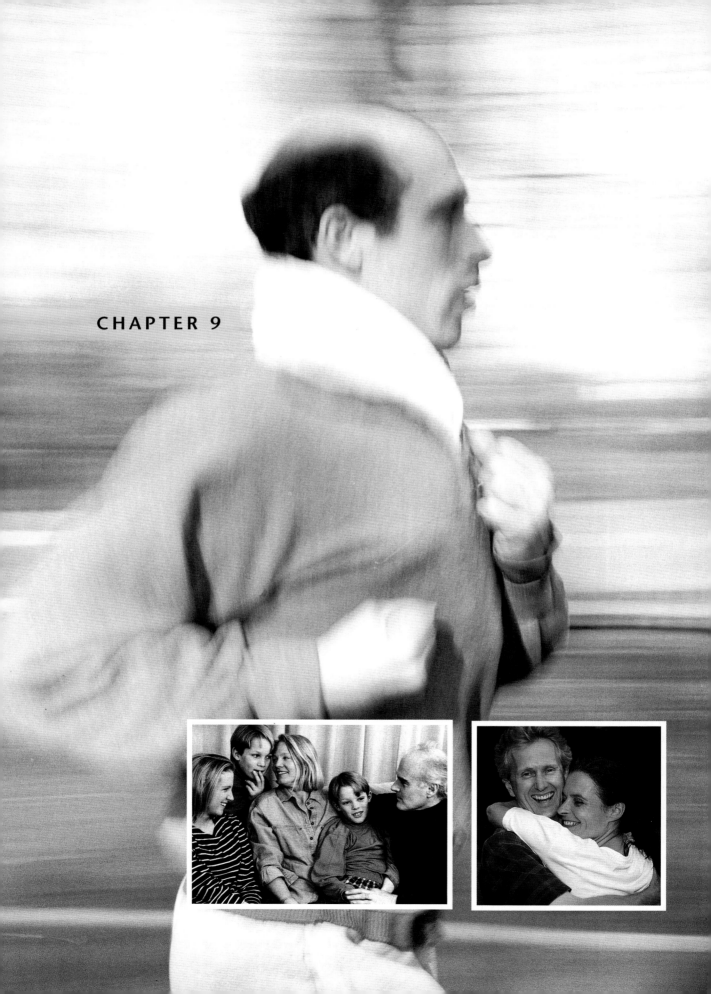

CHAPTER 9

The Middle Years

We may be too busy to notice that we have stopped being young adults and have reached the middle years of our lives, the period spanning our forties and fifties. Indeed, most people do not think of themselves as "older," since they have many of the same attitudes, desires, and expectations that they had 10 or 20 years earlier. Yet while we are focusing on establishing a home, bringing up a family, and pursuing a career, the more narcissistic attitudes of our twenties fall by the wayside as we adopt what we see as a more mature attitude toward life. This can be a very productive time: we have the benefit of experience, feel more relaxed about day-to-day challenges, and are usually more confident.

The middle years can also be a time of great change. Parents may see their children growing up and leaving home, causing them to redefine their family structure; they may find their relationship with each other is not working, perhaps to such an extent that they finally separate and start a new existence; or they may suffer the loss of a parent or find themselves looking after an elderly parent. Or occasionally, the transition from youth through middle to older age may pass with scarcely any upsets or upheavals.

In the middle years, the physical consequences of aging have yet to make any real impact. But it is important for individuals to be concerned about their health, however busy they may be. By eating well, exercising regularly, and enjoying general good health, men and women in their middle years can be nearly as fit and active as they were in their twenties. Establishing and maintaining a healthy lifestyle can pay great dividends in old age, by helping to reduce the chances of poor health. Being in good shape will also help a man or woman to look attractive and feel confident, both factors that will enhance their sexuality and help them enjoy a good sex life.

Many people feel in their middle years that any sign of aging will make them less attractive. In fact, aging has little effect on attractiveness to partners or would-be partners. For most people, especially as they get older, personality and intellect are more important than physical attributes.

Couples often find that their satisfaction with and enjoyment of sex increases in their middle years. As they become more experienced and confident in themselves, develop a greater understanding of their partner's needs and desires, and have had the time to explore their sexuality, men and women can feel more sexually fulfilled than when they were younger. Nevertheless, they may benefit from considering whether their sex lives could be improved if they tried new ways of making love and avoided the same old routines.

Advance planning for a longer life

Besides being a time for dealing with change, the middle years are also a time to plan for the future. Some people already have a healthy lifestyle, with a balanced, varied diet, plenty of exercise, limited alcohol, and no smoking or recreational drugs. But if they are not as healthy as they could be, they may wish to make changes. However, anyone in their forties or fifties who has not gotten regular exercise before, or who has had any major health problems, should consult their doctor before embarking on an exercise regimen, and should take it easy at first.

Smoking

People who smoke should stop immediately. Smoking is affecting their present health, and is almost certain to shorten their lives. Those who need help to stop should talk to their doctor, who may be able to prescribe a nicotine substitute to help wean them off.

Exercise plays a key part in maintaining good health and fitness. It can take the form of gym training (right) *or just a jog in the park. Stretching* (below) *helps keep the body supple and free of aches and pains.*

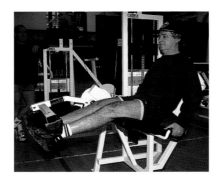

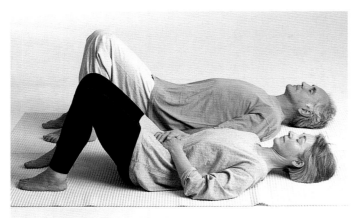

Keeping trim and slim

Keep trim with regular exercise and a healthy diet. An increasing proportion of men and women in the developed world are overweight, with a smaller proportion of them obese (they have a body weight 20 percent over the ideal maximum). But by keeping body weight within ideal limits (which can be determined by measuring body mass index or BMI—*see p.88*), and by maintaining the proportion of body fat at 15–20 percent for men or 20–25 percent for women, the body is under less strain from being overweight, and at much lower risk of disorders such as high blood pressure and joint problems.

Exercise

Exercise should be regular, and not less than three times each week. Each session should last for at least 20 minutes and the exercise should be aerobic *(see pp.88–90)*, such as walking, jogging, running, or swimming. Exercise does not need to be a formal workout in a gym. A brisk walk through a park, or to work, is a perfectly adequate form of low-impact aerobic exercise. Regular exercise keeps people trim by preventing fat accumulation, and by improving muscle tone so that the body's skeletal muscles perform a better job of supporting the body. It also improves cardiovascular fitness, helping the heart work more efficiently, and maintains bone mass, counteracting the effect of the bone loss that occurs naturally after the mid-thirties. Anaerobic exercise—such as weight training—can also be undertaken to increase muscle bulk, compensating for the loss of muscle tissue that occurs as people get older.

Stretching and flexibility

In addition to aerobic and perhaps anaerobic exercise, those in the middle years should try to do a range of stretching exercises as part of a daily routine in order to maintain flexibility, improve their posture, prevent aches and pains (including backache), and prevent muscle strains and tears during exercise. A regular program of stretching will help avoid postural and joint problems in later life.

Diet

A balanced diet *(see pp.88–9)* keeps the body in good shape; helps to avoid or protect against certain disorders, including cardio-vascular disease and cancers; and is essential to ensure that the body's defense system keeps working effectively.

Controlling alcohol intake

Recent research has shown that moderate intake of alcohol can have a beneficial effect on the body. But excessive alcohol—for example, long-term daily consumption of several glasses of wine, beer, or spirits—is damaging to health. And because alcohol consists of "empty" calories (it is not part of a food that contains other nutrients or fiber), it causes weight gain if consumed in excess. If an alcohol habit has developed by the middle years, it will probably continue in old age, so now is the time to act to control it.

Avoiding becoming a "couch potato"

Watching television, especially for prolonged periods, reduces the body's metabolic rate—the rate at which it consumes energy. Combine this with the tendency of many devoted TV watchers (so-called couch potatoes) to eat and drink while watching television, and you have an ideal recipe for weight increase and reduced fitness. The solution is to try to ration the amount of TV watched, or, if possible, exercise while watching it by using an exercise bike or treadmill.

In the majority of cases, a person's metabolic rate decreases as he or she gets older, as a natural consequence of aging. This means that the body requires slightly less energy (measured as calories) each day to keep it running normally. But if the same number of calories are consumed as before, there will be a tendency to put on weight. So it is wise to reduce daily calorie intake as we get older, while not compromising the range and balance of our diet. Also, regular exercise will help counteract the drop in metabolic rate.

As we live in the age of the car, it is only too easy to drive very small distances that we could easily walk. Try walking (or cycling) short distances to do some shopping or buy a

newspaper. Given a choice between elevator and stairs, take the latter if at all feasible; when taking an escalator or moving sidewalk, walk rather than stand still.

Preserving mental agility

There seems little doubt that staying mentally active in old age can do a lot to prevent some of the mental problems associated with aging. And it is useful for people in their middle years to think about exactly how mentally stimulated they are. How best to initiate a program of mental stimulation that will last into old age depends on each individual, but enrolling for an adult education course, reading, writing stories, keeping a journal, or taking up hobbies and games such as cards and crosswords will all exercise the mind.

Feeling good and looking good

Men and women who have been distracted from exercise or good diet by the all-too-absorbing demands of work or child care may decide to change their ways when they notice the first signs of aging. A healthier lifestyle will improve their fitness so that they look and feel better. It will also improve a person's self-esteem, make them look and feel more

FEELING CONFIDENT

Many of us in our middle years feel a loss of confidence because we feel less able to compete with younger people. Both women and men can experience an undermining of self-esteem caused by the thought of their youth disappearing over the horizon. It may be tempting to overcompensate by dressing to look younger, buying a "younger" (sports) car, adopting a younger lifestyle, competing directly with younger people in sports such as squash, or working extra-long hours at work to show that you can still make the grade. But the end result of all this may be the opposite of what was intended. By trying to look younger, you may attract the derision of the young; overdoing it in a demanding sport may cause an injury; and working too hard can cause stress and illness. It is far better to accept aging gracefully, while keeping the body healthy. The middle years bring with them an image of maturity that looks good when combined with good health. Why look back to your youth when you are more healthy, successful, and confident than you have ever been before?

PINCHING AN INCH

Body fat should make up 15–20 percent of a man's body weight, and 20–25 percent of a woman's body weight. A higher or lower proportion of body fat can cause health problems. In the middle years the body tends to lose muscle tissue and accumulate fat, although this can be controlled through diet and exercise. But how can you determine what proportion of your body is fat? One method that gives a rough indication is to "pinch an inch." Pinch a fold of skin around the waist, or the upper arm, between index finger and thumb. If this fold, without including any muscle, is more than 1 inch thick, you have too much body fat and should lose some of it. For a more accurate, quantitative measure of body fat, consult your doctor or a fitness expert; professionals will use calipers to measure skin-fold thickness at various parts of the body, and will then compute your overall percentage of body fat.

attractive and, therefore, make it much more likely that they will have a happy and fulfilling emotional and sexual life. Controlling body weight, giving up bad habits (such as smoking, or drinking or eating too much), getting plenty of regular exercise, and looking after the skin all help to maintain a positive self-image. Whatever one's past habits, it is not too late to create new habits at this stage.

How to lose weight...and not put it back on

A good proportion of men and women in the developed world are overweight and, at any one time, many of these people are trying to lose weight. This explains the financial success and popularity of the "miracle products" and weight-loss programs whose interest is in selling their products rather than ensuring that their clients' weight loss will be permanent. Unfortunately, most of those who do lose weight regain it within a few months or years, and may even end up heavier than they were before. But the following measures may enable a person to attain a body weight within healthy limits, and to keep it within those limits for a lifetime without their weight continually see-sawing up and down.
• Set a target weight by looking at a height-weight chart for your age and sex, or calculate the weight that will give you a BMI of about 24 (see p.88). Do not set a target weight that is too low. It may be difficult to achieve it without losing muscle mass, and may make you look skinny rather than healthy.
• Set a realistic target rate for losing weight—it should be a gradual loss of approximately 2 pounds per week to avoid losing the lean (muscle) tissue you want to keep along with the fat you want to shed.
• Eat small, regular meals each day consisting of a wide range of foods low in animal fats, especially fresh fruit and vegetables; avoid manufactured snacks and junk food. Contrary to popular belief, bread, potatoes, and pasta in reasonable amounts are not fattening, and provide an excellent energy source. Find foods that you will enjoy continuing to eat once you have reached your target weight.

QUESTIONS AND ANSWERS: WEIGHT

Q. I am 44. Up until my late thirties, my weight and my waist size remained exactly the same as when I was in my teens. Now my weight seems to increase year by year, and my waist size matches my increase in years each birthday. What can I do?
A. Increase in weight is not unusual at your age. Two things that will probably have an immediate effect are 1) get more exercise, even just by doing more gardening or walking upstairs instead of taking the elevator, and 2) eat less animal fat and drink less alcohol, while eating more fresh fruit and vegetables.

Q. I have had real problems in keeping my weight under control in recent years. Despite being on one diet or another, I don't seem to able to get rid of excess fat. Do weight-loss pills work?
A. While appetite-suppressant drugs may work in the short term, they are not effective in the long term. They do not allow the body to "reeducate" itself, as happens when one begins to eat more sensibly and exercise to lose fat tissue and gain muscle tissue. In addition, these drugs can be dangerous and in some cases have even caused deaths.

• Exercise regularly, at least three times a week—even a brisk walk. This will increase your metabolic rate, burn fat to release energy, tone muscles to give the body better shape, and make you feel better and less hungry. By maintaining and perhaps increasing your muscle bulk, you will burn more calories each day—muscle tissue consumes more energy than fat.

• Avoid fad diets—for example, single-item diets (such as grapefruit) or expensive diet products (such as liquid diets that provide unhealthfully small amounts of calories each day). Any weight lost this way will be at the expense of lean muscle tissue. These diets also cause the body's metabolic rate to slow because it "assumes" it is facing starvation and needs to conserve resources. As soon as the diet stops, the body stores as much food as possible as fat to provide a buffer against future bouts of starvation, so very often the ex-dieter ends up heavier than before.

• Avoid sugary foods (most processed foods contain hidden sugar), colas or other sweetened drinks, and junk food such as burgers, and limit your alcohol intake. Alcohol contains a lot of nutritionally empty calories.

• Avoid eating when you are not hungry, even if it is a mealtime.

• Use a smaller plate so that there is no temptation to fill the plate with more food than you actually need.

Anyone who sticks with this pattern of diet and exercise can be assured that they should be benefiting on a permanent basis.

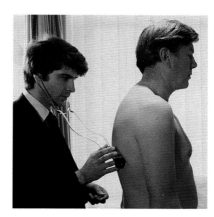

Before starting an exercise program in the middle years—especially if you are out of shape and have not exercised for years—it is important to have your health checked by your doctor to avoid possible injury or illness resulting from sudden exertion.

Drinking too much

Alcohol dependence develops gradually, so that by the middle years someone may not realize how much they are drinking, or how much they need a drink. Apart from liver damage, brain damage, and various cancers, long-term alcohol abuse *(see p.127)* also causes emotional and sexual problems that can put a relationship in jeopardy.

Answer yes or no to these questions to see if you may be damaging your health through drinking too much.
• Do you always look forward to having a drink and plan activities around drinking?
• Do you often drink alone, either at home or in a bar?
• Do you sometimes drink so much that you are unable to remember what happened?
• Do you feel uncomfortable or nervous if you do not have a drink each day?
• Do you drink as a way of unwinding at the

end of a day, to help you sleep, or because it gives you a special lift?

• Do you drink to forget emotional problems, or to overcome depression or anxiety?

• Have you been late for work, taken time off work, or missed an appointment because of drinking excessively the night before?

• Do you seem to be able to drink more than other people?

• Do you always look for a refill when your glass becomes empty at parties?

• Do you drink secretively and hide the evidence from relatives or friends?

• Do you set aside money and/or time for your drinking?

If you answer yes to three or more of these questions you may be, or be in danger of becoming, addicted to alcohol. Most people with an alcohol problem find this difficult to accept, but it is important to try to deal with alcohol dependence. Seek help from a doctor or counselor, or contact Alcoholics Anonymous or another alcoholic support group—numbers will be in the phone book. Relatives concerned about a family member can contact an Al-Anon Family Group.

How to drink in moderation

Consumed in moderation, alcohol may have a beneficial effect on health. But what is meant by "in moderation"? Common advisory limits are around 21 units per week for women, and 28 units per week for men, where one unit is equivalent to a 3–5-ounce glass of wine/an ounce of hard liquor/12 ounces of beer. The recommended level for women is lower than for men because women have a lower average body volume, and because a lower proportion of their total body weight is in the form of water, so they reach proportionately higher alcohol levels. The alcohol "allowance" should be spread through the week, not drunk in one session. If you are consuming more than this allowance and you want to moderate your drinking, try the following.

• Keep a notebook to record how much you drink every day and how many units you consume each week. Accurate knowledge of how much you are drinking may make you cut down immediately.

• When drinking at home, drink only with a meal. The body absorbs alcohol more slowly with food.

• When you go out for a drink, start with a nonalcoholic drink to quench your thirst. Also, instead of having one alcoholic drink after another, try alternating alcoholic and nonalcoholic drinks.

• Try alcoholic drinks that are heavily diluted with mixers, such as a spritzer (a mixture of wine and soda water).

• Drink slowly and put the glass down between sips.

• Work to have a number of alcohol-free days each week. Perhaps drink only (in moderation) on weekends.

Keeping drinking under control makes people feel more in control of life. You should also sleep better, be less prone to depression, and feel healthier and livelier.

Skin care

Covering the body like a protective overcoat, the skin is constantly exposed to wear and tear. Wrinkles and folds in the skin are one of the first indications that the body is aging, although, with care, some of these changes can be delayed. The major aging factor affecting the skin is exposure to sunlight and wind. Despite the many health warnings that over-exposure to sunlight also increases the risk of developing skin cancer, many people still fail to protect themselves against excess sun, especially during the summer months or while on vacation. Ideally, exposing the skin to sunlight, especially at the hottest times of day, should be kept to a minimum. Everyone should use a protective sunscreen or sunblock. Sunhats and protective, loose clothes should be worn whenever possible. Although moisturizing cream cannot get rid of wrinkles, if applied regularly it can help lessen the appearance of wrinkles caused by the aging process and the effects of sunlight.

Cosmetic surgery

Also known as esthetic plastic surgery, this is not carried out to cure an illness or deformity but to change, and hopefully improve, a person's appearance. Those women and men who choose to have cosmetic surgery in their middle years usually do so in order to give themselves a more youthful appearance and boost their self-image. Many other middle-aged people do not see cosmetic surgery as necessary because they do not believe that aging makes them less attractive.

Anyone seriously considering cosmetic surgery should realize that it may not necessarily produce the desired changes in their looks. Nor will surgery automatically remove any negative feelings a person has about their appearance or produce a new personality. Nevertheless, many people who have cosmetic surgery find the results worthwhile. It is important, however, to consider carefully the reasons for undertaking cosmetic surgery before going ahead with it. It is also important to find a plastic surgeon who has a track record of success. The following are some of the most commonly performed types of cosmetic surgery.

Facelift

Skin is removed from the side of the face in order to tighten the rest of the facial skin to remove wrinkles and folds. The results of a facelift are generally good, but it may need to be repeated within a few years, and the surgery can produce a tight-skinned, almost corpselike appearance in later life.

Liposuction

This involves sucking out excess fat from under the skin to change body shape. Carried out by an expert, the results can be very effective, although with a less proficient surgeon the procedure can leave a lumpy finish. The effects of liposuction may not last long, however, and it may be more effective to change the diet and exercise more in order to shape and tone the body naturally.

Breast enlargement or reduction

Breast enlargement is available for women who are concerned that their breasts are too small. Breast reduction can be of great benefit for women who feel weighed down and hampered by very large breasts.

Collagen replacement

Collagen is the name of the protein that gives the skin its natural elasticity. The amount of collagen present in the skin decreases with age. Collagen injections can therefore be used to give a more youthful appearance to part of a person's face or the hands, although these injections will need to be repeated when the collagen breaks down, in about two years.

BALDNESS

While male baldness can start in the twenties or even the teens, it tends to reach its full extent during the middle years. Male pattern baldness—the most common form of baldness—is an inherited condition that begins at the temples and progresses to the crown. There is no "cure" for male pattern baldness, although the drug minoxidil can be effective for some men if taken in the early stages of hair loss; however, it requires continuous treatment and is expensive. Hair implants also sometimes work. Some men become depressed at the thought of becoming bald and feel, wrongly, that it makes them less attractive. They are not helped by a common prejudice that equates baldness with aging and that sees a full head of hair to be more attractive. As a result, some balding men try to conceal their baldness by growing their hair long and sweeping it over their head, by undergoing painful hair-weaving procedures or hair transplants, or by wearing a wig or toupee. Often these devices only highlight the fact that the man is ashamed of his baldness and is trying to hide it—they can also make him look older.

QUESTIONS AND ANSWERS: COSMETIC SURGERY

Q. I am 41 and my husband is 38. Our relationship has not been too good recently, and I am sure this is because he thinks I look old. Could a facelift put some life back into our marriage?
A. This is most unlikely. If you think cosmetic surgery will revive your relationship, you will probably be sadly disappointed. It would be far better to talk to your partner about what is wrong between you so that you can start to work things out together. The only reason to undergo cosmetic surgery is because you yourself want it.

Q. I would like to have a breast lift, but I am worried that things might go wrong and I might end up being scarred. What can I do to minimize the risks?
A. If you are sure that you really want to have this operation, and have thought about *why* you want it, find a plastic surgeon—preferably by word of mouth—who has a successful track record with this type of operation. No surgery is risk-free, but using a good surgeon will considerably lessen the risks.

Blepharoplasty

This involves removing bags from under the eyes and reshaping the eyelids. A more effective remedy may be to drink less alcohol, get more sleep, or exercise more.

Sexual relationships and the middle years

As people age, their sexual relationships change. They may not make love as often as they did when they were younger. Some couples are happy and content with the amount of sex in their lives, whether they make love twice a week or twice a month. In other relationships, one person may feel unhappy because their partner does not want sex as often as he or she does.

IF CELLULITE EXISTS, HOW CAN YOU GET RID OF IT?

Cellulite is a controversial issue. A perennial favorite of women's magazines and the weight-loss industry, it is believed by some authorities to be a condition unique to women, and by others to be a complete myth.

Believers say that cellulite causes the bumpy, bulging appearance of the buttocks and thighs of some women, producing an "orange-peel" pattern on the skin of these areas. Proponents of cellulite describe it as a form of water retention within fat tissue, also involving the accumulation of toxins (poisons) resulting from sluggish blood circulation in a woman's buttocks and thighs, which, they say, gives rise to the characteristic dimpled appearance. Some businesses have taken advantage of this condition by manufacturing pills, creams, and specialized massage machines that are supposed to get rid of the cellulite. Others who do not have a financial interest suggest a good diet that is free of toxins (such as preservatives and alcohol), massage, skin brushing, aromatherapy, and exercise as ways of reducing cellulite.

Non-believers state that cellulite is simply body fat that gains its particular appearance because of the way it is stored under the skin. Fat cells are grouped in compartments separated by strands of connective tissue. In the buttocks and thighs, the fat compartments bulge outward into the skin from between the connective tissue strands, causing the characteristic bulges. This group believes that the only way to get rid of this kind of fat, like any other excess fat, is to get regular aerobic exercise and to eat a healthy, balanced diet.

But while the quantity of sex may have decreased, many couples who have a good relationship find that the quality of their sex life has improved over the years.

• As partners get to know each other better, and talk to each other about their feelings, desires, and fantasies, they become more in tune with what arouses them sexually.

• Partners are more relaxed about sex and have become more experienced.

• The nature of most men's interest in sex shifts as they get older. In his teens and twenties, when the physiological response was most rapid and potent, his main focus of sexual pleasure was his orgasm. By the time he reaches his late thirties and forties, a man is less orgasm-driven and more interested in the sensual pleasures of sex.

• By her thirties and forties, a woman will understand her body better than she did when she was younger, and will be much more capable of sexual arousal and orgasm.

Sexual compatibility and mutual enjoyment is an important factor contributing to the success of relationships. If both partners stay healthy, couples who have a successful, fulfilling, and interesting sex life in their middle years are likely to continue to enjoy sex into old age. If partners find that their sex life is going into decline, it may be that their

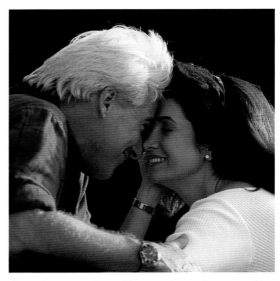

Open demonstrations of love are just as important in the middle years, when many couples find that the nature of their sexual relationship is changing.

relationship has been allowed to stagnate or that they feel themselves to be no longer sexually attractive; in this situation, the relationship could be enlivened by a few innovations. Alternatively, it may simply mean that the relationship is not working.

Keeping sex exciting

Without variety, anything in life can become boring and repetitive, and sex is no exception. If sex becomes a chore it is likely to happen less and less frequently, and a couple's relationship may suffer as a result. But there are ways, if both partners have the time and the inclination, to enliven flagging sex lives. However, it is important to remember that what may prove exciting for one couple, or for one partner within a couple, may be a complete turnoff for another individual or couple. Here are some of the ways that couples may choose to spice up their sex lives:
• talking to each other about what they enjoy doing sexually; this can be very arousing
• complimenting each other about how sexy they look, removing fears either partner has about losing their sexual attraction
• if sex has always been underwear-free, sexy underwear can add another dimension to arousal and lovemaking

• many men and women enjoy reading, looking at, or watching erotica in the form of books, magazines, or videos
• sex manuals can provide some new ideas
• sex toys such as vibrators may help. Women may find that using a vibrator to stimulate the clitoris produces a very intense orgasm
• meeting "secretly" at a new location, such as a hotel, to enjoy a sex session
• sharing sexual fantasies.

QUESTIONS AND ANSWERS: IMPROVING SEX

Q. While our sex life is satisfactory, there are some things I would like to try. I think my wife would enjoy them too, but I don't seem to be able to ask her. What should I do?
A. Lack of communication can be one of the biggest inhibiting factors in a sexual relationship. The only way to explore these new sexual avenues with your partner is to talk to her about them and ask her if she might enjoy them. Choose your moment—say, during a relaxing evening after a glass of wine, rather than before work on a Monday morning. Just talking about sex may be a turn-on for both of you, making it easier to explore new erotic territory.
Q. Does getting older mean our sex life will decline?
A. Not at all. Many couples in their middle years find sex more exciting, pleasurable, and satisfying than in their younger years. While you may take more time to get aroused, you will probably find that sex lasts longer and you both reach orgasm.

DESIRE DISCREPANCY

Desire discrepancy occurs when one partner in a relationship wants to make love more often than the other. Contrary to popular belief, this is not simply a matter of men wanting sex more often than women; just as many women as men desire sex more often than their partner does. However, this problem does not have to mean the end of a relationship. It can often be tackled by discovering its causes, and changing some lifestyle factors accordingly. Desire discrepancy may happen because:
• one partner is working so hard and for such long hours that he or she

just falls asleep when the other partner is feeling sexually aroused
• partners do not communicate, so neither knows about the other's sexual needs
• one partner feels anger toward the other, an emotion which overrides the desire for sex
• one partner is being unfaithful
• one partner feels so pressured to have sex that he or she becomes turned off as a consequence
• one partner is never satisfied by the sex offered by the other and therefore never looks forward to or initiates sex.
    In the case of working long hours,

the couple may be helped by adjusting their schedules and making more time for each other. In the other cases, communication is the key, and the couple may require help, perhaps therapy or counseling, to resolve their difficulties. However, some couples who apparently have desire discrepancy are perfectly content with their relationships. They find each other sexually attractive and arousing, but realize that while one may want to have sex daily, for example, the other is content to have sex once a week. Partners in this situation may find masturbation the simplest solution.

Losing interest in a relationship

Interest in partners can wane as a relationship matures, and a man or woman may seek, and perhaps find, a new sexual partner. There are various reasons why this may happen.

• One or both partners simply may not like the other anymore, in which case the relationship is probably doomed.

• One or both partners may be lazy and may make no effort to keep the relationship interesting and alive. In this case they may be helped by talking to each other or seeking support from a counselor.

• A partner may be feeling "old" and try to renew his or her youth by having an affair with a younger partner. If this is the case, the relationship can go either way—it may founder, or the couple may recover.

DECISIONS ABOUT EMPLOYMENT

Unlike our parents and grandparents, many of us no longer have careers that last for life. And the middle years, with their changing circumstances, can be the ideal time for women and men to seek a change.

• Freed from looking after families, women who previously had a career may return to their old line of work, or choose a new form of employment.

• Both men and women may seek to change work patterns, going against the training and ambitions of their youth. It is not uncommon for people to change direction altogether: a bank manager, for example, may decide to raise chickens.

• Learning does not cease when formal education ends. Informal education continues throughout life, but some people opt to resume formal education again in their middle years, either to train for a new career or to develop new interests.

In general terms it is important to maintain the dynamism of a relationship, keeping it alive by doing different things together, keeping sex exciting, and making a point of not taking each other for granted.

Midlife crisis—myth or reality?

The onset of middle age can be accompanied by a feeling of dissatisfaction about life. This may be caused by the realization that ambitions will never be attained, that old age is getting nearer, that a particular relationship is never going to work, or by fear of losing one's looks or sexual attractiveness. Not everyone experiences such feelings, and in those who do, they can range from mild discontent to serious depression. In recent years, some experts have gathered such symptoms under the general term "midlife crisis."

According to the proponents of the idea of the midlife crisis, men and women who experience it may feel that they are losing their youthful appearance and sexual vigor. Women who have spent much of their adult life caring for their children may be faced with a void in their lives when the children leave home. Aware that their "biological clocks" are ticking away toward menopause, some women may experience feelings of disquiet or even panic.

Both men and women may have affairs at this stage if they feel sexually dissatisfied with their partners. They may seek a clandestine

---

THE TICKING BIOLOGICAL CLOCK

Women's reproductive years extend to menopause, which is likely to occur in their late forties or early fifties. A woman in her late thirties who has not had children may feel anxious to have children before her biological clock has advanced too far and she is too old to conceive. If she is on her own, she may feel that she needs to find a partner quickly—and

perhaps unsuitably—in order to have a child before it is too late. If she is married and has a demanding job, she may worry about interrupting her career in order to have babies, as well as having to decide what to do about child care after they are born. If a woman, and her partner, want to have children in the middle years, they should go ahead and

have them, provided they are aware of the risks for older women. But if a woman is being pushed into having a child by friends or relatives, she should pause to consider what she herself wants. More couples are deciding that, because they do not really want children, they are not going to have them simply to please others.

relationship with a younger man or woman, believing that this will help bring back their youth. It should be noted, however, that statistically the number of extramarital relationships does not surge in this age group, although the incidence of affairs does increase gradually from the twenties to the fifties.

Whether or not a midlife crisis exists, many men and women in their forties do take stock of what they have achieved and what they want to achieve in the future. Men especially tend to be worried by the prospect or reality of losing their job, often because they have been brought up to see their role as a breadwinner. With more women in high-profile, highly paid jobs, men who are earning less or have lost their job may feel that they have also lost their significance. In this situation, it is often helpful for them to question their role and realize that they are still important as individuals, even if they have no job.

But if the future does appear frightening, it can be helpful to plan for it—as far as one can—by setting new but attainable goals. Most of all, try to adopt a positive approach. Look to the future, not the past.

• If you are not happy with your current career and do not see much future in it, then think about what you would really like to do, and investigate the possibilities of doing it. It is probably not too late! Discuss your thoughts with your partner.

• Consider the advantages of getting older if you have children. When they are in their late teens or twenties, you should find that you can have a more mature, adult relationship with them. And when they have left home you will have more space and time for your partner and yourself. If children are younger, think about their education and future; plan things that you want to do with them.

• Think about parents. As they reach old age, will you be able to provide them with help or care if they need it? A little advance planning now can help you avoid feelings of guilt and anxiety later on.

• Plan what you want to do with your partner —places to visit, where you want to live. Write down when you want to achieve your goals by, and check them off as you do them.

Contraception in the middle years

Although a woman's fertility decreases in her thirties, early forties, and, most dramatically, late forties, she and her partner should continue to use contraception until she is certain she has reached menopause *(see Chapter 10)*. Until then, there is always a risk of pregnancy if a couple has sex without contraception; if a woman embarks on a new relationship without adequate protection she also risks catching a sexually transmitted disease. Some couples in their middle years prefer to stay with a contraceptive method they have been using, while others decide it is time to change. *(Contraception is covered in Chapter 5.)*

The combined pill

For women who are healthy nonsmokers, low-dose combined pills provide good protection in the middle years. The estrogen in the pills can also offset initial menopausal symptoms. At present, pill use declines sharply in women over 35 in the US, perhaps because many women prefer not to continue using a hormonal method for prolonged periods.

Progestin-only pill (minipill)

The minipill is also effective in this age group, although some women experience irregular periods or loss of periods. The same applies to hormonal implants and injections.

QUESTION AND ANSWER: CONTRACEPTION

Q. I am 38, my wife and I have two young children, and I would like to have a vasectomy so that we can forget about using contraception in the future. My worry is this: if for some reason we want another child later, could the vasectomy be reversed?

A. Vasectomy can be reversed, but there is no guarantee that a man will then be able to father children. The reversal uses microsurgery. Its success depends on the skill of the surgeon, and on the length of time since the vasectomy was performed—the longer the time lapse, the lower the chance of success. If there is any doubt in your mind as to whether you want more children, do not have a vasectomy.

Condoms

Condom effectiveness tends to increase with age, as couples become more proficient in their use and women's fertility decreases. In the United States, 11 percent of couples in their thirties and forties use male condoms.

Intrauterine device (IUD)

The IUD is appropriate for women who have had their families. It is highly effective and can remain in place for long periods.

Natural methods

Although natural methods are more effective at this age, because of greater experience and diminishing fertility, they are only used by a small proportion of couples. Natural family planning is not recommended once a woman's periods become irregular.

Sterilization

In Western countries, female sterilization is the most popular form of contraception in the middle years, followed by male sterilization (in the United States, 47 percent of women and 21 percent of men). Both are effective, and mean that a couple does not have to think about contraception ever again, but many people prefer to opt for methods that do not involve surgery and are reversible.

Parenting

At some time duirng their forties and fifties, many people face the prospect of their off-spring leaving home to go to college, travel, live on their own, or get married. Some parents react to the departure of children happily, relishing the feeling of autonomy and freedom. Others feel grief and loss, which in their most profound form are akin to bereavement and are sometimes described as empty nest syndrome.

Because advance planning, both practically and emotionally, can be invaluable, it is worth considering some of these factors.

• Women who have spent their adult life bringing up their family may find children leaving home hard to bear because they have invested all their emotional energy in their children and have defined their life in terms of motherhood. Finding new interests or work before the children leave home can alleviate feelings of loss.

• Although women are typically seen as the ones who experience empty nest syndrome, it can also affect fathers and other members of the family. Open discussion about changes in the family structure can be invaluable in sorting out conflicts and anxieties that may occur when children leave.

• The home environment will change, because it is not only the child that departs but also their noise, untidiness, friends, and liveliness. This is the time to reorganize the household.

• Younger children who remain at home will probably seek substitutes for the older siblings who have left, resulting in a shift in family dynamics. Parents need to take everyone's feelings into account when a child leaves home: their own, those of the departing child, and those of children remaining at home.

• When older children return home for visits, both parents and children need to establish new ground rules so that the parents do not drive their children away by nagging them. At the same time, the children should not treat the parental home like a hotel.

THE EMPTY NEST: A TIME FOR RENEWAL?

The sense of loss caused by the departure of children from the family home may shock a couple into reappraising their relationship. The children's presence may have provided a focus that masked the fact that individual partners were growing apart.

• Partners may find that in the void left by their children's departure they have time and space to rediscover each other and rebuild their relationship.

• Partners may decide that, once the commitment to their children has been fulfilled, they should separate in order to find new identities, and possibly new partners.

• A couple may discover that they have grown apart while bringing up their children, and have developed in different ways, but that they can continue to live together while pursuing their own interests. This allows their children, and perhaps their grandchildren, to have a physical and emotional base.

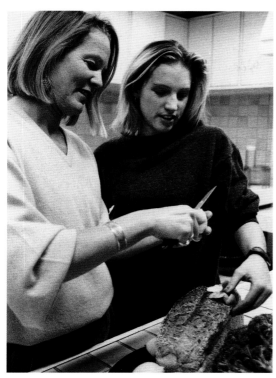

Relationships between single parents and their children are often very close, and when daughters or sons leave the parental home their departure can leave a big gap in the parent's life. That gap needs to be filled.

Letting go for single parents

For mothers or fathers who have brought up children on their own, the departure of a child from the family home can be a particularly devastating loss. Children obviously require more attention from a single parent than would be expected from either partner within a two-parent family. This means that the child or children often effectively defines the structure of the single parent's life, a structure that can disintegrate rapidly when the child leaves home. While some single parents, like other parents, may be overjoyed at the prospect of the new freedom that will come with the release from parenting, many—although wishing their offspring well—experience grief and depression. Remember that in these circumstances it helps to talk and be open about worries. Talk over your feelings—and this may be easier for women than men—with friends who are in, or approaching, the same situation, or with any children still at home. You may find support from a single parents' group. It is also important to remember that the investment a single parent has put into his or her child does not come to an end just because the child has left home: he or she will still be much in demand for help and advice.

Being an older parent

For increasing numbers of couples, parenthood does not arrive until they are in their late thirties or early forties. The first problem for many is that they may feel more tired taking care of a new baby than younger parents do. Then, as children get older, parents come to recognize the considerable age gap, and may need to adjust their lifestyle to cope with their children's demands. By the time the children are adolescents, parents may be approaching their sixties, and be in the age bracket that is more traditional for grand parents than parents. But despite these possible problems, being an older parent can be very satisfying. Maturity may prove advantageous, equipping couples to cope more calmly with the stresses of parenting, and the bond between children and parents is likely to be just as strong as it is with younger parents.

QUESTION AND ANSWER: EMPTY NEST SYNDROME

Q. I took my 19-year-old son to college last week to start his freshman year. Driving home afterward I was so upset I had to stop the car. I just burst into tears, and have done so once or twice a day since then. My son, on the other hand, seems to be happy and settled at college, and does not seem to be missing home at all. Is there something wrong with me?

A. No, not at all. You are simply grieving for the "loss" of your son. If possible, talk to your partner about the way you feel and ask him how he is feeling. You may find, in time, that if you talk about your feelings, the sense of loss will pass, and you will be able to continue with the next phase of your life. And don't resent your son's lack of emotion. He has embarked on the next part of his life and is enjoying himself in a new environment with new interests and relationships.

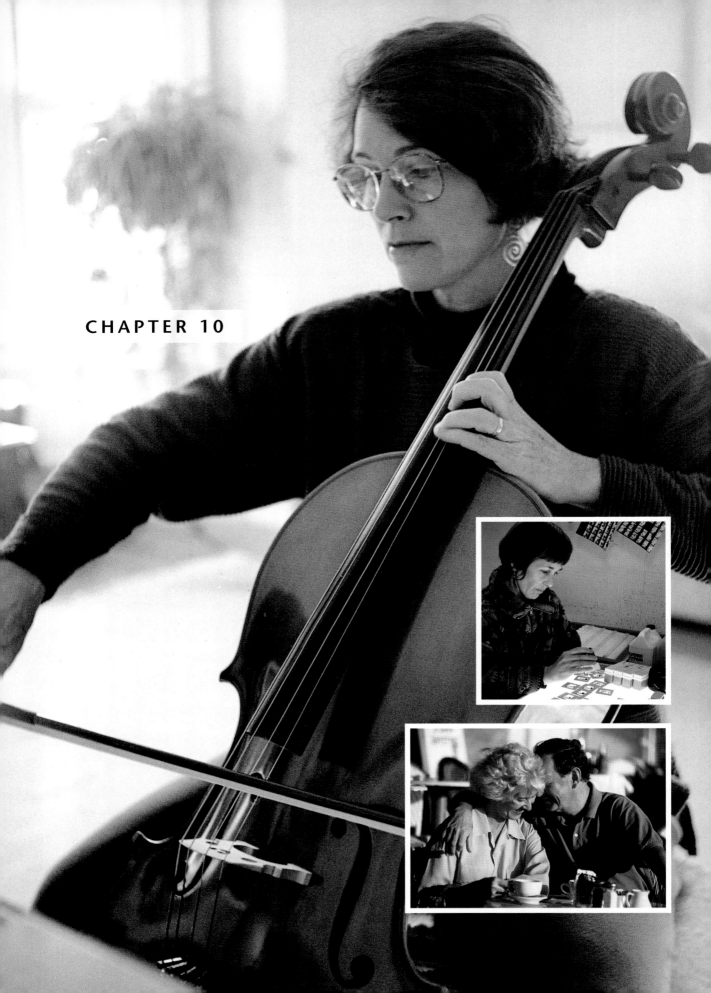

CHAPTER 10

Menopause

Menopause is the phase of a woman's life that marks the end of her fertile years. Like puberty, menopause is initiated by changing levels of estrogen and other hormones inside a woman's body. As a woman progresses through her forties, estrogen production by her ovaries gradually goes into decline. Eventually, usually sometime between the ages of 45 and 55, her periods cease and her ovaries no longer release eggs. The falling hormone levels also produce other changes inside the body.

At first, it is unlikely that the woman will notice that she is approaching menopause, but eventually she will become aware that her body is changing. For some women the changes will be slight, perhaps no more than the cessation of periods; for others, menopause will be accompanied by a variety of physical and emotional symptoms that she may find unsettling and upsetting.

Some of the changes experienced during this phase of a woman's life may be due not to menopause itself but to other events that can occur during these years. The late forties and early fifties are a time when many women reassess their lives, careers, and relationships. If their children have left home, they may be feeling unsettled, or be conscious of the need to restructure their daily life. It is certainly a phase of life when a woman, and her partner, will be experiencing the early symptoms of aging. This combination of life changes can make menopause a difficult time for a woman and her family, a time when she needs maximum support from those around her.

Many women worry about the onset of menopause. The usual cause of their concern is the old stereotype of the menopausal woman—someone who is ill, irritable, and asexual. This negative attitude also reflects the low status afforded to older women in Western society. In some parts of the world, postmenopausal women have high status and play an important part in decision-making. Indeed it appears that the more older women are revered by the society they live in, the fewer menopausal symptoms they suffer. Only in Western countries has menopause traditionally been regarded more as a medical condition than a natural part of life.

Fortunately, times and attitudes are changing. As women become more aware of what is happening to their bodies, and learn to adjust to the changes, many find that menopause is not only liberating but also the beginning of a new, positive phase of their life.

Furthermore, menopausal women soon realize that not only does their sexual life continue after menopause, but it is often enhanced by freedom from monthly periods and the need for contraception.

What is menopause?

Although the word menopause means specifically the time when a woman's periods stop, the term is commonly used to describe the changes that happen to a woman as her reproductive years come to a close. The end of menstruation is just one event during a long period of physical adjustment called the climacteric, which can last up to 20 years, from about the age of 40. During the climacteric, the production of the sex hormone estrogen by the ovaries declines as these organs gradually stop releasing eggs. While their bodies adjust during the climacteric, women notice outward symptoms of the changes occurring inside them, most notably in the years just before and after their last period.

The climacteric is a transitional phase that can be divided into three stages:

• **Premenopause** is the early part of the climacteric, when the menstrual cycle is still regular and ovulation is still occurring on a monthly basis.

• **Perimenopause** is a time of fluctuating hormone levels and irregular menstrual cycles that lasts for several years between premenopause and menopause itself. The time between each period may shorten and periods may become lighter, or there may be longer spaces between periods, with heavier bleeding each time. Some woman may stop having periods altogether, only to find that they start again later. Despite the irregularity of periods, it is still important for sexually active women to use contraception, because there is still a risk of pregnancy. During perimenopause, a woman may start to experience characteristic symptoms such as hot flashes and emotional changes *(see pp.266–71)*.

• **Postmenopause** is the phase of life that begins with the cessation of periods during menopause and continues until the end of a woman's life. During the early years of

---

PREPARING FOR MENOPAUSE

Perhaps influenced by negative attitudes about menopause, some women simply wait for events to overtake them and put up with what they perceive as the unavoidable symptoms of menopause. Yet there is plenty of evidence to show that women who take control of their lives and adopt a positive attitude toward menopause find this period of change much easier to pass through than those women who react passively to menopause and regard it as an inevitable consequence of aging. There are several ways in which women can prepare for menopause.

• Read the latest books about menopause—especially those that approach this phase of a woman's life in a positive way.

• Become aware of how your reproductive system works, and how it will change during menopause.

• Find out what symptoms you may experience during menopause so that you are not taken by surprise.

• Assess your general health and lifestyle—do you exercise enough and eat a balanced and nutritious diet?—and make changes as necessary.

• Talk to your partner about the years ahead so that he is aware of the changes that may occur during menopause, and how it may affect your relationship and sex life.

• Investigate the therapies currently available that may help you during menopause and the postmenopausal years. Ask your doctor for advice.

HISTORY OF MENOPAUSE

Menopause is a uniquely human phenomenon. Other female animals do not experience a phase of infertility at the end of their lives. Human females do because our cultural development enables us to live to an old age. This was not always the case. Our Stone Age ancestors had a life expectancy of 20 or 30 years—just long enough to grow up, breed, and then die. By the end of the nineteenth century, our average life span was no more than 50 years. It is only during the twentieth century that most women have lived long enough to experience menopause. In the past, the study of menopause has been carried out by men who portrayed it as a medical condition that transforms women from fertile, feminine beings into aging, asexual figures. Such negative attitudes still survive unquestioned in some quarters because menopause is regarded as a taboo topic. Fortunately, because of the growing proportion of women who are over 50, and because of the increasing interest in women's health issues, attitudes toward menopause are changing considerably, and a range of menopausal management strategies is now available.

postmenopause, a woman may continue to experience the symptoms that began in the perimenopause phase, as well as new symptoms that reflect continuing changes within her body. The postmenopausal period can occupy up to a third of a woman's life, and is a time of change and adjustment, but not "the beginning of the end."

Why and when does menopause occur?

By the time a woman has reached her forties, the supply of eggs inside her ovaries is starting to run out. As a consequence, during the climacteric the number of egg-containing follicles that ripen each month inside the ovaries declines. And the fewer follicles that are produced, the smaller the amount of estrogen manufactured by the ovaries. As a result of this, ovulation ceases to occur, preventing the formation of the corpus luteum—the body that forms in the ovary from a ruptured follicle after ovulation—which produces the hormone progesterone. As estrogen and progesterone levels fall, the levels of FSH and LH —hormones produced by the pituitary gland to stimulate the ovaries—increase. The immediate effect of these hormonal fluctuations is that a woman's fertility declines rapidly, and both her menstrual cycle and menstrual flow become erratic. But, because these hormones, especially estrogen, affect many other body activities, a woman will probably start to notice symptoms of these inner changes, such as hot flashes. Eventually, levels of estrogen and progesterone become so low that menstrual activity ceases altogether and the periods cease. This is menopause. The average age for menopause is 51, but it generally occurs between the ages of 45 and 55. Determining whether or not menopause has occurred may be straightforward: the cessation of periods for at least six months and at an appropriate age; and, possibly, hot flashes or other menopausal symptoms. If there are any doubts as to whether or not menopause has happened, blood tests can be taken to see whether levels of the hormones FSH and LH are elevated.

PREMATURE MENOPAUSE

This is usually defined as menopause that happens before the age of 40, and there are various reasons why it may occur. Women who experience premature menopause can be more at risk of developing osteoporosis (see pp.269–70) or heart disease, and may wish to seek their doctor's advice about having hormone replacement therapy (see pp.271–5).

- **Hysterectomy (removal of the uterus)**
If a hysterectomy (see pp.108–9) is performed on a younger woman, and the ovaries are left in place, they will continue to produce hormones as normal, so the hormonal effects of menopause will not be experienced yet. However, there is evidence to show that the ovaries in a woman who has had a hysterectomy may stop functioning some years before the ovaries in a woman who still has her uterus.

- **Oophorectomy (removal of the ovaries)**
The removal of the ovaries in premenopausal women is the most common cause of premature menopause. Once the ovaries have been removed, the production of estrogen and progesterone will cease immediately. Women who have had an oophorectomy are usually advised to use HRT to counteract the effects of the sudden, premature onset of menopause (see also pp.108–9).

- **Illness**
There are some disorders that may lead to premature menopause. These include autoimmune conditions, in which defensive chemicals called antibodies, normally produced by the body to destroy disease-causing microorganisms, fight instead against parts of the body, which stop working normally; and, more rarely, diseases such as mumps, which if they occur in adult life may damage the ovaries.

QUESTION AND ANSWER: TIMING

Q. I am 45 years old and have yet to experience any signs or symptoms of menopause. Is there any way of predicting when my menopause will happen?
A. The average age for menopause is 51, but there is no proven method for predicting when your last period will occur, although your menopause may occur at around the same age that your mother experienced hers. Timing may also depend on when your periods started: the later they started, the later your menopause may occur. However, since you show no signs of change as yet, your menopause should not happen for several years.

Menopausal changes and symptoms

The hormone estrogen influences the activities of many organs and tissues throughout a woman's body *(see pp.20–3)*. As estrogen production by the ovaries goes into decline during menopause, so the activities of these parts of the body start to change. This is a natural part of menopause, and many of the changes are minor.

Major body changes during the menopause

During menopause women can seem forgetful, find that their movement is less well coordinated, and experience emotional symptoms such as mood changes, depression, and loss of sex drive. As ovarian production of estrogen decreases, so the labia and the walls of the vagina, uterus, bladder, and urethra tend to become thinner. The ability of the vagina to produce natural secretions tends to become reduced, and this may lead to sexual problems because of vaginal dryness. Estrogen has a

protective effect on the heart and blood vessels, so that premenopausal women are much less likely to suffer heart attacks or strokes than men of the same age. However, after menopause, this protective effect is lost and the risk of developing cardio-vascular disease equalizes between the sexes. This risk can be reduced by a number of factors: eating a healthy diet that is low in saturated fats from animal sources, getting regular exercise, avoiding obesity and keeping weight in the recommended range, and not smoking.

One of the consequences of menopause is that muscles tend to become weaker and lose their tone, and bones lose mass *(see osteoporosis, pp.269–71)*. Women may also experience joint problems and pains. All of these changes can be reversed, at least partially, by regular exercise and by stretching and strengthening activities such as yoga.

Various changes in body metabolism can occur during menopause. Distribution of fat alters somewhat so that it comes to resemble that in males, accumulating more around the abdomen and breasts than the thighs and hips. However, weight increase is not an inevitable result of menopause, especially if a woman exercises regularly and eats a balanced diet. Another metabolic effect of menopause is a change in the control of body temperature, which can cause hot flashes *(see opposite)*. Decreasing estrogen levels affect the condition of the skin, reducing its suppleness, as well as making hair drier and nails more brittle. A woman's waist can thicken, as more fat is laid down in the area, while her breasts may flatten and sag.

Symptoms of menopause

While some women go through their menopause without really noticing it, others may experience a number of symptoms, including, most commonly, hot flashes and night sweats, vaginal dryness and emotional changes. Some symptoms, such as hot flashes, are transient, lasting from a few months to several years. Others, such as vaginal dryness and urinary symptoms, are also signs of aging—although ones that can be overcome.

POSSIBLE MENOPAUSAL SYMPTOMS

This list of symptoms encompasses those that a woman may, but will not necessarily, experience. Each woman's menopausal experience will depend on physiology, physical and mental fitness, and attitude toward and awareness of her body. And, of course, it depends on whether she is using any treatments such as hormone replacement therapy. All the symptoms listed here are caused by fluctuating levels of hormones.

• Early perimenopausal symptoms that occur as periods become less regular may include: hot flashes and night sweats, loss of or reduced sex drive, vaginal dryness, vaginal irritation, pain during sexual intercourse, loss of self-esteem and feeling of being less sexually attractive, mood swings, anxiety, irritability, depression, forgetfulness, palpitations, headaches, and insomnia.

• Later symptoms that occur around the time periods stop, or afterward, may include: a frequent or urgent need to urinate, pain or a burning feeling when urinating, incontinence, vaginal dryness, irritation or pain during sexual intercourse, slower sexual arousal, joint pains and muscle aches, dry and/or itchy skin, and thinning hair.

Hot flashes and night sweats

These are commonly the earliest signs of menopause. During a hot flash, a woman feels a sudden rush of heat moving across her face and neck, or the upper part of her body. The sensation can last for one minute or more, as skin temperature rises. The intensity of hot flashes varies considerably: they can be mild, with just a slight feeling of warmth; or they can be intense, causing discomfort and disrupting a woman's normal activities. They may be accompanied by sweating, palpitations, and an increase in heart rate. Night sweats are simply hot flashes that occur while a woman is in bed. They may be so intense that sheets and sleepwear become soaked in sweat. Regular night sweats can cause insomnia and exhaustion.

Over 80 percent of women have hot flashes. In two thirds of cases, these start months or years before periods cease, and tend to get worse as menopause takes place. Some women experience mild, occasional hot flashes over a few months, while others have regular, intense hot flashes several times daily for many years. The most effective treatment is hormone replacement therapy, although there are also self-help remedies *(see box)*.

Why do hot flashes occur? Under normal conditions the body maintains a steady temperature by losing heat when it is too hot and conserving heat when too cold. Heat loss under hot conditions is achieved by sweating, and by increasing the diameter of the tiny blood vessels that run near the surface of the skin so that they act as a radiator releasing their heat to the outside air. Evidently, in many perimenopausal women, the brain—which controls body temperature—lowers the normal "set point" for body temperature so that it "thinks" body temperature is too high when it is in fact at normal levels. The brain therefore attempts to cool the body by causing the blood vessels under the skin to open wide, resulting in the characteristic flash and, sometimes, in excessive sweating. There also appears to be a connection between hot flashes and the increase in levels of certain hormones such as LH that occurs before and during menopause *(see p.21)*

QUESTION AND ANSWER: HOT FLASHES

Q. I have started experiencing hot flashes and find them extremely uncomfortable. But my fear is that everyone around me can see what is happening. It makes me so embarrassed. Can I do anything about this?
A. It is likely that worrying about how you look is making the experience of a hot flash feel worse than it really is. Try looking in a mirror next time you have a hot flash and you will see that there is no outward sign that you are having one. Getting advice about self-help techniques for dealing with hot flashes should also help you.

SELF-HELP FOR HOT FLASHES AND NIGHT SWEATS

There are several ways in which women may find relief from hot flashes.
• If possible, try to relax, breathe regularly and deeply, and let the hot flash sweep over your body. Some women find practicing meditation helps as well.
• If you are indoors, and it is very hot, try to move to a cooler room; if you are outside, find some shade.
• Avoid food and drinks that can trigger hot flashes. These include coffee, tea, alcohol, chocolate, and highly spiced dishes.
• If possible, exercise. By improving the blood circulation, exercise appears to reduce the incidence and effects of hot flashes. It is worth noting that the blood circulation is adversely affected by smoking, so giving up cigarettes often helps to make hot flashes less intense.
• Take a cool or tepid shower to cool off.
• Wear lightweight, loose-fitting clothes—preferably not made from synthetic fabrics—that can be removed if necessary.
• Keep a bottle of iced water, a moist sponge or towel, and an electric fan by the bed to deal with night sweats.
• Keep rooms, especially bedrooms, well ventilated to stop them from becoming too warm and stuffy.

Vaginal dryness

This is the main symptom for one fifth of menopausal women, and one of a number of symptoms caused by changes affecting the urinogenital systems. As estrogen levels fall, the vaginal wall becomes thinner and less secretory. This means that during sexual arousal the vagina may produce less of its lubricating secretions and may produce them more slowly than before. Vaginal dryness can lead to pain and soreness if a couple attempts intercourse without allowing time for the vagina to become lubricated. Understanding vaginal dryness and the strategies that can be used to alleviate it may help avoid the discomfort that women may feel during intercourse, and that may put them off sex altogether.

Overcoming vaginal dryness

Ways of overcoming vaginal dryness include the following.

• Hormone replacement therapy (HRT) can alleviate vaginal dryness and irritation, along with many other symptoms of menopause, such as night sweats. For women who prefer not to take HRT in tablet or patch form, there are hormonal creams and suppositories available by prescription that can be applied directly inside the vagina. As an added advantage, local vaginal application can also help reduce urinary problems such as frequent urination and slight incontinence. However, it does not help with hot flashes or night sweats.

• Take care of your adrenal glands. The adrenal glands—one sits on top of each kidney—release small amounts of estrogens after ovarian estrogen production has ceased. Stress, poor diet, and lack of exercise can all combine to decrease the activity of these glands. Conversely, exercise, a balanced diet and a strategy of stress reduction should help alleviate vaginal dryness and other menopausal symptoms.

• Regular sexual activity, including masturbation, can help keep the vagina lubricated. This is because the increased blood flow to the vagina during sexual arousal helps keep it in a "younger" state, and because sex may stimulate the adrenal glands to secrete more estrogens. Pelvic floor exercises *(see p.209 and p.221)* may help as well.

• Vaginal lubrication during sexual arousal does not generally cease after menopause; it may simply take longer. Spending more time than before arousing, and being aroused by, a partner, can produce as much lubrication as experienced before menopause.

• Water-soluble gels, such as K-Y Jelly, applied inside the vagina, or on the fingers or penis of a partner, will relieve vaginal dryness and painful intercourse if natural lubrication is difficult. Water-soluble gels are preferable because they are less likely to lead to any vaginal infections.

• Avoid using perfumed soaps, bath oils, foams or sprays, or tissues near the vulva, as perfume chemicals can irritate the vagina and make sex even more uncomfortable.

• Avoid, unless prescribed by a doctor, using antihistamines and decongestants. These will dry out mucous membranes throughout the body, including the walls of the vagina.

Urinary symptoms

The urinary system—especially the bladder and the urethra—experiences the same type of changes that affect the vagina, with their walls becoming thinner and drier. These changes can cause a variety of symptoms, including the need to urinate frequently and with some urgency, even if there is little urine actually inside the bladder; a feeling of discomfort during urination; and varying degrees of incontinence, resulting from a weakened sphincter muscle at the base of the bladder, ranging from an occasional dribble to stress incontinence, in which urine is forced out of the bladder if, for example, a woman coughs or is carrying a heavy weight.

These symptoms are distressing, especially if they are unexpected, although there are some self-help remedies that may be of assistance. Like other menopausal symptoms, urinary symptoms are generally alleviated by treatment with HRT, or by the use of a hormonal cream applied locally in the vagina. However, women who choose not to use HRT but who are having urinary problems may be able to help themselves by practicing pelvic floor exercises in order to strengthen control over the bladder sphincter. Drinking plenty of fluids, especially water, will help reduce urinary discomfort.

Skin and hair

Another consequence of menopause is the effect that it can have on a woman's skin, hair, and nails. Skin derives its natural flexibility and suppleness from two proteins—collagen and elastin. During menopause, decreasing amounts of these two proteins, coupled with a thinning of the skin and a weakening of the underlying muscles, tends to make the skin less supple and more wrinkled, especially on the face and neck. Around 20 percent of women also experience a periodic but intense itching or tingling feeling in the skin called formication—often described as like the feeling of insects crawling over the body—which can be distressing, especially if it occurs at the same time as a hot flash. Changes that affect the skin also affect related body structures, including hair, which can become dry, and nails, which can become brittle and chipped. The condition of the skin, and of hair and nails, will improve if a woman uses HRT, although there are other ways of helping to reverse or control these symptoms.

Self-help methods for maintaining healthy skin

Although menopause will change the structure of skin, hair, and nails, there are ways of "fighting back" to minimize these changes.
• A healthy, balanced diet, including an adequate supply of vitamins and minerals, is as vital for maintaining good skin, hair, and nails as it is for counteracting other menopausal symptoms.
• Using soap to wash the skin removes the natural oils that keep it supple. Instead, use cleansers that remove dirt from the skin without removing these oils.
• Moisturizing the skin on a daily basis can help temporarily to prevent dryness and wrinkles. (There is no need to buy expensive creams that purport to contain collagen or elastin; these will not be absorbed by the skin to replace the naturally occurring proteins that have been lost.) However, no moisturizer can permanently halt the wrinkles that come naturally with age.
• Sunlight damages the skin at any age, drying it and making it more wrinkled. But this is especially true after menopause because the drying effect of sunlight accentuates the loss of suppleness in the skin. The remedy is to avoid overexposure to sunlight by wearing protective clothing and a sunhat; by using

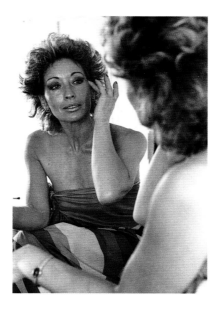

Taking care of the skin can do much to counteract the increased tendency toward wrinkling that occurs after menopause. Regular use of a skin moisturizer is one way to keep the skin feeling supple and looking good.

sunscreens and sunblocks with an SPF of at least 15; and by avoiding exposure to the sun during the hottest part of the day when sunlight is most intense, or by staying in the shade. Avoiding intense sunlight is also important because the amount of melanin—the skin pigment that protects the body against the damaging effects of ultraviolet light—in the skin decreases, so that the skin is more likely to be damaged by ultraviolet light, with the increased risk of developing skin cancer.

Osteoporosis

Osteoporosis is a condition that weakens the bones. It poses the most significant health hazard for postmenopausal women (it is less commonly found in men). The condition is not caused by menopause itself, but is a serious side effect encouraged by the drop in estrogen levels that is associated with menopause. So how and why does osteoporosis occur?

The bones of the skeleton form a strong framework that supports the body and its organs, and to which the muscles that move the body are attached. Bones themselves consist of two basic components: a matrix of protein fibers that makes them strong and flexible; and minerals—primarily calcium phosphate—that, deposited on the protein matrix, make bones rigid and hard. Bones are being constantly broken down, built up, and reshaped by an "army" of bone-building cells called osteoblasts. As we get older the renewal and repair service becomes less efficient, resulting in a loss of the protein matrix from the bone, and with it the calcium salts normally deposited on the matrix. The bone becomes less dense and more brittle. Usually, a woman's bone mass peaks at around the age of 35, and then declines at a rate of about 1 percent per year, although this rate of loss decreases in women over 60. But in a sizable minority of menopausal and postmenopausal women, this natural aging process is accelerated as estrogen levels fall, and bone mass decreases severely—resulting in osteoporosis. Estrogen helps maintain bone mass by stimulating the osteoblasts to do their job, and by preventing excessive loss of calcium from the bone. If osteoporosis occurs, the inner, microscopic structure of the bone becomes riddled with small holes and increasingly weak, so that it is less able to fulfill its functions of support and movement.

How do women know that they are developing osteoporosis? In its early stages, there are few signs that the condition exists. By the time that bones have reached the state described above—usually between 10 and 15 years—there is little that can be done to reverse the process, although occasionally it can be reversed with high-dose estrogen patches or implants, and to a lesser degree with tablets. Severe osteoporosis reveals itself when unexpected fractures occur, especially of the wrist and top of the thigh bone (hip fractures); or when one or more vertebrae of the backbone become partially crushed, causing height loss and severe pain. If osteoporosis is suspected, it can be confirmed by a medical test that determines bone density.

This account of osteoporosis may sound depressing, but preventative measures can be taken, and treatments may alleviate and even partially reverse symptoms. Although all postmenopausal women can develop osteoporosis, it is more likely to occur in:
• women who have had a hysterectomy with oophorectomy (removal of the ovaries)
• women who, when younger, experienced

amenorrhea (cessation of periods – *see p.98*) because they had low body fat—such as athletes, dancers, or those with anorexia nervosa
• women who experienced a premature menopause before the age of 40
• women who have thyroid problems;
• women who smoke heavily
• women who are on long-term medications such as heparin and prednisone
• women whose mothers have suffered from osteoporosis.

The chance of developing significant osteoporosis can be minimized, even in high-risk groups, by preventative measures such as:
• regular exercise for at least 20 minutes a session, three times a week. Exercise naturally strengthens bones as muscles pull on them. The exercise program does not have to be sophisticated or complex—brisk walking is perfectly adequate
• making sure that the diet is rich in calcium-containing foods—and this applies well before menopause begins. Calcium-rich foods include dairy products, such as milk and cheese; green leafy vegetables; eggs; canned fish with edible bones, such as sardines and salmon; shellfish, such as clams and shrimps; citrus fruits; and nuts, dried peas, and beans. Foods rich in vitamin D are also important for bone maintenance because the vitamin helps calcium absorption. These foods include dairy products, fish, vitamin-enriched margarine, leafy

CALCIUM SUPPLEMENTS

It is recommended that the daily diet of a woman over the age of 40 should include 1,500mg of calcium (1,000mg if she is using HRT); and 1,200 mg if she is over 60. A varied and balanced diet that contains the calcium-rich foods mentioned in the main text should provide sufficient calcium. If a woman feels that she may be at increased risk of osteoporosis, or if she feels that her diet may not be sufficiently rich in calcium, she should seek advice from her doctor about whether she needs a calcium supplement and what type she requires, according to her age and general health. However, no supplement can be guaranteed to prevent osteoporosis.

green vegetables, bread, and whole-grain foods. Vitamin D is also produced in the skin under the influence of sunlight *(for details on healthy diet, see pp.88–9)*;

• hormone replacement therapy (HRT), especially for women whose ovaries have been removed, or who have experienced premature menopause. Increasing estrogen levels is believed to maintain the activity of the osteoblasts and can reverse the decrease in bone mass. However, HRT may not be suitable or acceptable for all women

• the use of drugs. Alendronate sodium, recently approved in the United States, used to help treat osteoporosis of the hip and backbone, helps prevent bone loss and may help women at risk who are unable or unwilling to use HRT. It may also help alleviate the effects of osteoporosis in other parts of the skeleton as well as the backbone. Use of a nasal spray containing calcitonin, a hormone normally produced by the thyroid gland, can stimulate calcium uptake by the bones.

Emotional symptoms

While there is no doubt that most women experience emotional symptoms during their menopause, it is unreasonable—although not unusual—to blame all behavioral changes on menopause. Certainly, decreasing estrogen levels alter the activity of the parts of the brain that control a woman's feeling of well-being. But emotional symptoms may also be evoked by other changes that are happening in a woman's life at the same time as menopause. Her relationship with her partner may be changing or may have ended; older children may be leaving home, while adolescent children may be the cause of stresses and conflicts; or she may be concerned about the direction her life and career are taking.

Common emotional symptoms experienced during menopause are feelings of anxiety, irritability, and depression, interspersed with mood swings and tearfulness. These may lead to a woman losing some self-confidence and having a lowered sense of self-esteem, and can result in conflicts and arguments with family and colleagues.

Women experiencing any or all of these symptoms may find it helpful to talk to their partner, and perhaps their children, about how they feel. HRT and/or some complementary remedies may alleviate the feelings. Exercise often helps as well because it causes the release of calming chemicals called endorphins into the bloodstream.

In addition to emotional symptoms, a woman may also notice that her mental processes are changing as well. During menopause, some women find that they have such unsettling symptoms as forgetfulness, or a temporary inability to concentrate on tasks. Once again, HRT may help remove these symptoms. A woman may also benefit from "exercising" her brain by developing new interests or leisure activities.

Managing menopausal symptoms

Menopause is not a disease and should not be treated as such. However, there are a number of strategies that can help women manage the symptoms they may experience during menopause. Conventional medicine offers HRT, while complementary therapies are used to remove the underlying causes of menopausal symptoms by taking a holistic approach. In addition, a healthy lifestyle that includes exercise and a balanced diet, plus an avoidance of health-damaging habits such as smoking and excessive alcohol consumption, is believed in many cases to reduce or eliminate menopausal symptoms.

Hormone replacement therapy (HRT)

Hormone replacement therapy, or HRT, has become, over recent years, both the most popular and the most controversial medical treatment for the symptoms of menopause. HRT introduces estrogen, and frequently progestin as well, into the body in order to restore the levels of these hormones that prevailed before their secretion by the ovaries went into decline.

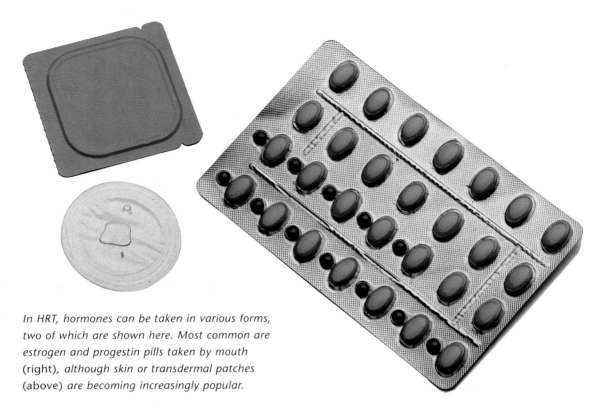

In HRT, hormones can be taken in various forms, two of which are shown here. Most common are estrogen and progestin pills taken by mouth (right), although skin or transdermal patches (above) are becoming increasingly popular.

HRT can be administered in a number of ways *(see above)*. The driving force of the treatment is estrogen, which, on introduction into a woman's body, reverses many menopausal symptoms. Originally, HRT consisted of giving estrogen alone until it was realized that this increased the risk of developing endometrial cancer *(see p.107)*. Today, progestin, which has a protective effect on the uterus, is usually given as a supplement to estrogen to reduce the risk of cancer (unless a woman has had a hysterectomy—*see pp.108–9*). Progestin is only given for part of each month, and when a woman stops taking progestin each month she will probably experience withdrawal bleeding, much like a period. There are also types of no-bleed HRT that supply estrogen and progestin throughout the month.

HRT is undoubtedly effective in reversing the most common menopausal symptoms— hot flashes and vaginal dryness—and often relieves other symptoms including irritability and depression. It also produces an increased sense of well-being. However, some women who have not experienced any particular menopausal problems now use HRT because of the research showing that it can slow or prevent osteoporosis and can reduce the risk of heart disease.

Despite these apparent benefits, some authorities argue that HRT is an unnecessary intrusion into a woman's life that puts her under the control of the medical profession and drug companies for the rest of her life, and treats the menopause as a disease rather than a part of life. *(The arguments for and against HRT are summarized on p.274.)*

Some women experience side effects from HRT, including migraines, bloating (water retention), weight gain and breast tenderness. Side effects such as these, as well as the unwelcome return of monthly bleeding and fears about possible long-term health problems, are responsible for many women "dropping out" of HRT. However, side effects that last for more than one or two months can usually be relieved by changing to a different dose level of hormones, or by changing the type of HRT—from pill to patch, for example. Stopping HRT usually means that menopausal symptoms will return.

Before being prescribed HRT, all women are interviewed and given a thorough medical examination to assess how suitable it is for them. Women who have had undiagnosed vaginal bleeding, a history of breast or endometrial (uterine) cancer, or a strong family history of breast cancer will need careful assessment and may be advised not to have HRT. The same applies to women with heart problems or high blood pressure, or those who are at risk of developing a thrombosis, who are very overweight, or who smoke, although these women may actually benefit from HRT *(see box on long-term effects, below right)*. Because HRT slightly increases the risk of breast cancer, women who are prescribed HRT should be sure to examine their breasts monthly *(see pp.100–1)*, as well as having regular mammograms *(see pp.101–2)*. They should also report to their doctor as soon as possible any unusual symptoms, such as unexpected vaginal bleeding, dizziness, or muscle pains.

The issue of HRT frequently arouses strong feelings. While some people see it as wholly beneficial, others view it as a form of disempowerment engineered by the medical profession. Most doctors now agree that HRT can help in many cases, especially as a preventative measure to reduce the risk of osteoporosis and heart disease. However, it should be seen not in isolation but as an adjunct to a good diet, a healthy lifestyle, a positive attitude toward the body, and the other natural factors that are known to reduce the impact of menopause.

Types of HRT

There are several ways in which HRT can be administered. The choice of different types of HRT means that if one form is not appropriate, another one can be tried to match the individual needs of the woman. Most forms of HRT, apart from suppositories and creams, alleviate the majority of menopausal symptoms, and confer a degree of protection against osteoporosis and heart disease in most women. However these forms of HRT may also cause breast tenderness, nausea, and bloating as side effects, although with a number of different products available within each type of HRT, it should usually be

DIETARY SUPPLEMENTS

Although a balanced diet rich in fresh fruit and vegetables should provide adequate amounts of vitamins, the following supplements may help some women cope with menopausal symptoms. Recommended doses are indicated here as IU (International Units) or mg (milligrams). Vitamin supplements can be obtained from drugstores and health food stores.
• Vitamin B6 (50–100mg daily) may reduce the bloating and depression that can occur as side effects of HRT.
• Vitamin C (500mg daily) helps the body's defense system and may help slow the appearance of wrinkles.
• Vitamin D may improve absorption of calcium into the bloodstream from the small intestine and help reduce the risk of osteoporosis. Vitamin D deficiency is rare, however.
• Vitamin E (400 IU twice a day) may help reduce the effects of hot flashes and night sweats, although large doses of the vitamin should be avoided by women with high blood pressure or a heart condition.

LONG-TERM EFFECTS OF HRT

There have been few long-term studies of the effects of HRT, although one American study, published in 1995 in the *American Journal of Obstetrics and Gynecology*, appears to indicate considerable health benefits for women using HRT long-term. Comparing a group of HRT users with a group of nonusers, the study concluded that those who used HRT had a 60 percent reduction in risk of dying from coronary heart disease and a 73 percent reduction in risk of dying from a stroke. However, there was a slightly higher risk of death from breast cancer. Overall, the mortality rate for women who used HRT was 46 percent below that of women who did not.

possible to find a form and dose of hormones that does not produce any side effects.

Tablets (oral HRT)

These are hormone-containing pills, taken daily or with a seven-day break each month. Typically they contain estrogen, with some also containing progestin, but women who have had a hysterectomy can take estrogen-only pills. Tablets allow a woman to control her therapy, and to stop treatment immediately if she wishes. Oral HRT may be unsuitable for woman who have a history of cardiovascular disorders, such as thrombosis or high blood pressure, and those with liver problems, because the hormones are "processed" by the liver after being absorbed from the intestine.

Skin patches (transdermal HRT)

These are plastic patches containing estrogen that are applied to the skin, usually on the thigh or buttock. The hormone is absorbed steadily through the skin and into the bloodstream. Patches are replaced every three or four days, or once a week. Women who have not had a hysterectomy may also be prescribed progestin in tablet form for part of each month. Like oral HRT, skin patches give a woman control over her therapy, enabling her to stop it at any time. They also appear to have fewer side effects, although they can cause local inflammation of the skin at the site of the patch.

Skin implants (subcutaneous HRT)

This technique (which is not available in the US) involves a tiny incision being made in the skin of the abdomen or buttock under local anesthetic, and the insertion of a pellet containing estrogen into the subcutaneous ("under the skin") fat. Each pellet lasts about six months, during which time estrogen is slowly released into the body. Women who have not had a hysterectomy are also usually advised to take progestin tablets for between 10 and 12 days each month. The advantage of skin implants is that there is no need to remember to take pills or replace skin patches; the disadvantages are that it requires minor surgery, that a woman has no control over the therapy, and that if the dose of hormones is not correct and causes side effects it cannot be modified. However, women experiencing a reduced sex drive may benefit from an implant that also contains small doses of the hormone testosterone.

Creams and suppositories (local hormonal treatment)

Estrogen applied locally to the vulva or vagina can be used to relieve vaginal dryness, one of the most commonly experienced symptoms of menopause. Creams are applied to the vulval area or inside the vagina, and suppositories are inserted into the vagina itself. Such local application not only stimulates vaginal lubrication but also alleviates urinary discomfort. However, these treatments are not effective against other menopausal symptoms, such as hot flashes, nor do they confer any protection against osteoporosis or heart disease. In addition, these suppositories and creams should not be used to aid lubrication during sex —estrogen can be absorbed by a partner through the skin of the penis or fingers during foreplay or intercourse, with possible detrimental effects on the partner's health.

HRT: miracle remedy or interfering with nature?

HRT is an issue that has given rise to considerable controversy.

Supporters of HRT claim that:
• by replacing and keeping constant the estrogen levels inside the body, HRT reverses symptoms associated with lack of estrogen during menopause, including hot flashes and vaginal dryness
• HRT empowers women by allowing them to escape from the female stereotype associated with the "change of life"
• HRT delays or prevents osteoporosis, and can reverse it
• HRT reduces the risk of developing cardiovascular disease, including heart attacks and strokes
• HRT gives a woman a feeling of well-being and extra energy that improves her self-esteem and self-confidence
• HRT enables women to avoid the problems of memory loss and loss of concentration associated with menopause
• some side effects experienced when using HRT can be dealt with by changing to a different type of HRT.

Detractors of HRT claim that:
• use of HRT implies that the menopause is considered a disease to be treated long-term by hormonal drugs
• HRT is not the "answer" to menopausal problems, nor is it a "cure" for old age nor an elixir of youth
• HRT makes a woman a patient, preventing her from having control over her own body
• HRT produces symptoms such as depression, bleeding, and migraines that force many women to stop using it
• the long-term health risks of using HRT are

not fully known

• the claims that HRT can alleviate all menopausal symptoms—including the prevention of osteoporosis—cannot be substantiated

• many menopausal symptoms are the result of lifestyle factors such as lack of exercise and eating poorly. Addressing these factors can alleviate menopausal symptoms without the use of hormonal drugs

• there are many complementary therapies, such as herbalism and yoga, that are as effective in managing menopausal symptoms as HRT

• the driving force behind the popularization of HRT comes from the multinational pharmaceutical companies that manufacture the drugs, whose sole concern is to maximize their profits.

Other drug treatments

For women who do not wish to, or cannot, use HRT, there are other drug treatments available that may be effective in dealing with certain symptoms.

Clonidine
Otherwise used to treat migraine and high blood pressure, this drug may be effective in treating hot flashes and severe headaches.

Propranolol
Normally used to treat high blood pressure and migraine, propranolol may be helpful in dealing with hot flashes.

Antidepressants and tranquilizers
Depression, irritability, and anxiety may arise as side effects of menopause, or as a result of other life changes that are occurring at the same time. In the past, antidepressants and tranquilizers have been prescribed to women to treat such symptoms. It is now recognized that very often these symptoms can be relieved, either by HRT or through complementary treatments, adjustments in lifestyle, or counseling or therapy. Only in a few cases are such drugs needed, and then generally only on a short-term basis. Doctors are nowadays aware that there are no grounds for regarding menopausal symptoms as signs of female neurosis.

Complementary therapies

There are treatments and therapies that lie outside the boundaries of what is conventionally recognized as orthodox medicine. Although they may be used as alternatives to orthodox medical treatments, these therapies are also commonly used to complement orthodox medicine. Traditionally, most complementary therapies were regarded by many doctors with suspicion and disdain. However, there is now a much greater interest from the medical profession in using complementary methods, and in adopting a holistic approach to treatment, in which the whole person is treated rather than simply the "diseased" part. Described below are some of the complementary therapies that menopausal women may find helpful.

Acupuncture
This ancient Chinese therapy is based on the belief that a life force, or Qi (pronounced "chee"), flows around the body along invisible energy channels called meridians. If the flow of this life force along a meridian is blocked, this will cause a disorder. However, the "blockage" may be some distance away from the part of the body that shows signs or symptoms of a disorder. Having ascertained what the problem is, and determined the general health of the patient, the acupuncturist inserts fine acupuncture needles a short distance into the skin at certain points along a

QUESTION AND ANSWER: DRUG-FREE THERAPY

Q. I am 52, and find myself becoming increasingly tense and anxious. I don't want to take HRT or any other drugs. Is there anything else I can do to combat the way I feel?
A. There are various strategies that you may wish to try. First, try talking with a partner or friend about the way you feel or, failing that, see if there is a local support group that you can join. Second, try increasing the amount of exercise you do, or join a yoga or meditation class. Third, try a herbal remedy, such as passionflower, that has a calming effect; seek advice from an herbalist or an herbal remedy book about which remedies are appropriate for you.

particular meridian and rotates the needles between finger and thumb. The purpose of this is to restore the normal flow of Qi along the meridian, thereby removing the disorder. Some women have found that acupuncture is effective in treating their symptoms. Before consulting an acupuncturist, however, it should be established that he or she is fully trained and qualified.

Aromatherapy

This form of complementary therapy uses highly concentrated oils extracted from petals, leaves, and other parts of plants. These oils, known as essential oils, exert their healing effect on the body by being detected as odors or by being absorbed through the skin. The effect of these oils may be mood-altering or may relieve sickness or pain. Each essential oil is used to treat one or more conditions. For example, sage, cypress, rose, lavender, geranium, lemongrass, and ylang-ylang are among the oils believed to help alleviate some menopausal symptoms.

There are various ways of using essential oils. Women who are interested in using aromatherapy may prefer to visit a qualified aromatherapist, or, alternatively, may learn self-help techniques and administer the oils themselves— aromatherapy oils are now available in many drugstores and health food stores. Essential oils, suitably diluted with a base oil to avoid any damage to the skin, are commonly massaged into the skin. They can also be inhaled, or used as a compress (the oil should be diluted, as with massage), or a few drops of the oil can be added to bath water.

Herbalism

The use of herbs to treat disorders is an ancient practice, and although its importance declined as orthodox medicine became more prevalent, it is now seeing something of a revival. Herbalism involves the use of plants, often administered in teas or infusions, as treatments for disorders. If prescribed by herbalists, such treatments may be specifically tailored to an individual's needs. Alternatively, herbal remedies can be obtained from health food stores or natural drugstores. Women who use herbal remedies are advised to seek professional advice, and not to take them in excess or for long periods. Herbal remedies that may be useful in managing menopausal symptoms include chaste tree (also known as *vitex agnus-castus*); wild yam and black cohosh, which both have natural estrogen-like properties; sage, which is believed to be especially effective in dealing with hot flashes and night sweats; and motherwort. Chamomile and hops also act as general relaxants.

Homeopathy

Homeopathy uses natural remedies to enhance the body's built-in healing mechanisms. Each natural remedy produces the same symptoms as a particular disorder, but if administered in a very dilute form it will help the body to resist and overcome that disorder. Homeopathy is also holistic in its approach: each patient is given treatment appropriate for her own physical and emotional makeup. The homeopathic view of menopausal symptoms is that they represent imbalances within the body that need to be addressed. Among the homeopathic remedies that may be prescribed for menopausal symptoms are *lachesis* (the venom of the bushmaster snake, which, if administered undiluted, causes severe hot flashes and palpitations), which helps alleviate hot flashes, and calendula cream, which can reduce vaginal dryness when applied. For advice about homeopathic remedies it is probably best to consult a recognized homeopathic therapist, or a doctor who also has homeopathic qualifications.

Hydrotherapy

Hydrotherapy is treatment with water, most commonly with alternating hot and cold water. One type of hydrotherapy is the sauna. Sitting or lying in the heat of the sauna increases the circulation of blood to the skin, and encourages sweating. This is followed by a cold shower or bath, which reduces blood flow to the skin and increases it to the body's organs. The overall effect is, apparently, to improve circulation and to induce a feeling of well-being. Other forms of hydrotherapy include a steam bath, a sitz bath—where part of the body is immersed in hot water and part immersed in cold—and simply lying in a hot bath to relax the muscles.

Massage

If performed properly, this ancient art, which involves one person stroking and pressing the skin and muscles of another, is an ideal way to relax and calm the mind.

Meditation

Meditation is a self-help technique in which a person "empties" their mind and cuts off the troublesome thoughts that cause stress and tension. The technique has to be learned, and many people find that joining a meditation group with a teacher is the easiest way to do this. There are various meditation techniques, but all involve using the powers of concentration and controlled breathing to focus the thoughts and calm the body. To be effective, meditation should be practiced every day for between 10 and 20 minutes. Its immediate effects are to lower the blood pressure and pulse rate. In the longer term, by helping her gain control over her body, meditation can give a woman the power to manage her life more effectively.

Naturopathy

Naturopathy is a complementary treatment that aims to help the body to treat itself. Rather than looking for a symptom and attempting to alleviate it, a naturopathic therapist will adopt a holistic approach. Each person is treated according to their mental, physical, and social circumstances: the naturopath seeks first to determine the underlying causes of a disorder, and then remove them. In the case of menopause, symptoms are indicative of imbalances within the body, but since symptoms vary from one woman to another, so will the treatment. Diet is regarded by naturopaths as being foremost in aiding recovery, along with therapies that promote a relaxed mind and body, including meditation, yoga, massage, hydrotherapy, and exercise. However, all naturopaths emphasize that success in dealing with disorders depends totally on the patient's recognition of the need

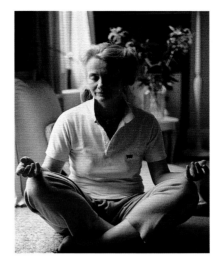

Practicing relaxation techniques such as these, which remove tension from the muscles and "empty" the mind, can be very helpful for many women in providing relief from some of the symptoms commonly experienced during menopause.

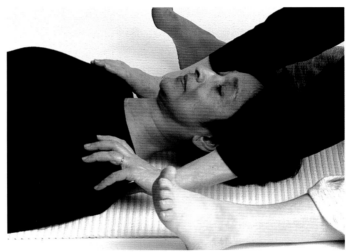

to feel positive about good health, and on her desire and ability to help herself.

Yoga

Yoga is a system of mental, physical, and spiritual training that aims to improve posture and balance and make a person feel relaxed and calm. This is achieved by a series of postures that stretch the body and breathing exercises that relax the mind. As well as increasing suppleness, yoga makes those who practice it more aware of their body. Most menopausal women who use yoga find it helps to lessen or eliminate their symptoms. Those wishing to take up yoga should take lessons with a qualified teacher, who will show them how to work slowly at achieving suppleness without damaging the body.

Diet, exercise, and a healthy lifestyle

It is much easier for a woman to adopt a positive attitude toward menopausal symptoms if she is feeling healthy and generally good about herself. Adopting a healthy lifestyle that will benefit both mind and body, and may help to reduce the impact of the more unwelcome symptoms of the menopause, is straightforward and inexpensive.

Diet

A healthy balanced diet, as described elsewhere in this book *(see pp.88–9)*, should contain a wide range of foods, plenty of fresh fruit and vegetables, and not too much fat, especially not saturated animal fats. Ideally meals should be prepared from raw produce, to ensure that their vitamins have not been lost, and processed and junk foods should be avoided. Menopausal women are often advised to increase the amount of calcium in their diet by eating, for example, skim milk, leafy greens, and canned oily fish with bones, such as salmon, to counteract the calcium that is lost from their bones *(see osteoporosis, pp.269–71)*. Oily fish is also valuable because it contains polyunsaturated fats that help protect against heart disease.

Exercise

Aerobic exercise for 20 minutes or more, three times a week, is beneficial for various reasons. First of all, it increases cardiovascular fitness and reduces the risk—in combination with a lowfat diet—of heart disease or a stroke. Second, it improves muscle tone and bone strength, both of which would otherwise naturally decrease in women of this age (muscle tone and strength can also be enhanced by anaerobic exercise such as weight training). Third, exercise relaxes the body, so it will counteract any feelings of tension and anxiety. Fourth, people who exercise usually sleep better and feel rested when they wake up. And finally, exercise makes people look and feel better, improving their body shape and giving them a healthy glow. Women do not have to join an expensive gym in order to get exercise—both swimming and brisk walking provide good, low-impact aerobic exercise.

Mental stimulation

Brain fitness can be seen as being comparable to muscle fitness—the more the brain is stimulated, the stronger and healthier it will become. Menopause and other changing circumstances in a woman's life can give her the opportunity to exercise her brain by, perhaps, taking up new activities or beginning new

---

LOOKING GOOD AND FEELING GOOD

Although a woman's self-esteem may be dampened during menopause, most women find that their morale can be boosted by one or more of the following strategies, designed to make them feel and look good:

• doing regular exercise, to keep the body toned and at its desired weight
• trying a new hairstyle, or at least making regular visits to the hairdresser
• spoiling oneself by having a special beauty treatment
• having a massage and/or aromatherapy session
• buying some new clothes
• buying attractive and feminine underwear
• going away for a romantic vacation
• enjoying a fulfilling sex life.

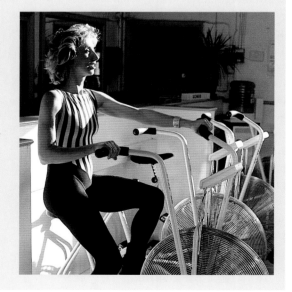

studies. By avoiding boredom or stagnation, a woman should find that she is not only busier but also happier.

Halting body abuse

There are various ways in which many men and women choose to abuse their bodies, thereby making them function less efficiently and, possibly, reducing their life span. Favorite among these abuses are smoking and excessive alcohol intake, both of which can have a deleterious effect on a woman before and after menopause.

Alcohol and menopause

In small quantities (a glass or two of wine a day with meals), alcohol may be beneficial to health. But regular drinking on a long-term basis that exceeds these levels can be harmful. Because some people drink to relax and escape from the stresses and strains of everyday life, it may be tempting for some menopausal women to use alcohol as a way of escaping their anxieties and tensions. However, they should be aware that alcohol can help set off hot flashes, causes depression, stops the body from absorbing certain vitamins, and often prevents women from benefiting fully from a healthy diet or doing exercise. Over longer periods, alcohol can give a woman a bloated, puffy appearance, make her overweight, affect her mental functions, and damage her liver.

Smoking and menopause

Smoking cigarettes is dangerous at any age, and there are numerous reasons for quitting. As far as older women are concerned, those who smoke tend to start menopause earlier, experience more intense menopausal symptoms, and have skin that is in poorer condition and more wrinkled than that of a nonsmoker. And while the risk of having a heart attack, a stroke, or osteoporosis increases in all women after menopause, smoking will increase the risk even more. Add to these factors the greatly increased risk of lung cancer, bronchitis, and emphysema, as well as a number of other conditions, and the

arguments for stopping smoking seem overwhelming. Once withdrawal symptoms have faded, an ex-smoker will feel immediate benefits such as lack of breathlessness. Women who want to stop smoking but are finding it difficult may benefit from seeing their doctor in order to obtain nicotine patches to help wean them off cigarettes.

CHECKUPS DURING MENOPAUSE

Good health does not just depend on a healthy diet and exercise. Preventative medicine also has a part to play, in the form of regular medical checkups. In addition to regular checks of breasts *(see pp.100–1)* and cervix *(see pp.107–8)*, menopausal women should have a yearly physical to assess their general health, including a measurement of blood pressure.

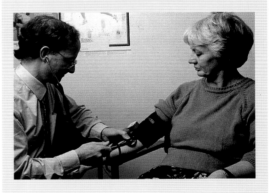

QUESTION AND ANSWER: SEEING A DOCTOR

Q. Do menopausal symptoms always need to be treated? When I experience symptoms, should I automatically see my doctor?
A. No, treatment by conventional or complementary medicine is not automatically required by all women as they go through menopause. Some women experience few if any menopausal symptoms, because of the way their body works and/or because of their lifestyle, and they continue as normal. Other women may experience menopausal symptoms that are severe enough for them to seek help. But the best form of "treatment" for all women is an awareness of what menopause is, knowing what changes are going on inside the body, and having control over their body.

Q. I have been married for 26 years. My relationship with my husband has never been very strong, but we stayed together for the sake of the children. Now that they have left home, I feel tempted to leave my husband and start again. I am going through menopause at present, and I wonder if this feeling is just the result of "the change"— or should I act on my impulses?

A. Many women face this kind of decision in midlife. What you feel is unlikely to be due purely to your being menopausal, although it may be triggered by it. Reaching the menopause milestone gives women the opportunity to reflect on life and relationships. It may help you to talk to your partner about your relationship, and perhaps to consult a marriage counselor. You may find there are other ways to improve your quality of life. But if ultimately you're sure that your relationship is the root of the problem and can't be significantly improved, it's not too late to start a new life.

Q. I seem to have experienced few changes during menopause, and find that my relationship with my husband is going from strength to strength. In many ways we both feel younger every day. But I feel guilty. My good friend, who is about the same age as me, has felt very run down because of menopause, and finds that her relationships with her husband and children are very negative. Should I feel guilty? Am I unusual?

A. The answer to both questions is no. Every woman's experience of menopause is different. It depends on her body physiology, her attitudes, and her relationships. But it may help your friend if you talk through some of her problems with her. It may be that many of them are easy to solve.

Menopause can be an especially difficult time for women who have been unable to have children or have put off having children until it is too late. Now that she is no longer fertile and the possibility of having children is gone forever, a woman may find herself dwelling on lost opportunities and the thought of a future without any children or grandchildren. As with so many worries and anxieties, the best way to overcome them is to talk about them. It helps, of course, if partners can be warm, sympathetic, and comforting. Other members of the family can also provide support. Talking to other couples and single women who have not had children can help remove the feeling of isolation and the sense that there is a norm in society of everyone having children to give meaning to their lives and care for them in old age.

Relationships during menopause

Menopause can be a worrying time for women who are unprepared for what is happening to them, or whose knowledge of this landmark in their lives is based on negative images passed on from an older generation. Even if she is totally aware of the physical and mental changes occurring to her as her body passes through its menopausal phase, a woman may well be exposed to the types of relationship pressures that tend to arise at this stage of life, but which can make her anxious and tense. If she has children, they may be passing through a particularly difficult period of adolescence, or be worried about exams, or looking for work. Alternatively, they may have left home, leaving her with an "empty nest" *(see pp.260–1)* and thereby removing a large part of her maternal role. Her relationship with her partner may be going through the doldrums, for no other reason than that they have been together for so long. If she has a job, she may feel that her colleagues are becoming increasingly younger, and seem to view her as being out of touch and useless. This is also an age when elderly parents may be making ever greater demands on her time and her emotions.

It is therefore vitally important that menopause, and other pressures, do not combine to interfere with a woman's relationships by undermining her confidence in herself and her abilities. It helps enormously if a woman is prepared for menopause by knowing what is happening to her, and if she can discuss her situation openly and in an informed way with her partner and her children. Friends who are also going through menopause, and support groups, can provide vital support: it is often a huge relief to talk with other women who may be having the same problems. Some women seek help from professional counselors to help them put their life into context, and couples may look for assistance in the same way to improve or stabilize their relationship. Communication and knowledge are the keys.

Sex and menopause

Menopause may mark the end of a woman's reproductive life, but it does not mean that her need and desire for sex come to an end. Many women find that their sex lives continue as before both during and after the menopause. Indeed, some woman find that the liberation from contraception and periods is a positive bonus that increases their enjoyment of sex. In the period leading up to menopause it is important not to forget contraception, even when periods are irregular.

Contraception

Although a woman is less fertile in her forties than she was in her twenties, contraception should still be considered an important issue for both herself and her partner. Despite her declining fertility, a woman in her early forties who is sexually active still has a 20 percent chance of becoming pregnant within 12 months if she and her partner neglect to use any contraception. Furthermore, the early signs that menopause is on its way, such as irregular periods and hot flashes, do not mean that a woman has become infertile. During the perimenopausal phase ovulation still occurs, so there is a chance, albeit a small one, that a woman may become pregnant.

If a woman does become pregnant at this age, and the pregnancy is not wanted, she and her partner will need to make some hard decisions. She could opt for a termination, but this may not be acceptable to her for moral or religious reasons. If the pregnancy is terminated, she may have to deal with feelings of guilt and loss. If she is considering proceeding with the pregnancy, she and her partner should think about the greater risks and complications for the older mother (see box, p.206). In addition, if they decide to have a child, they should consider the realities of coping with an adolescent when they are in their sixties! To avoid the risk of unplanned pregnancy and to feel reassured that the woman is fully protected, couples should ensure that they have suitable contraception. Extra reassurance is provided by the fact that as a woman becomes less

fertile during the perimenopausal stage, contraceptive methods become more effective. A couple should keep using contraception until ovulation has definitely ceased.

Contraceptive choices for older women

The contraceptive options open to women during the perimenopausal period are much the same as those available to younger women. However, certain forms of contraception may be more appropriate at this time. An ideal perimenopausal contraceptive would be one which is not only effective but helps to alleviate symptoms such as vaginal dryness; which provides estrogen as protection against osteoporosis (see pp.269–71); and which does not mask symptoms of menopausal onset such as the cessation of periods. There are both advantages and disadvantages associated with any method of contraception that a woman might consider during the menopause (for more detail on contraception, see Chapter 5):

• The combined pill is considered by many doctors to be an appropriate contraceptive for menopausal women (apart from those for whom it is not suitable—see p.145), not only because of its effectiveness but also because the estrogen it contains supplements the declining amounts produced naturally by the body. These supplements can also relieve sexual symptoms associated with the decline in estrogen levels that occurs during the perimenopause, such as vaginal dryness and

WHEN CAN WOMEN SAFELY STOP CONTRACEPTION?

If a woman is sexually active and she or her partner has not been sterilized, they should continue to use contraception until they are sure she is no longer fertile. Generally speaking, women over 50 can stop using contraception if they have not had a period for more than a year, and if they are showing some menopausal symptoms. For women under 50, the "waiting period" should be extended to two years before they can consider it safe to abandon contraception. Another indication is provided by measurement of the hormones FSH and LH (see pp.20–3) in the blood. If these are elevated above the levels normally expected, they generally indicate that a woman is no longer fertile and can stop using contraception. However, if a woman experiences amenorrhea (see pp.98–9) under the age of 40, she should consult her doctor.

reduced libido, as well as acting as a contraceptive. The pill can prevent manifestations of menopause such as hot flashes, and reduce the effects of early-onset osteoporosis. It also reduces the risk of developing conditions such as ovarian and uterine cancer and endometriosis (see pp.105–8). However, because of its effects, the pill does mask menopausal symptoms, as well as causing regular bleeding. Many doctors advise women of 50 to stop taking the pill, and to switch to an alternative nonhormonal contraceptive method. If they then show menopausal symptoms, such as hot flashes, they can decide whether or not to proceed with HRT.

• The progestin-only pill or minipill is a highly effective alternative for older women who want to use a hormonal method but for whom the pill is not suitable. But, because it contains no estrogen, it does not confer any of the pill's beneficial side effects. The same applies to other hormonal methods such as implants and injections.

• Barrier methods such as male and female condoms, and the diaphragm and cap, are much more effective in older women because their fertility is lower. However, they are not usually popular with couples who have not used barrier methods before. And they do not provide any hormonal benefits.

• The IUD (see pp.152–5) is a highly effective contraceptive device in perimenopausal women. While this is used as a contraceptive, HRT can also be given at the same time to alleviate perimenopausal symptoms.

• Natural family planning methods are not usually recommended for a woman in her late forties because menstrual cycles tend to become more erratic at this age.

QUESTION & ANSWER: CAN HRT BE A CONTRACEPTIVE?

Q. If HRT is used to introduce hormones such as estrogen into the body, why can't it be prescribed before menopause as a contraceptive?

A. Most of the forms of HRT in current use do not have a contraceptive effect. Unlike the pill, which contains synthetic estrogen, HRT uses "natural estrogens" that alleviate perimenopausal symptoms but are not "strong enough" to prevent ovulation.

• Male or female sterilization has, in many countries, been the most popular option for couples over 40. However, with more effective methods of contraception now available—made still more effective at this stage in a woman's life because of her reduced fertility—and with the possible risks of sterilization, more couples are being advised to opt for contraception rather than sterilization. Sterilization for women over 45 is thought to be ill-advised since they will become naturally "sterile" within a few years anyway.

Enjoying sex during and after menopause

Every woman is different in the way menopause affects her sexuality and desire. A majority of women find that there is little change in their sex life, while some find that their desire for sex increases, and others experience a loss of interest in sex. The way in which a woman responds is not solely related to her hormonal levels, however. Sexual desire is both learned and innate. If a woman had a pleasurable sex life with her partner before menopause, and she is healthy, it is likely that sex will continue as normal after menopause. On the other hand, if a woman did not particularly enjoy sex before menopause, or if she had a poor relationship with her partner, or if she finds that she is losing her self-esteem and no longer feels sexually attractive, her interest in sex may decline further, unless she and her partner make an attempt to change the situation and deal with any problems that may have been exacerbated by her changing hormonal levels.

The postmenopausal period, freed as it is from the worries of pregnancy and periods, may give women more time to enjoy and explore sex. A woman and her partner may find that their sexual activity involves greater enjoyment, subtlety, and variety. Nongenital contact, such as massage, as well as extended foreplay, oral sex, and mutual masturbation can all form part of a wider range of sexual activities. Sexual enjoyment will, obviously, depend on how openly partners communicate with each other, and how close they are.

At the same time that his partner is going through menopause, a man may also be experiencing midlife changes that affect his emotional and sexual life. He may find that his sexual drive is decreasing and he has erection difficulties. But if partners care about each other, and can talk about these worries, then problems can usually be overcome.

Male menopause: myth or reality?

Do middle-aged men experience a "change of life"—an andropause—analogous to a woman's menopause? Most doctors would respond with a firm "no" to that question. However, there is no doubt that some men in their forties, fifties, and sixties experience troublesome and upsetting symptoms that can include lethargy, mood swings, depression, loss of sex drive, and erection problems. Moreover, it appears that these symptoms are caused by a decrease in the influence of testosterone, the male sex hormone that affects sex drive and erections as well as a man's feelings of well-being and zest for life.

Most experts believe that there is no andropause as such, but that the symptoms experienced by middle-aged men—sometimes described as andropausal symptoms—are the result of either a decrease in production of testosterone or a lessening of its effectiveness in the body. But why should this decline happen? Certainly, the testes (the source of male sex hormones) do not "switch off" as do the ovaries (the source of female sex hormones). And although there is usually a steady decrease in testosterone production in the later years, this is probably not sufficient to produce changes in the middle years.

In many cases it is believed that andropausal symptoms can be attributed to a continuously unhealthy lifestyle. For example, heavy smoking and excessive consumption of alcohol both contribute to decreased libido and impotence; heavy drinking increases the production of a chemical called sex-hormone-binding globulin that lowers the effectiveness of testosterone. In these circumstances, adopting a healthier lifestyle by quitting smoking, drinking in moderation, managing stress,

RESTORING DIMINISHED SEX DRIVE

The sex drive in both women and men is controlled by hormones called androgens, the most common of which is testosterone. Women who find that their sex drive has diminished after menopause, or after the removal of their ovaries, may well be candidates for hormone replacement therapy using testosterone. This form of HRT can be administered as an injection or in tablet form. Women should be prescribed the lowest dose possible to increase their sex drive. In excess, testosterone will produce masculine characteristics such as some facial hair growth or a lowering of the voice, and may have longer-term effects, including the increased risk of heart disease.

exercising regularly, losing excess body fat, and eating a balanced diet with plenty of fruit and vegetables may well cause a disappearance of any symptoms and a return to better health and sexual vigor.

However, in some cases injury or illness may be the cause of irreversibly lowered testosterone levels. If this is the case, and blood tests confirm a hormone deficiency, some specialists opt to give their male patients hormone replacement therapy (HRT) in the form of testosterone supplements. When used properly, male HRT, which can be administered orally or by injection (see p.274), has a high success rate. However, some doctors fear that male HRT may lead to an increase in the occurrence of prostate cancer (see pp.111–13) because testosterone stimulates the growth of any existing prostate tumors. And although doctors who administer HRT usually also give their patients a blood test for prostate-specific antigen (a chemical marker for prostate cancer), and cease prescribing HRT if the test proves positive, there are as yet no studies on the long-term effects of HRT in men.

Certainly, most men who experience andropausal symptoms should not see HRT as a cure-all but should look first at the emotional and lifestyle factors that may be affecting their emotional and sexual happiness. It will obviously help if they have a secure and trusting relationship with their partner in which they can discuss matters openly and sympathetically.

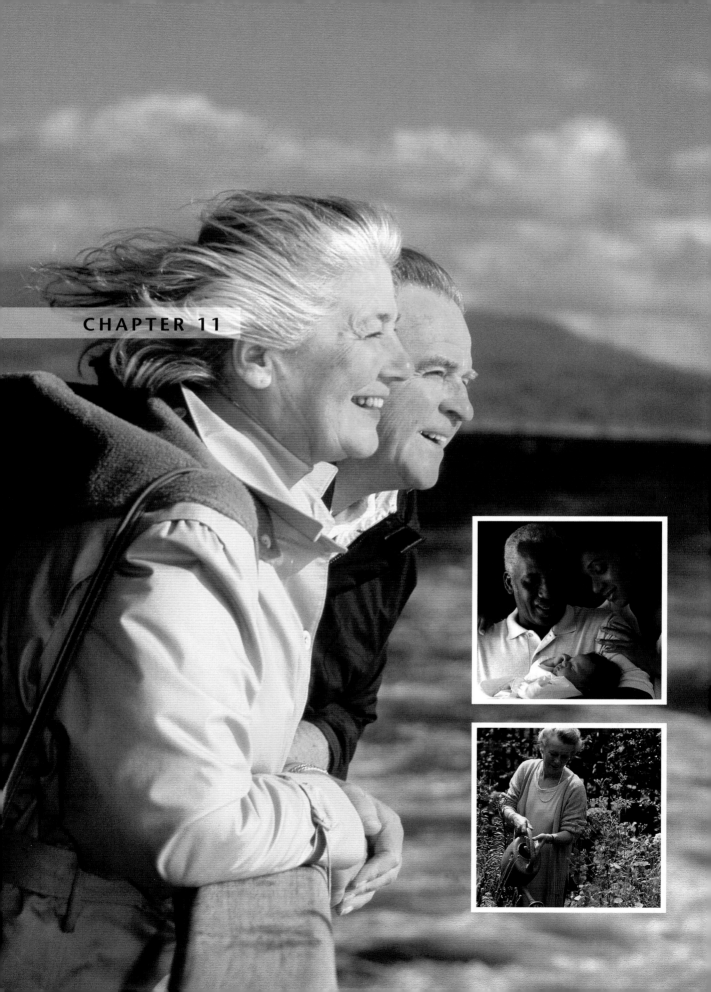

CHAPTER 11

The Later Years

The later years are marked by many milestones. Women reach the end of their reproductive years. Men and women who have been employed for much of their adult life are usually anticipating retirement, sometimes with apprehension, but frequently with pleasure. Couples who have had children will probably have seen them leave home and set up home on their own. And whether married, in a relationship, or single, people become aware in their late sixties and seventies that they are beginning the later years of their life. In many ways these milestones are advantageous. Freed from the constraints of work and raising children, many older people find that they can enjoy a new lease on life—provided that they have an informed and proactive attitude toward aging.

Many people view the prospect of becoming old with trepidation. Fortunately, times are changing and agism is being challenged. The conventional image of the old as frail and dependent is being cast aside as people realize that a healthy 65-year-old can be in better shape than an unhealthy 35-year-old. Increasingly, older men and women are showing that they can live full, productive, and independent lives, especially if they exercise regularly, eat a healthy diet, and keep mentally stimulated. And despite continuing widespread ignorance about sexuality in the later years, there is a growing recognition not only that many older couples enjoy an active sex life, but that good sex helps maintain a happy relationship, and contributes to a sense of well-being.

Understanding the physical, emotional, social, and economic changes that are likely to occur from their sixties onward can empower older people to take control of their lives by planning for the future and making the most of their later years. They are also usually confident enough about themselves to no longer worry about other people's opinions and to resist social and family pressures. By coping successfully with these changes—such as menopause, becoming grandparents, retirement, or bereavement—older people can devote their time to developing new interests, grasping new opportunities, and enjoying the rest of their life.

A new lease on life
Average life expectancy for both men and women has increased considerably during the twentieth century. In the US, by the mid-1990s a woman of 60 could expect to live on average another 22.6 years and a man of 60 on average another 18.2 years. Certainly most people in the developed world now can expect to be living active lives well into their seventies and eighties.

Myths about aging

Many people in their later years have active, interesting lives and make valuable contributions to their community. Here some of the commonly held falsehoods about old age are listed—and dismissed.

• "As they get older, most people's mental facilities go into decline until they eventually become senile."

False. The majority of older people retain their mental ability and agility, especially if they "exercise" their brains with activities, such as reading, study, hobbies, and volunteer work, that are intellectually stimulating. Only a minority of people in their later years—in the US just one in five people over 80—develop a general decline in mental ability.

• "Everyone should retire at 60 because, after this age, they are no longer fit to cope with the demands of work."

False. Although many jobs, in both public and private sectors, have retirement ages set at 60 or 65, there is no reason why people should not continue working after this, provided that they are able. In fact, retirement at a set age

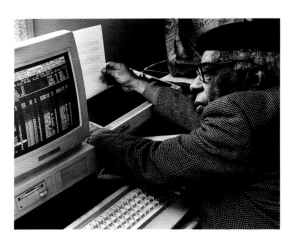

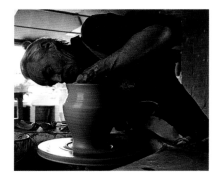

Getting older does not mean enforced idleness. Many people in their later years enjoy learning new skills like computing (above) *or developing hobbies such as pottery* (right).

may have a deleterious effect on a person's health and confidence if he or she feels that they have been pushed out of work prematurely. Some employers are now hiring people over retirement age because they make better workers than their younger counterparts, with more common sense and reliability. Indeed many people continue to be or become self-employed or start their own business after retirement.

• "Old people are incapable of leading independent lives and need outside support."

False. Most older people lead an independent existence and care for themselves in just the same way that they have done all their lives. It is only a minority of older people who, for reasons of physical or mental health problems, require help or need to move into a hospital or nursing home.

• "People in their later years are no longer capable of enjoying a sexual relationship."

False. A majority of men and women continue to enjoy sex and intimacy well into old age, sometimes with a new partner.

• "Old people are content to sit back and think about the past."

False. Just because they are old does not mean that older people do not experience the same joys, anxieties, pleasures, and setbacks that everyone else does. Many older people have no desire to dwell on the past, preferring instead to look to the future and enjoy a variety of new experiences.

Later years—golden years?

In contrast to those negative myths, some writers have idealized the later years of life as a golden age, when people move happily to the end of their life, content with everything and surrounded by a loving family. In reality, older people can face loneliness and illness, as well as many of the other problems that the rest of us have. However, providing we remain healthy, adopt a positive attitude, and adapt to the changes that inevitably take place within our families, we are perfectly capable of taking on the challenges of the later years and enjoying an enjoyable and fulfilled—if not golden—phase of our lives.

Retirement

Retirement from work should not mean a withdrawal from life in general. Freedom from a daily timetable can give you and your partner time to do all the things and visit all the places that you previously had no time for. But there is no point sitting at home waiting for things to happen. You need to take the initiative to make your retirement as enjoyable and productive as you want by making plans before you stop working. This will help ensure a smooth transition from full-time work to full-time retirement.

• Seek advice from a reputable financial consultant or attend a preretirement seminar, if there is one available to you.

• Discuss retirement plans with your partner. She or he will be spending more time with you, so you need to make sure that you both have a positive attitude about embarking on this new phase in your lives.

• Try to ensure that you have a firm financial footing so that you can continue to enjoy a quality of life similar to that which you had when you were working. Consult a financial planner if you feel you need more advice on any aspect of your finances.

• Make a list of all the things that you want to achieve, and when you want to achieve them. It is very easy to procrastinate; if you leave things until tomorrow, they never get done.

• You might investigate the possibility of future part-time work, either to supplement income from your pension or to exercise your skills on a volunteer basis—for example, by working for a charity.

The downside of retirement

Retirement can mean, for many men and women, a new lease on life, freed from the constraints of a daily pattern of work. But for a sizable minority of retirees, especially men, work was such a major part of their lives, that their reason for existence seems to have disappeared. Most men in this position have spent their life working long hours, with few outside interests, and, perhaps, with minimal involvement with their partner and children. Now they have nothing to do and limited

THE "RIGHT" TIME TO RETIRE

If you are thinking about when to retire from your job—and if you have the choice—it may help if you ask yourself some of these questions.

• Do you really want to stop working, or do you have to because there is a set retirement age in your job? If it is the latter case, and you want to keep on working, look around to see if there is another job you can do—perhaps part-time, or even volunteer work—so that you can keep busy.

• Will you have a pension to live on, and will it be sufficiently large to support you and your partner, if he or she does not have a pension of their own? If your future finances are not secure, then resolve them before you retire.

• Have you done any planning ahead to decide what you are going to do on a day-to-day basis when you stop working? Have you discussed plans with your partner, and taken her or his views into account?

QUESTIONS AND ANSWERS: RETIREMENT

Q. My husband retired from his job a year ago. Since then he has spent most of his time sitting around the house reading the newspaper or watching television, and generally getting in my way. He has also lost the vitality and cheerfulness he had when he was working. What can I do to help him?

A. When you say that your husband is "getting in your way" you may have put your finger on one of the problems. If, in the past, work was his domain, and the home was yours, he may now feel he has no control over his surroundings. Try to make him feel that he is not a nuisance; share some of the household chores with him, perhaps allocating him his own tasks, so that he feels useful; go out for meals or day trips or take a vacation together, so that you get out of the house and share new experiences on neutral territory; and suggest that he find a part-time job or a new interest.

Q. Now that I have retired and have more free time I would like to improve my fitness, but I am too embarrassed to join the local health club because I am worried that everyone there will be much younger than me. What can I do?

A. There is no need to join a gym in order to get into shape. Exercises such as jogging and running are good for improving fitness, and so are swimming and tennis. But if you want to join a health club, go ahead. Health clubs are not restricted to young people, and most have a broad age range in their membership. If you do join, nobody will be staring at you! In health clubs most people are too busy admiring themselves!

ideas of how to occupy their time. This will also affect their partner, who now finds that she has a depressed and underoccupied man under her feet all day.

But it is not just men who can be adversely affected by retirement. A busy career woman can retire to find that her partner expects to have gained a cook, a cleaner, and a gardener.

In either of these scenarios a couple may start to feel trapped together, a feeling often aggravated by a drop in income that prevents them from enjoying the same standard of living as before.

Another possible negative aspect of retirement can be that a man has such a loss of self-esteem when he retires that it results in sexual problems such as impotence. Women may become so depressed that they lose interest in sex.

Couples who are concerned about the effects of retirement, and who dread its arrival, should talk about how they are going to deal with this life change, and perhaps attend classes on retirement, or even seek counseling, before it happens.

Looking good and feeling good

Aging does not mean decaying. While it is true that the body slows down and undergoes the irreversible changes of aging—such as wrinkling skin and stiffer joints—as we get older,

there are many ways in which people in their later years can delay or slow these changes by looking after their general health so that they feel healthy and alive. Feeling good not only helps to maintain self-esteem, it can also help partners to retain the liveliness of their relationship, allowing it to grow and develop rather than stagnate. By keeping fit and eating well, and by adopting a positive attitude toward aging, older people are also less likely to suffer from the health problems that become more prevalent in the later years, and are more likely to be active and optimistic.

Body changes and health problems

Once we get into our fifties, general wear and tear starts to take its toll on our bodies and we start to age visibly.

However, many of the physical and mental changes associated with age can be delayed by leading an active lifestyle. Eating well and exercising can slow physical changes such as decreasing heart efficiency or loss of muscle tissue, while mental stimulation such as doing crosswords or even playing trivia games can combat mental changes. In many cases being old does not mean that a person's quality of life has to be downgraded by reduced vitality, provided that measures are taken to keep the body healthy.

The standard of health care in the developed world is improving all the time, and regular health tests, such as mammograms and pap smears for women, prostate examina-

---

SKIN AND HAIR CARE IN THE LATER YEARS

Healthy-looking skin and hair are essential parts of looking good. Although, as we age, the skin tends to become less elastic, more wrinkled, and drier, and the hair grayer and thinner, there are ways of making these changes less obvious.

• Moisturizing cream used daily on the face, neck, and hands can improve the condition of

the skin enormously and lessen the apparentness of any wrinkles that develop.

• Skin is easily damaged by sunlight. Protect it from overexposure by wearing sunscreen, a hat, and loose clothing, and by not walking or sitting outside during the hottest parts of the day.

• Put bath oil into your bath water to prevent excessive

drying out of the skin. (Be careful getting out of the tub!)

• Cosmetic surgery (see pp.254–5) may be an option.

• Having your hair cut and styled regularly will keep it in good condition and allow you to change your look as necessary. Remember that unwashed, unkempt hair looks just as bad on a man as it does on a woman.

EXERCISING FOR BETTER HEALTH

Exercise makes you feel healthier, more supple, and relaxed, and can help prolong your life. As many people get older they find that they switch from strenuous sports, such as squash, to less strenuous ones, such as swimming. Unless they have a severe disability in old age, most people can find a type of exercise to suit them. There are two important points to remember: first, never overdo it; and second, if you are starting to exercise, begin slowly and build up gradually. Here are some exercise suggestions.

• Walking, especially brisk walking, is an excellent form of aerobic exercise.

• Golf is good for flexibility and has the benefit of being sociable as well.

• Swimming provides all-around exercise for fitness, strength, and suppleness without straining joints.

• Tennis is enjoyed by some people well into old age; it has the benefit, like golf, of being a sociable sport.

• Yoga is an excellent way of maintaining suppleness and of finding inner peace.

• Exercise classes especially designed for those over 60 can be ideal. Many health clubs and senior groups provide free classes.

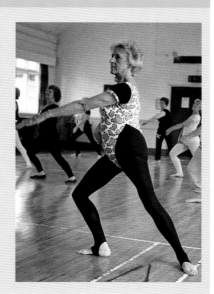

tions for men, and blood pressure monitoring for both sexes, provide early warning of treatable diseases. *(The possible effects of these conditions and of the drugs used to treat common disorders are described in detail in Chapter 4.)*

Diet and exercise

A balanced diet and exercise are just as important in the later years as at any other time in life. As the body ages, its metabolic rate—the rate at which it uses energy to power its life processes—slows down. As a consequence, some older people may put on weight, especially after retirement when they tend to become less active. Anyone who finds that they are putting on weight can do something about it by slightly reducing their daily intake of calories, by eating less fat and sugar, and, if possible, by getting more exercise. Staying well by eating healthfully and exercising also boosts the immune system—the body's system that protects it against disease.

Sensible eating in the later years

A healthy diet *(see pp.88–9)* should contain a variety of foods, preferably fresh and not processed. Some older people, especially if they are living on their own, eat a poor diet because they "can't be bothered" or because they are physically unable to shop for fresh foods or prepare and cook them. In either case, older people can find that a balanced, varied diet will help them feel and look better. Also, fresh foods often cost less than processed foods. Eating unrefined foods such as brown rice, vegetables, and fruit adds fiber to the diet and helps prevent constipation. To improve their diet older people can take some of the following measures.

• Avoid eating too many processed foods; these usually contain hidden fats and sugar.

• Eat carbohydrate in the form of pasta, rice, or potatoes as the main energy source.

• Avoid too much fat, especially animal fats; eat lowfat dairy products because these provide vitamins and vital calcium without extra fat. Try broiling or steaming foods rather than frying them.

• Eat fresh fruit and raw or lightly cooked vegetables every day. Both provide vitamins and minerals, as well as the fiber needed to keep the digestive system working efficiently.

• Choose fish and poultry rather than red meat, which is rich in saturated fat. Oily fish eaten regularly as part of a balanced lowfat diet can help to protect against heart disease. Canned oily fish with soft bones, such as sardines and salmon, provides a handy source of calcium, a mineral essential to older people for the maintenance of strong bones (see osteoporosis—pp.269–71).

• Drink plenty of nonalcoholic fluids (preferably eight glasses per day). Avoid coffee and tea, because of the effects of the caffeine contained in them. With adequate fiber in the diet this will help prevent constipation.

• Avoid drinking excessive amounts of alcohol. Tolerance to alcohol decreases steadily with age, and excessive consumption can result in malnutrition—because the person does not eat sufficient food—as well as an increased risk of developing certain diseases. It is best to limit yourself to one or two measures of alcohol a day, preferably consumed with food.

QUESTION AND ANSWER: DIET

Q. I have decided at the age of 66 to become a vegetarian, and will no longer be eating any animal products apart from eggs, milk, yogurt, and cheese. How can I make sure that I am receiving all the vitamins and minerals I need?
A. Provided your diet is varied and balanced, you should have no problem obtaining all the minerals and vitamins that you need. Apart from plenty of fresh fruit and vegetables, include foods rich in complex carbohydrates such as rice, bread, and pasta, for energy; and protein-rich foods such as beans, nuts, textured vegetable protein (TVP), and tofu, for repairing and maintaining the body. However, take particular care that you get enough of the following minerals and vitamins, because these are not as abundant in a vegetarian diet as in one that contains meat and fish—take supplements if necessary.

• Calcium is found in dairy products, dried fruits, nuts, broccoli, leafy green vegetables, and dried peas and beans. Calcium is needed for healthy bones and is especially important in the later years because bones tend to become weaker as they lose some of their mass.

• Iron is found in beans, dried fruits, leafy green vegetables, nuts, egg yolks, and whole-grain flour and bread. Iron is an essential component of hemoglobin, the chemical found in red blood cells that carries oxygen around the body. Lack of iron results in anemia.

• Vitamin B12 is found in milk, eggs, and some breakfast cereals (read the ingredients list for confirmation). While Vitamin B12 deficiency is rare, it can cause pernicious anemia and neurological problems. B12 is necessary for red blood cell production and for a healthy nervous system.

Sex in the later years

In most societies, sex is perceived to be the domain of the young. Sex in the later years may be seen by both young and old people as being either unbelievable—many children cannot imagine that their parents have any sort of sex life—or something of a taboo subject, with the only acknowledged physical contact being a kiss or a hug. But in practical terms, there is no reason why most people should not be sexually active well into old age, and the main constraint in actuality is that many elderly people have no partner because of death or divorce.

In fact, survey after survey has revealed that, in spite of what the younger generation may believe, older people who are healthy often enjoy an active and interesting sex life into their sixties, seventies, and later. One recent study revealed that in the 60-to-70 age group, over three quarters of men and women enjoyed regular sexual activity—sexual intercourse, oral sex, or masturbation. In fact, while the intensity and frequency of sex often decline with age, sexual activity and interest only ends if severe illness or bereavement intervenes. If the quantity of sex decreases, the quality of sex can increase because many of the contraceptive and menstrual constraints that interfere with sex in the younger years are no longer present. And, since people are living longer, enjoying sex into old age can and does significantly enhance the quality of life.

The pattern of sexual behavior experienced by a couple in the later years depends very largely on how often and how much they enjoyed sex previously. Couples who have always enjoyed uninhibited sex, and found their sex lives to be fulfilling and fun, should continue to enjoy active sex. They may well increase their sexual repertoire and become better lovers in the process. On the other hand, couples who in their younger and middle years found sex distasteful or a chore are unlikely to experience a surge in sexual interest in their later years. Women or men who tolerated sex as part of their "matrimonial duties" may see the onset of old age as a way of escaping their obligations, particularly if they can exaggerate a health problem into an excuse for avoiding sexual contact.

Why sex can get better as you get older

For many couples, sex may actually improve as they get older, especially if they have enjoyed a good sex life earlier in their relationship. Couples may find that they discover new ways of making love, perhaps because they are feeling innovative, or perhaps because they are looking for positions that are more comfortable for them. There are various reasons why this may happen.

• When children have left home, a couple can enjoy leisurely sex without the worry of being interrupted.

• A couple can enjoy sex at any time of the month because the woman is no longer having her periods.

• There is no longer any need to think about contraception, or to worry about the possibility of becoming pregnant.

• If one or both partners have retired from full-time work, they have more leisure time in which to enjoy sex.

• Freed from many of the pressures that interfere with the sex lives of younger and middle-aged people, older couples can spend longer arousing each other and talking about what gives each of them pleasure. They also may feel less stressed and less tired than they did in their middle years.

Sexual changes and aging

Changes in the reproductive system and the other parts of the body involved in sex are as inevitable as other changes to the body in older age. Described below are sexual changes that commonly occur during aging, as well as ways of adapting to these changes by changing patterns of sexual behavior.

Sexual changes in men

As they age, all men experience changes in the way their body performs sexually. Overall, there tends to be a decrease in the feeling of sexual urgency. Men often find that, unlike in the past, their penis does not leap to attention at the first hint of sex but takes time to

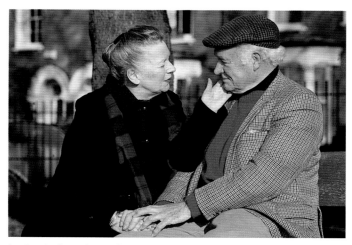

Loving feelings do not have to dim with age. Affection and tenderness are just as important in the later years as in the first years of a couple's relationship.

become erect, and may need some direct stimulation—either from the man himself or from his partner—to help things along. Once erect, the penis may not be as stiff as it used to be, and it may spend some of the period of arousal in a state of partial erection. A man may also notice that he loses his erection once or twice during sex even though he is feeling very aroused. Ejaculation may change as well. Most older men find that they experience fewer contractions during ejaculation, and that the actual amount of semen squirted out of the penis during ejaculation decreases, as does the force with which ejaculation takes place.

Older men may also find that they do not ejaculate every time they have sex. A man's refractory period—the time he needs to wait after one sexual episode before he feels sufficiently interested in sex to embark on another one—increases steadily with age.

If he is unprepared for these changes, a man may feel that he is on the way out sexually. Many men wrongly equate rapid erection and stiffer erection with greater arousal. And by not recognizing that the physiological changes associated with aging are perfectly natural, a man can feel inadequate, resulting in a loss of interest in sex and possibly impotence. This explains why many men in their mid-fifties and older feel that they have lost their virility. In fact, nothing could be further from the truth. In the majority of cases, an older man will feel just as sexually aroused as he did before, except that his sex organs are behaving in a slower and more gentlemanly manner!

Sexual changes in women

After her menopause, a woman usually experiences sexual changes caused by falling levels of female sex hormones *(see Chapter 10)*. The most common of these changes affects the lubrication of the vagina during sexual arousal. Vaginal dryness may be alleviated by the use of hormone replacement therapy (HRT —*see pp.271–5)*, or possibly by prolonging sexual foreplay *(see box, below)*. On the other hand, the clitoris and nipples normally retain their sensitivity, and clitoral response and orgasmic contractions are similar to those experienced in earlier years. Some women find after menopause that their sex drive decreases, while others find it increases. The main reason for any decrease is a fall in the level of androgens, hormones that control sex drive in both men and women. Should this occur, a woman may wish to seek advice from her doctor about using HRT in the form of testosterone to boost her androgen levels.

Tips for sexual happiness in the later years

Developments in a person's sexual interests and activities as one gets older depends very much on individual expectations and experiences (assuming the person is in good health). There are, however, various ways in which couples and individuals can enhance their sexual satisfaction in their later years.

Exercise and a healthy diet

By staying in shape through regular exercising and eating a well-balanced diet rich in vitamins and minerals, a person will feel more confident about their looks and more relaxed, which in turn can only help to enhance sexual arousal and enjoyment of sex.

Communication

It is still important to discuss feelings and needs with a partner, so that neither of the two takes the other for granted. Also, talking about sex with a partner can be just as arousing and exciting as it was when both of them were younger.

Attitude

If older people become brainwashed by the old-fashioned notion that getting older automatically means that the body is in steep decline, then their sexual activities may well go into steep decline as well. Taking a positive

ADAPTING TO SEXUAL CHANGES

While it is true that a man and woman often take longer to become sexually aroused as they age, they also have greater control over their sexual responses and can, if they wish, delight in long, lingering sessions of sensual pleasure. But to do this successfully, each partner must be aware of any changes in the way their partner is functioning sexually. This will enable both to be most effective in helping each other to achieve sexual pleasure.

● **Helping a woman**
A man can help his partner enjoy sex by spending more time arousing her. Touching, holding, stroking, and kissing are all important in arousal, and the man should pay special

attention to his partner's breasts, nipples, vulva, and clitoris. Prolonged foreplay of this type may well produce sufficient lubrication in the vagina to allow comfortable and satisfying intercourse to take place, should the couple desire it. If vaginal dryness remains a problem, even though the women is sexually aroused, a lubricating gel will usually help.

● **Helping a man**
A woman can help her partner enjoy sex by spending time stroking or kissing his penis and scrotum to provide direct stimulation, appreciating the fact that he may take longer to get an erection. It may help if they adopt new positions

for intercourse—for example, if the woman is on top during intercourse, she can control the movement of his penis inside her vagina and stimulate the penis by hand if necessary. Another suitable position for intercourse might be for the couple to lie side by side, facing each other. They can stay in this position for prolonged periods—without getting tired—so that lovemaking can be slow and sensual. Both partners can benefit from the fact that the man now takes longer to become aroused, because he will also "last longer" during intercourse or oral sex, so he will be able to delay his orgasm until his partner has achieved her orgasm.

attitude toward aging, and realizing that it is feasible for many men and women to remain sexually active into old age, can not only prolong but even improve your sex life.

Imagination and variety

Trying new ways of enjoying sex, finding different times of the day to enjoy being intimate, and perhaps changing the location for sexual encounters may help improve a couple's sexual relationship.

Alcohol

It is wise for older people to limit the amount of alcohol that they drink, and to have some periods when they avoid alcohol altogether. Alcohol is a drug that depresses the central nervous system. One or two drinks may have a beneficial relaxing effect. But taken in excess—meaning more than a couple of glasses of wine, beer, or hard liquor—alcohol can delay or completely inhibit arousal in both men and women.

Troubleshooting

If problems do arise, such as vaginal dryness or taking longer to get an erection, recognize that these are natural changes which you can handle with self-help techniques. If they are not dealt with, or not discussed, the smallest problems can become intensified to the point that they inhibit sex completely. Don't be put off by any disappointments along the way.

Use it or lose it

Just as regular exercise helps tone muscles and maintain cardiovascular fitness, so regular sex—and regular means as often as you both want to have sex, as well as masturbation—will help keep the reproductive organs in good condition and counteract the effects that aging normally has on sexual arousal and response.

Sex and those over 80

Sex has no age limit, providing the participants are healthy. In 1988 the results of an American survey on the sexual interests of a group of women and men in good health between the ages of 80 and 102 were published in the *Archives of Sexual Behavior*. Although the most frequent type of sexual activity involved caressing and touching, one third of the women and nearly two thirds of the men said that they still enjoyed having

sexual intercourse. Only a quarter of the men complained of having difficulties with erections, with the same proportion of women reporting that they had a lowered libido. In fact, one quarter of the older people interviewed complained that their main problem with sex was the lack of sufficient opportunities for sexual contact.

Sexual problems in the later years

Sexual problems, either transient or long-term, may occur at any time in a man or woman's life. Most people experience, at some time or another, a loss of interest in sex for reasons of stress, tiredness, or illness. As we age, however, the occurrence of chronic problems increases—although having a long-term sexual problem is certainly not an inevitable consequence of getting older, and such problems can often be overcome. Sexual problems may be physiological in origin—the result of changes happening to the reproductive system or other body systems as we get older, or as a side effect of some other health problems—or they may have a psychological cause, occurring in situations where the woman or man is otherwise apparently perfectly healthy. Some sexual problems that may be experienced by older people are described below (*a fuller description of sexual problems can be found in Chapter 6*).

Erectile dysfunction (impotence)

The incidence of chronic impotence—the long-term inability to achieve an erection—increases with age, from around 20 percent of 55-year-old men to over half of 75-year-olds. Between 50 and 75 percent of these cases of impotence have a physiological cause. The most common cause is the side effects of drugs used to treat, for example, high blood pressure or angina. Other causes include excessive alcohol consumption; the effects of long-term smoking; medical conditions such as diabetes or cardiovascular disease; or changes in the nerve or blood supply to the penis that preclude erection. In many cases chronic impotence can be treated by changing a man's medication or avoiding harmful habits. Where

SEX AND THE SINGLE OLDER PERSON

The proportion of single people in any adult age group steadily increases with age. While the majority of 50-year-olds are married or in partnerships, the majority of 70-year-olds are single—perhaps they have lost their partner, or perhaps they never had one. Most of these older single people are women. Whether their sexual interest wanes or continues depends very much on the individual. Some may find that the loss of a loving partner removes all desire for sex. Others may find an outlet for their sexuality in masturbation, occasional liaisons, or new relationships with other single people. Whether sex remains of interest or not, many older people find alternative forms of physical contact to be relaxing and beneficial. The easiest way to experience this is through massage or aromatherapy, both techniques that use the stimulus of touch to relax the body, but without sexual arousal.

QUESTIONS AND ANSWERS: SEX IN OLDER YEARS

Q. I am 63, apparently free from health problems, exercise regularly, and have always enjoyed an active and varied sex life with my partner. But I do have one nagging problem. In the past, my penis would become erect at the slightest hint of sexual activity, even if it was just kissing. Now, even if we are being very intimate with each other, it takes some time for me to become fully erect, and then it happens only after my wife has touched and stroked my penis directly. Can I do something to improve matters?
A. What you are experiencing is a consequence of getting older but it does not mean in any way that your sex life is coming to an end. Yes, your responsiveness is changing but, as you may have noticed, you may be feeling sexually excited but not have a full erection. This needn't be a problem. Discuss the situation with your partner, and perhaps ask her to focus more on your penis and scrotum during foreplay so that they receive more direct stimulation.

Q. In the past my husband has always become aroused— he's gotten an erection—when he sees me undressing before we have sex. But recently he seems to take ages to get erect, sometimes not becoming fully erect at all. I feel worried about this because I think he may not find me sexually attractive any longer. I am 60. Should I worry?
A. You should not be surprised if he does not have an erection when he sees you naked. It does not mean that he is not attracted to you, just that his responses have slowed a little. Talk to your husband about this, because he may be worrying that his penis is not "indicating" the way he feels about you. A rock-hard penis is not essential for satisfying sex.

such strategies cannot work, because the physical cause of impotence is irreversible, treatments such as penile injections or prostheses (see p.195) may be of benefit.

Chronic impotence may also have psychological causes. Some men who experience erectile dysfunction during sex find that they still get an erection when waking from dreaming or first thing in the morning. This means that the erectile mechanism itself is functioning; it is just being inhibited when it is most needed. There are various reasons why this may happen in older men. Impotence may be initiated by loss of self-esteem after retirement. The crisis in self-confidence can result in impotence as well as an overall loss of interest in sex. Talking things over with a partner and developing new interests in life can help to restore flagging sexuality. Another common psychological cause of impotence is a side effect of treatment for problems of the prostate gland (see p.113). Without adequate counseling, men may fear—because of what they have heard—that prostate surgery will mean an end to their sex life. Armed with such misinformation, they recover from their operation and find, by virtue of their self-fulfilling prophecy, that they cannot achieve an erection. However, effective counseling before and after prostate surgery, and the help and the reassurance of a caring partner, will ensure that in most cases there are few sexual problems after the operation.

Loss of or reduced libido

This can affect both men and women, and has a variety of causes. Libido (sex drive) in both sexes is driven by hormones called androgens, the most abundant of which is testosterone; fluctuation in androgen levels can depress the sex drive in people who are otherwise healthy. Some men also experience sharply decreasing testosterone levels as they get older, with a resultant loss of interest in sex. If their loss of libido is the result of low testosterone levels— and this can be confirmed using blood tests —they may benefit from hormone replacement therapy in the form of a testosterone patch, which is now available from some doctors. There are, of course, other reasons why a man's sex drive may be affected. They may well find themselves impotent with a partner they do not love, but be potent with a new partner.

After menopause some women may also find that their interest in sex fades as a result of falling androgen levels. They may find that their libido is restored as a result of hormone replacement therapy, if they are using it. Alternatively, some women receive testosterone by injection or implant to treat their reduced sex drive.

For both men and women, chronic illness, such as Alzheimer's or Parkinson's diseases, or the effects of a serious stroke may result in the complete removal of the desire for sexual activity or closeness, and treatment may be impossible or considered inappropriate. Another reason for the sudden disappearance of libido is that people who have lost long-term partners—especially women, who outnumber men by four to one at the age of 65, and have less chance of finding a new partner—may effectively switch off their interest in sex as a result.

Maintaining relationships

Despite the saying "familiarity breeds contempt," long-term relationships do not automatically go into decline in the later years. Obviously, the state of a relationship, whether it has lasted for four weeks or 40 years, depends on the attitude of the individual partners toward each other, how much mutual respect they have, and the degree to which they value each other.

Without respect and genuine love and affection, there is no chance of a couple being close and intimate, and it is likely that the relationship has lasted for purely practical reasons. But in many other relationships, the partners are happy and content with each other, and enjoy each other's company. However, even relationships such as these may start to get stale if partners are taking each other for granted. To avoid the relationship becoming stale, it may help older couples to try taking some of the following steps.

FRIENDS

Keeping active and stimulated during the later years is essential for mental health, especially for people who have lost their partner. One of the ways to be active and stimulated is by seeing friends. Old friends can be ideal companions to go on vacation with, or for a trip to the theater or movies, or to stay at home and have dinner with. Good conversation and laughter are the ideal natural medicine to lift depression and induce a positive attitude to life; during difficult times they can provide comfort and consolation. Old age does not mean that you cannot find new friends, either, perhaps by joining a club or society with the deliberate intention of meeting new people. Friends do not necessarily have to be of your own age group: many older people

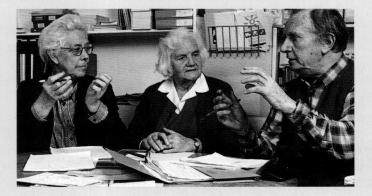

also enjoy spending time with slightly younger people.

Those men and women in their later years who have been living alone might consider creating a new home with other people who are in the same situation. Some people may have thought of this but been put off because, although they welcome companionship, they do

not necessarily want to initiate a sexual relationship. The solution might be for two men and two women to establish one household. In this way they will always have someone to talk to and have meals with, someone who will be there if they are ill, and someone with whom to share the ups and downs of their everyday life.

- Treat your partner as an individual who has his or her own thoughts and aspirations, rather than as your "other half."
- Be thoughtful and considerate about your partner's needs.
- Organize surprises, such as a bouquet of flowers or a candlelight dinner.
- Share thoughts and ideas and try to understand how the other person feels.
- Never show contempt or deep resentment toward your partner.
- Comfort each other, especially in times of crisis or illness.
- Develop new interests together, such as travel or sports or leisure activities such as bowling, hiking or dancing.
- Continue to see each other as sexual beings and tell your partner that she or he is both desirable and attractive.

New relationships

One life crisis that many men and women will inevitably face in the later years is the death of their partner. Or they may lose their partner through divorce. It may be that the loss and sense of bereavement is so great that the surviving partner feels no need for or interest in a new relationship. But some widows and widowers, especially those who are in their fifties and sixties, do start new relationships,

and many get married again. However, a new relationship does not have to be sexual; some couples choose to enjoy each other's company within a committed but celibate relationship.

A higher proportion of men than women remarry after their partner dies. This is partly because women have a longer life expectancy and therefore gradually outnumber men in larger and larger numbers. If a man finds a new partner who is loving, caring and has the same interests, he may find that he can build up a successful new relationship. But some men, especially those who had a long, faithful relationship with their late wife, find that a new relationship brings with it sexual difficulties sometimes described as "widower's syndrome." Men who experience this find that although they feel aroused by being sexually active with a new partner, they are not achieving an erection or are attaining only a partial erection. Erectile problems of this type are probably the result of guilt and anxiety generated by the man sleeping with a woman who is not his wife, even though the wife is now dead. Such feelings are not only distressing but can also revive feelings of loss. If the new partner is sympathetic and willing to talk things through, the problem may pass. Alternatively, a bereavement counselor may help alleviate the man's feelings.

Women who have lost their partner and start a new relationship after a period of sexual abstinence may find that arousal does not occur automatically. In the later years—and this applies equally to men—ceasing sexual activity means that the sex organs can go into decline in terms of function and responsiveness. Such decline is not necessarily irreversible, however, if the woman or man chooses to become sexually active again. Older women and their new partners should be prepared to be patient, taking plenty of time with sexual foreplay, so that in time they can gradually overcome any problems with arousal. Understandably, some men and women who have been in long-term, loving relationships with their late partners may choose, with a new partner, to remain celibate, although they can still enjoy a caring, close relationship.

A changing family role

As we get older our roles within the family usually change. Parents whose children have left home and had children of their own may find themselves in the position of being grandparents. People who retire from full- or part-time work find themselves having to adapt to spending more time at home and more time with their partners. Women or men who lose their partners have to adapt to living alone, and may experience a role reversal with their children, being cared for by sons or daughters instead of caring for them. Recognizing that these changes are taking place, and adapting to them, can go a long way toward maintaining a good relationship with both partners and children.

Becoming grandparents

Becoming grandparents in their later years means new interests as well as a new outlook on life for older couples. Their children are now responsible for children of their own: a shift of responsibility has taken place from one generation to the next. This does not mean, however, that grandparents should not continue to have responsibilities. Grandparents can be of invaluable assistance in helping their children to bring up and look after their own children. But they must always remember to treat their children as adults with their own lives, as well as to tread carefully and avoid interfering too much with their children's family affairs. Here are a few do's and don'ts for grandparents.

• Do offer to take care of your grandchildren so that their parents can have a break.

• Do play games with your grandchildren as well as reading with them.

• Do provide help and assistance—financial or otherwise—to your children, provided that they agree and approve.

• Don't contradict your children's instructions to their children.

• Don't actively try to impose your values on your children and grandchildren.

• Don't expect your children to run their home the same way that you ran yours.

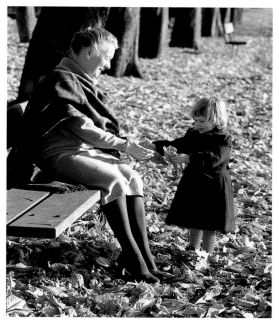

Grandchildren and grandparents often have a special relationship that greatly benefits both of them.

QUESTIONS AND ANSWERS: ELDERLY PARENTS

Q. My father died last year, and my mother has now moved in with us. At first things were fine, but recently she has started criticizing everything. She doesn't like the way we run our house, how we talk to the children, what we buy in the supermarket, or what we read to our two children. This is causing a great strain in our relationship. How do we cope with this delicate situation?

A. If your mother is mentally healthy, there is only one thing you can do. You must talk to her calmly but firmly, explaining what she is doing and why it is upsetting your household. It may be that she has never received any feedback from you about the way she fits into the family. However, if she will not adapt or compromise, you may have to talk about alternative living arrangements. It is difficult to do this—she is your mother, after all—but you cannot allow an uncompromising parent to ruin relationships within your family.

Q. I lost my wife three months ago. My daughter's family live nearby and we have always been very close. I would like to help them, perhaps by baby-sitting (they have three young children) or by doing some odd jobs, but I am worried that I will be intruding. What should I do?

A. If you are close to your family, they will probably appreciate the offer. However, talk to your daughter and her husband first to make sure that they would really welcome your help. And set some limits with them so that you don't do too much, or do things that they see as being too personal.

CHAPTER 12

Sexual Offenses and Counseling

Every culture controls the sexual activities of its citizens to some degree, and people who break that culture's rules are regarded either as suffering from a psychological disorder or as depraved and criminal. However, cultures differ widely in the rules regarding the sexual acts they prohibit and, within any culture, the rules are likely to change over time. Thus in Western society, masturbation, oral sex, and homosexual acts were regarded as "perversions" until quite recently, but are now widely accepted as normal variations of sexual expression.

Changes in what is regarded as permissible reflect wider cultural developments, but they also reflect increased knowledge about human sexual behavior. The results of large-scale surveys conducted by the pioneering sexologist Alfred Kinsey in the 1940s revealed that many men and women had participated in homosexual acts, that many couples had engaged in oral sex, and that a large majority of adults had masturbated by the time they reached adulthood. Such revelations led to a fundamental reevaluation of human sexual norms and made it untenable to regard certain "deviant" behaviors as uncommon and perverted. Kinsey's findings had an extraordinary impact. Indeed, many would claim that the work of Kinsey and those who followed led to a major revision of sexual values within Western culture and had an indirect influence on the liberalization of many laws regarding sexual behavior.

Of course, many forms of sexual activity are still regarded as "abnormal" and "disturbed," and many are still prohibited by law. Some are illegal because they offend the legislators' sense of morality. Thus in some countries it is illegal for a husband and wife to engage in anal intercourse. But in most Western countries the principle underlying most of the legislation in this field appears to be that the only illegal sexual activities are those that involve some form of victimization, in that one or more participants do not consent to the sexual activity or cannot fully consent either because they are too young or because they are mentally disturbed.

Sexual offenses are often extremely damaging to victims, both immediately and in the long term. One reason why there are so many victims of these crimes is that many sex offenses are "serial crimes"—the offender will go on to engage in the same offense repeatedly, often in a compulsive fashion and despite a high risk of prosecution. Most sex crimes are committed by lone offenders, but there are also examples of collusion in sex crimes, of gang rape and of sex rings—groups of people who conspire to entice children into sexual activities.

Sexual harassment

The term sexual harassment covers many different forms of inappropriate behavior—actions or words—and is usually applied to behavior at work or in a school or college setting. Some forms of sexual harassment involve sexual contact, but others are gender-related acts of degradation, disparagement, or humiliation.

The more abusive and offensive types of sexual harassment are easily recognized, but there is often some problem in deciding whether a particular action does or does not constitute sexual harassment. Men often have little idea of how their behavior affects women, and may be surprised when they find that a woman has been distressed and offended by what they had intended to be a compliment, a joke, or a mild flirtation. Many men also misinterpret women's friendly gestures as signs of sexual interest.

Some men feel that the increasing allegations of sexual harassment reflect an oversensitivity on the part of some women, and some suggest that there is now a "witch hunt" against men in the workplace. However, many of those who deliberately engage in obscene or intrusive behavior use the excuse that they were "only joking," and men are well advised to avoid any behavior that might possibly cause offense. Some commentators suggest, as a rule of thumb, that a man should behave toward a female colleague or student only as he would if his boss or his wife were present.

Sexual harassment is all too common, with around one third of working women having been subjected to serious sexual harassment at work. Women employed in factories and offices, and those working within many professions, often report unwelcome touching as well as offensive and sexist remarks. In academic settings, too, many male teachers act in inappropriate ways toward their female students. Most victims of sexual harassment have a lower status in the workplace than the person who harasses them, and sexual harassment often involves an abuse of power. Harassment frequently includes an element of bribery, with promotion, increased salary, or higher academic grades being implicitly (and sometimes explicitly) offered in return for sexual favors. Another form of power abuse occurs when a superior persecutes a woman who fails to comply with, or who complains about, harassment.

Some forms of harassing behavior do not involve any attempt to gain sexual favors. Risqué comments, or remarks about a woman's physical attributes, for example, are sometimes made in an attempt to put the woman "in her place." Men sometimes use this strategy to assert their superiority over women, or to demonstrate to other men "what they can get away with." The display of pornographic posters in an office or at a workbench can be an indirect way of deprecating and humiliating women in the workplace. Sexual harassment can also be used in an attempt to undermine a woman who is in a powerful position; some men regard any woman who occupies a senior position as a personal threat or even as an anomaly, and will seek to demean such a woman by making explicitly sexual remarks, using sexual innuendo, or even by attempting to start a sexual relationship with her as a way of attaining control over her.

Even male academics, who might be expected to know better, often attempt to use their power to gain sexual favors from

TYPES OF SEXUAL HARASSMENT

- unwelcome physical contact: e.g., groping, pinching, patting, or unnecessary touching
- unwelcome invitations and comments: suggestive invitations and explicit comments (for example, about a woman's physical appearance)
- unwelcome pressure for social contact: e.g., persistent requests for dates
- use of demeaning/sexist gestures: wolf-whistling, leering
- use of demeaning/sexist terms: use of "bimbo," "sweetie," or similar terms as a form of address
- sexist social environment: sexually suggestive jokes, sexist remarks, or sexual innuendo
- gender-oppressive physical environment: e.g., the display of sexually suggestive or pornographic pictures and calendars in the workplace

students. On the other hand, some male students sexually harass their female teachers. They may seek to embarrass the teacher by making explicit personal remarks in front of other students, or they may attempt to seduce her as a way of undermining her power. It should also be recognized that some female students make sexual approaches to their male teachers, perhaps seeking to embarrass them, to compromise their position, or to gain academic favors. In some cases, sexual harassment is homosexual.

In an attempt to prevent sexual harassment, many industries, public services, and educational establishments are now adopting antiharassment policies. These usually specify acts that contravene the expected code of conduct and outline procedures to be taken if there is cause for complaint. Some academic institutions, for example, insist that no male teacher should ever be alone in a closed room with a female student, and others stipulate that staff must notify the head of their department if they are having an affair with a student. Some companies now make provisions for any woman who wishes to make a complaint about sexual harassment to report to a female superior rather than having to speak to a male boss.

When is sexual harassment illegal?

In the United States and in most European countries, the number of cases of sexual harassment reaching courts of law has increased dramatically in recent years. The vast majority involve a woman making a complaint about a man's behavior. Such cases usually involve a chronic pattern of abusive behavior, rather than a single dramatic incident, and the man involved will usually have received many clear signals from the woman that his remarks or actions are unwelcome and distressing. A court case may indicate a failure of any disciplinary procedure that would normally operate within the company or institution.

Some types of sexual harassment are illegal because they constitute forms of sexual assault. Other types (especially verbal harass-

ment) are usually regarded in law as infringing either civil rights or sex discrimination legislation, and most cases are dealt with under civil rather than criminal law. Because sexual harassment generally occurs when two people are alone together, there is rarely any hard evidence and most cases involve judgments about which of the two people is telling the truth. Cases of false accusation appear to be very rare.

Many victims suffer considerable psychological distress as a result of sexual harassment. Such treatment can lead to sharp decreases in self-confidence and work morale. Some victims become severely depressed or anxious. Victims may attempt to cope with the harassment by trying to ignore it, suffering in silence, or resigning from the job. More assertive strategies include protesting and making a formal complaint, but although these are sometimes effective in putting an end to the harassment, in many cases the victim finds that she receives little support from colleagues and managers. She may find herself branded as "neurotic" or "oversensitive," and may be ostracized until eventually she leaves.

Rape

Rape is the most serious of all sexual offenses. Legal definitions vary across countries and states, but rape always refers to sexual intercourse without the partner's consent. Rape may occur by means of physical force, threat of physical violence, or the use of drugs or intoxicants. Intercourse with a victim who is deemed incapable of giving full consent, because she is intellectually handicapped, mentally ill, or below the legal age of consent, is usually classified as "statutory rape." The laws differ between countries as to whether rape can only be committed by a male (the age at which a boy can be convicted of rape also varies), whether the victim of the rape must be female, and whether a man who forces his wife to have intercourse against her will is guilty of the crime of rape. However, the relevant laws are changing in many countries, and marital rape is now increasingly specified as an offense, homosexual rape is more widely recognized in law, and women are increasingly acknowledged as possible perpetrators of rape.

Cultural factors

Rape reflects prevailing social conditions and social attitudes, and the incidence of rape varies widely across cultures. Anthropological studies have found that relatively high rates of rape occur in those societies in which the sexes are sharply segregated, in which women have a particularly low status, and in which male dominance and aggressiveness have a high cultural value.

Types of rape

Cases of rape can be classified in a number of different ways. For example, it is useful to distinguish between marital rape, rape which occurs in the context of a dating relationship ("date rape"), and rape by a stranger. While the majority of rape incidents involve only a single perpetrator, there are many cases in which two or more men are involved in an assault on a woman.

Rape can also be classified in terms of the perpetrator's motive. Although the principal motive is often assumed to be sexual, anger and hatred appear to be more significant for many rape attacks than any desire for sexual gratification.

Opportunistic rape

This type of rape is unplanned. A man takes advantage of a situation in which rape is possible and the chances of detection or prosecution are assumed to be very low. In such cases, the motive is usually that of immediate sexual gratification. Many cases of date rape fall into this category.

Power rape

The principal motivation behind power rape appears to be a wish to intimidate the victim. Such men often threaten extreme physical harm, and their sexual violation of the woman is a deliberate act of degradation. Few of the men who commit power rape have ever had a satisfactory close relationship with a woman. Many lack social skills and feel socially inadequate.

Vindictive rape

Those who engage in vindictive rape appear to be motivated by a desire for revenge. Many offenders have a profound hatred of all women, or of women of a particular type. Such men seem to derive little or no sexual satisfaction from the assault but use violence and verbal abuse as a way of expressing their resentment.

Sadistic rape

Relatively rare, this type of rape is committed by men who derive sexual gratification principally by imposing extreme suffering on their victim.

The rapist

Despite many theories attempting to explain why some men become rapists, none can be said to offer a satisfactory account (probably because there are several types of rape, and several types of rapist). One extreme view is that the majority of men are potential rapists, and that if an opportunity presented itself in which a rape would go undetected or unpunished, most would commit the offense. The alternative extreme view is that rapists are deviant and different from other men, and so we do not therefore need to offer an explanation of why the minority become rapists.

REACTIONS TO RAPE

Trauma following rape is often heightened by other people's reactions to the victim and by the victim's self-blame. There may be some suspicion, even from the victim herself, that she somehow encouraged or stimulated the rapist, that she was not careful enough, or that she offered too little resistance. These thoughts may be more conspicuous in cases of date rape (or marital rape) than in cases of rape by a stranger. One aspect of help and therapy typically given to rape victims is to relieve them of any such erroneous and damaging views. The woman needs to accept that she was the victim and in no way the collaborator in the sexual assault. She then needs to develop a view of herself, in the present, not as a rape victim, but as a rape survivor.

It has been found that many rapists have particularly negative views of women. They tend to have highly sexist or "macho" attitudes, and as well as having little or no respect for women, they lack insight into women's attitudes, feelings, and responses. Regarding women as objects for men's sexual gratification, rapists also tend to believe various myths about rape (for example, the idea that many women enjoy being forced to have intercourse). It is not surprising that many rapists have never been successful in forming a close attachment with a woman. In addition, men who rape tend to be highly impulsive, with little respect for moral values.

The rape victim

About one third of rape victims sustain a physical injury as a result of the rape, but a much higher proportion experience severe psychological distress. Sometimes the trauma takes the form of immediate extreme distress, high levels of fear and anxiety, and crying. In other cases the woman shows an initial controlled response before her apparent calm gives way to profound shock and distress. Women who have been raped often remain intensely fearful. They may experience frequent intrusive thoughts about the rape, flashbacks, and recurrent nightmares, and many strive to avoid any situation that might bring back memories of the rape.

The rape victim's judgments about the nature and the causes of the rape will affect her emotional response. Sometimes victims feel in some way responsible for the rape, and such feelings will often lead to a sense of guilt. Although most victims return to normal functioning some months after the rape, some remain in a chronic state of fearfulness and are unable to recover their trust in other people. Some of those who have been raped become very depressed, and some begin to abuse alcohol and other drugs. Various forms of sexual dysfunction may also arise, and the woman may find it impossible to relax sexually, even with a loved partner.

Rape victims need help. Immediately after the rape they need medical attention. They may have sustained injuries during the attack, and they need to find out whether they have contracted a sexually transmitted disease or been made pregnant. There is also a need for immediate and sustained emotional support, particularly from close friends and relatives. Initially, they may need to be helped to report the attack.

Until relatively recently, rape victims were often treated with a lack of respect and sympathy by the police. Despite substantial improvements in police attitudes and procedures in recent decades, the legal process, involving a medical examination, a full police investigation, and a trial, often remains extremely traumatic. If the case reaches the trial stage, the woman will need to appear in court, to face the rapist once more, and to give a detailed account of the attack. She will also have to submit to cross-examining by the defense lawyer, who may suggest that rather than being an innocent victim she is a woman who agreed to intercourse and then "cried rape" after the incident. Until recently, the legal procedures in many countries also allowed the woman's previous sexual history to be examined in detail in court. Following the lengthy, arduous, and highly distressing

QUESTION AND ANSWER: RAPE

Q. Since my wife was raped we have not been able to resume a normal sex life and I feel rejected. Is this normal?
A. Many women who have been raped find it difficult to have intercourse for a long time afterward, even with someone whom they love very much. It is important to be very understanding and patient, because any pressure to have sex may reawaken the feelings your wife had during her trauma. Your wife should contact a counselor to help her overcome the distress that she still feels. In due course it might be appropriate for both of you to receive marital help. It is important for you to reestablish, in very gentle stages, some kind of physical intimacy (kissing and hugging, for example) but you should agree with your wife that this will not lead to any sexual act until she tells you that she feels ready. This is a difficult time for her, and for you, but it is a time when your wife needs you to stand by her and not to show any signs of impatience. Appreciate that these difficulties are common, and that you are not being rejected as a person (or, permanently, as a lover).

legal procedure, the rapist may then be found not guilty and such a verdict often constitutes a shattering blow to the victim.

Considering the emotional trauma experienced by the victim as a result of the rape and fears about police intervention and possible legal proceedings, it is not difficult to understand why many rape victims fail to notify the authorities of the fact that they have been raped. It is generally estimated that less than a quarter of all rapes (excluding marital rape) are ever reported to the police.

Many rape survivors benefit from counseling. Talking through the incident with a therapist can often help a victim to identify and express their fears, anxieties, and anger. Many women who have been raped also find it particularly helpful to talk with other women who have undergone a similar trauma, and rape survivors' support groups exist in many areas.

It is important to recognize that some women manage to cope with rape without becoming traumatized, and that most do recover from the most severe psychological effects within months of the assault. Although they are very unlikely ever to forget what happened to them, and may remain emotionally scarred for a long time, most women refuse to remain permanent victims. Relatives, friends, and professionals should do what they can to aid the coping and recovery processes, and should avoid obstructing emotional recovery by treating the victim as someone who has become permanently psychologically disabled.

Finally, it should not be forgotten that some men are also rape victims. Men who have been raped by another man are often severely traumatized by the attack, and often feel stigmatized, especially if they are homosexual. They may also feel humiliated by the fact that they were unable to defend themselves and that their sexuality may have been questioned. Overall, the psychological aftermath of male rape appears to be similar to that of female rape, except that more male rape victims feel extremely angry with their assailant and engage in fantasies involving retributive violence.

Voyeurism

The voyeur (or "peeping Tom") becomes sexually aroused when he observes people without their permission when they are naked, undressing, or engaged in sexual activity. The term voyeurism is not applied to normal curiosity about sexual activities or sexual responses to pornographic movies or strip shows. The invasion of other people's privacy and the forbidden nature of the activity are essential to the voyeur's pleasure.

The voyeur seeks out places where he might observe strangers undressing or engaged in sexual activities, and may wait for hours in the hope of witnessing an arousing scene. Most voyeurs are aroused more by their illicit spying activities than by having sexual intercourse with a consenting partner. They gain sexual satisfaction by masturbating while observing a "forbidden" event or by incorporating scenes from their peeping expeditions into their masturbation fantasies.

The vast majority of voyeurs are male, most are relatively young, and most are single. Because they are usually very apprehensive about any direct sexual contact, they rarely make any physical approach to the unwitting victim or commit a serious sexual offense. Although prosecutions for voyeurism are fairly common, it is likely that only a minority of peeping Toms are ever caught.

Exhibitionism

An exhibitionist (colloquially a "flasher") is a man who derives pleasure by displaying his genitals to an unwilling audience. Many exhibitionists seek out particular types of victim (women who are alone, for example, or groups of schoolgirls). Some expose themselves whenever an opportunity arises, but others commit the offense only when they are feeling particularly stressed. The majority of offenders are aged between 16 and 30 (although some begin to engage in this kind of behavior much later in life, often following the onset of senility). Despite the fact that many exhibitionists have poor social skills, are often emotionally immature, and tend to lack assertiveness, most are married.

Exposure can take on a compulsive quality, so that many exhibitionists seem oblivious to what is happening around them. Many do little to reduce the risk of arrest. A fairly high proportion of offenders are eventually caught, and indecent exposure cases account for around one third of all prosecutions for sex crimes in most Western societies.

Although some exhibitionists masturbate while exposing themselves, very few attempt to touch their victims or incite a victim to touch them. This suggests that the behavior is generally not to be understood as a sexual invitation. Some exhibitionists hope that the victim will react by showing some sign of pleasure or admiration, but most seem particularly gratified when the victim registers shock, fear, or indignation. Most feel disappointed and frustrated if the victim remains composed and appears unruffled.

One explanation for the development of exhibitionism links the behavior pattern to some chance event that occurred when the person was fairly young. Some exhibitionists recall with considerable excitement the shock and embarrassment shown by someone who

inadvertently disturbed them when they were either masturbating or urinating, so that any sign of another person's shock or disgust has become a powerful sexual stimulus.

Various methods have been used to treat exhibitionists, although most meet with only partial success. The most effective approach involves training the person to identify particular circumstances that lead to temptation and then helping him to employ strategies to avoid dangerous situations and thus preempt the sequence of actions that is likely to result in exposure.

Pedophilia

It appears that a sexual interest in children is not confined to just a few men. Many children are sexually abused, there is a considerable market for child pornography, and child prostitution is prevalent in many parts of the world. One study of male students in the United States found that around 20 percent admitted to having had sexual feelings about young children. For the vast majority of these, however, children were not the principal focus of erotic interest, and they would probably never actually engage in any sexual activity with a child. On the other hand there are some people (mostly men), known as pedophiles, whose sexual interests focus exclusively on pre-pubertal children. Pedophiles obtain sexual gratification by fantasizing about or engaging in sexual contact with children. Although many children fall victim to these men (an active pedophile may victimize several hundred children), it must be stressed that the majority of adults who sexually abuse children are not pedophiles. Many adults abuse children simply because a child is judged to be "available," "amenable," or in some other way an easy target for sexual attention.

Most pedophiles are sexually attracted to children between the ages of 8 and 12, and while some are principally heterosexual or homosexual in their orientation, many are attracted to both boys and girls. Many pedophiles are law-abiding citizens with no

OBSCENE TELEPHONE CALLS

Some people derive sexual gratification from making obscene telephone calls. The most common form of such a call is colloquially known as a "heavy breathing" call. The caller attempts to engage the woman victim in an intimate conversation (asking her, for example, about the color and style of her underwear) while he masturbates. As he does this he will typically inform his victim about his sexual fantasies. Other obscene callers pretend to be conducting a survey and try to elicit information from the woman victim about her sexual habits. Some of these callers are highly sophisticated in their approach, and many women have been deceived into believing that they are being interviewed by a journalist or researcher. The true nature of the call emerges only when the enquiries progress to frank obscenities. Many callers derive gratification from any shocked response or reprimand. Therefore the recommended method for dealing with obscene telephone calls is to make no verbal response, to leave the telephone off the hook for 10 or 15 minutes, and then to replace it, again making no response.

history of psychiatric disorder. Some are married, and many have a good employment record. Many obtain jobs, or positions with volunteer groups, that bring them into close contact with children, while others make strenuous efforts to become accepted as a friend of a family in which there are children. When they have gained a position of trust and authority, they then use their power over children to engage them in sexual activities. Other pedophiles "cruise" for their victims in parks and other places where children may lack adult supervision. The approach to the child is usually playful, rather than threatening, and most pedophiles "groom" children in order to gain their trust and acquiescence. The child victims are often given gifts, or may be bribed or tricked into participating in sexual acts.

Some pedophiles merely expose themselves or show children pornographic material. Some entice groups of children to join them in sexual activities, and some persuade the children to act together sexually or to pose for pornographic pictures. Other pedophiles fondle their child victims, or engage in masturbatory acts, but there is rarely any attempt at intercourse. Many are not concerned with reaching orgasm while they are with a child, but gain their sexual satisfaction later when they recall their contact with the child in masturbation fantasies.

Few pedophiles behave aggressively toward their victims; most insist that they love children and would never hurt them. They are usually friendly or seductive in their manner, partly because this is often effective in gaining the child's compliance, but partly because they often have a genuine affection for the child.

Many pedophiles regard themselves as kind-hearted and childlike and claim that they are attracted by the child's gentle and trusting nature. They generally have no wish to frighten their victims, and also realize that a distressed child is likely to draw attention to the abuse. Nevertheless, following the abuse, the pedophile may threaten the child with a frightening picture of the possible consequences of disclosure.

The sexual abuse of children is fiercely condemned, but whereas some people regard pedophiles "merely" as criminals, others see pedophilia as a psychiatric condition and feel that pedophiles have little control over their sexual preference. Despite the views of legislators, law enforcement agencies, mental health professionals, and the general public, some pedophiles refuse to accept that their actions are either immoral or disturbed. Such men insist that sexual contact between a "caring adult" and a child is not harmful and argue that such contacts should be permitted within the law.

Why does someone become a pedophile?

Pedophilia can develop in a number of different ways. Some pedophiles appear never to have matured emotionally. They continue to think of themselves as children and claim that they feel at ease only when in the company of "other" children. In some cases, a person who initially resorted to sexual contact with a child (because no suitable adult partner was available, for example) will eventually come to prefer sex with children. Other instances of

PHYSICAL TREATMENT FOR SEX OFFENDERS?

When horrendous sex crimes are reported in the media, many people suggest that repeat offenders should be castrated. The ethics of this as a form of punishment can be debated, but it is clear that despite its severity castration would not necessarily end the person's sexual offenses. There is only a very weak association between levels of circulating sex hormones and human sexual behavior, and sexual offenses can very rarely be attributed to an excessive sexual appetite. Certain drugs may be used to reduce the level of an offender's sex drive, but this form of intervention appears to have little effect unless the drugs are used as part of a comprehensive program in which psychological interventions are the major element. Although continued use of hormone-related drugs may help the sex offender curb his antisocial responses, such preparations are certainly not an easy answer to the problem of sex crimes.

pedophilia seem to have developed when a man who has continually fantasized about his own childhood sexual experiences (with peers or with an adult) becomes highly aroused when he is alone with children and eventually acts out his fantasies. A relatively high proportion of pedophiles appear to have been victims of sexual abuse during childhood, but only a very small minority of victims of child sexual abuse later become pedophiles.

Child sexual abuse

Over the past few decades there has been a growing awareness that child sexual abuse (CSA) is not a rare phenomenon but that a substantial proportion of children are sexually victimized. The alarming rise in known cases probably reflects a growth in the awareness of the problem by professionals, parents, and victims themselves, however, and there is little to suggest that the problem itself has been increasing.

The nature of sexual abuse

Child sexual abuse is not a legal term, precisely defined in law in the way that "incest" and "rape" are. Although definitions vary (in terms of what kinds of behavior constitute abuse, the age of the child involved, and so on), it is generally agreed that CSA involves a sexual act between a child and someone substantially older. The act may be intercourse, although this is relatively rare, at least with younger children. More often it is one of fondling, petting, or oral-genital contact. Non-contact behaviors, such as masturbating in front of a child, or showing pornographic videos to a child, may also be forms of CSA.

An abusive incident may be an isolated event, especially if the perpetrator is a stranger to the child. But many children are abused repeatedly by the same perpetrator, who may be a member of his or her family. In some cases the offender will continue to abuse a child over a period of several years, and the child may be subjected to literally hundreds of abusive incidents. Repeated abuse often involves a gradual progression from casual fondling to more serious forms of abuse. Such chronic abuse may end as a result of disclosure by the victim, pregnancy, or the diagnosis of a sexually transmitted disease. However, in the majority of cases it ends when the victim reaches an age when he or she feels powerful enough to resist the abuse.

Although few countries have laws which specifically prohibit child sexual abuse, all have laws which can be used to prosecute adults who abuse children sexually. Prosecutions may be brought under laws relating to rape, intercourse with a minor, or indecent assault. A child's compliance in any sexual activity with an adult is not a defense, because it is assumed that a child cannot consent to any kind of sexual relationship with an adult.

Why are children sexually abused?
It is a common assumption that adults who interfere sexually with children must be psychopathic, psychotic, or retarded in some way, but this is not the case. Relatively few offenders are pedophiles and most do not have a criminal record for any other type of sexual offense. In many ways child abusers represent a cross-section of the male population (most abusers are male, whether the victims are girls or boys) in terms of their personality, level of education, social class, religious affiliation, and so on.

Offenders do not engage in sexual abuse because they wish to inflict pain or trauma on children. In the majority of cases CSA is a selfish act in which the offender uses a child to satisfy some personal hunger. The motive is usually sexual, but some perpetrators use sexual contact with a child to satisfy their craving for tenderness, intimacy, or power.

Adults are able to gain sexual access to a child because they have power, and abuse is an exploitation of the power, respect, and trust that children are encouraged to place in adults. Some of those who are in a privileged position of power and responsibility (and this includes parents, teachers, baby-sitters, and youth leaders) betray the trust that others (including the children themselves) place in them and use their access to a child as a means of gaining sexual pleasure. Although some offenders claim that their victims were "seductive" in their manner, it is clear that whatever a child's behavior, adults must refrain from any sexual contact with a child and that the blame for any sexual contact lies entirely with the adult.

Child abuse within the family

Although the motive of sexual gratification can explain most cases of child sexual abuse, some offenders have developed an inappropriate romantic inclination toward the child whom they abuse. In some cases of father –daughter abuse, for example, the father's parental love for his daughter becomes sexualized. While close father–daughter relationships are normal, particularly at certain ages, it is dangerous for a father to think of his daughter more as a girlfriend than as a daughter, and fathers should avoid the kind of interactions that may blur the generation gap in this way. A father's romantic feelings toward his daughter, whether or not these feelings ever lead to any sexual overture, may result in extreme sexual jealousy of the daughter's boyfriends.

One reason why so much sexual abuse takes place within the family is that relatives may have many opportunities to be alone with the child, behind closed doors. Some adults (relatives or others) deliberately create opportunities in which abuse might occur, but it is likely that most adults who are tempted to behave toward a child in a sexual and inappropriate way find the idea of actually making any sexual overture simply "unthinkable." Thus many potential abusers may inhibit their inclination, perhaps because they think that any approach would be immoral, or because they have fears of possible consequences for the child or for themselves.

Inhibitions against approaching a child sexually are sometimes weakened as a result of stress, alcohol, or various rationalization strategies. Thus some sexually abusive fathers convince themselves that sexual contact between fathers and daughters is natural, or they may justify their abuse by claiming that

WHEN ABUSE IS SUSPECTED

What should parents do if they discover that their child may have been abused? Parental responses to disclosure are not always helpful. Some parents react with shock and horror, which is likely to frighten the child. Others refuse to believe the child, and some accuse the child of being partly responsible for the abuse. Some parents also feel a sense of guilt because they feel that they have failed to protect the child. An adult who suspects that a child may have been abused should remain as calm as possible. Any bid to encourage disclosure should not be forced. Help is needed, and as a preliminary move, contact might be made with a relevant agency which offers telephone advice. Depending on the circumstances, other people who may be contacted are the family doctor, the social work department, a teacher, or the police. Many parents avoid contact with all "officialdom," fearing that such contact might further distress the child. However, it is essential that the child be protected from any further sexual exploitation by the perpetrator, and it must be remembered that failure to report suspected abuse may lead to other children being victimized.

because the abuse does not involve intercourse it is "not really abuse" or "not harmful."

Inhibitions may also weaken when an abuser finds that the victims appear to accept the abusive behavior. Most children are relatively passive when they are sexually abused, and this might allow a perpetrator to convince himself that "she is enjoying it," "she doesn't mind," or "she won't be harmed."

Despite apparent passivity, many victims experience a complex and diverse assortment of emotions. Many are confused because, in addition to feeling guilt, shame, fear, anger, and resentment, they may also experience some physical pleasure, a feeling of special closeness with the abuser, and loving feelings toward the offender.

Most abusers act as careful seducers rather than as attackers, and violence is rarely used. There is usually no need to use physical coercion because persuasion, bribery, or threats will often be sufficient to gain a child's compliance. CSA perpetrators also realize that injuring, marking, or traumatizing a victim will increase the likelihood that the abuse will be revealed. A need to prevent disclosure by the victim, however, may lead to threats and warnings following the abuse. Abusers often frighten their victims into silence by warning them about the possible catastrophic consequences of disclosure.

Relatively few victims disclose abuse to a relative, teacher, or other adult. Various factors contribute to this silence. Young children might not understand that they have been abused, particularly if the offender treated the abuse as a game. Older children may be embarrassed, or might feel guilty and ashamed about the abuse. Some are afraid that they will be blamed, and punished, and many worry about the possible consequences for the offender (especially if he is a relative). Some victims repress memories of the abuse.

The effects of abuse on the victim

The experience of sexual abuse can be severely traumatizing, both immediately and in the long term. No uniform picture can be presented of the typical aftereffects of CSA

PREVENTING CHILD SEXUAL ABUSE

Most efforts to protect children from sexual exploitation have focused on increasing children's awareness of sexual abuse, so that they can recognize inappropriate behavior by adults or older children. Such prevention programs also empower children so that they learn to say no and feel free to disclose abuse if it should occur. Among the various methods used to convey such messages, in the home and in the school, are comic books, videos, posters, and play presentations. Such methods have been shown to increase children's knowledge of abuse, although it is not clear how far such knowledge actually protects them from exploitation. Abusers often work in subtle ways, and take great pains both to undermine the child's inhibitions and to ensure non-disclosure. It is very difficult to teach children to differentiate between friendliness and potential exploitation and to recognize adults who are safe and those who are dangerous. Early prevention programs emphasized "stranger-danger," but more recent programs also mention potential threats from relatives. There is clearly a danger that children might develop an undue wariness and fear of all adults, and parents should therefore examine the content of any prevention program carefully and judge whether or not it is suitable for their own child.

because there is no post-sexual abuse syndrome and the effects are highly varied. They may include anxiety, depression, an abnormal interest in sexual matters, and various forms of behavioral difficulties. In adult life, those with a history of abuse are more likely than other people to experience anxiety, depression, difficulties in forming and maintaining intimate relationships, and sexual dysfunction. A relatively high proportion of the adults who abuse children were themselves victims of child abuse, and it is also true that many women who become prostitutes have a history of sexual abuse during childhood.

The psychological damage that results from CSA is not simply a result of the child's experience of the sexual element of the abuse, but may also reflect the child's awareness of powerlessness and the fact that the secrecy imposed by the abuser tends to isolate them from other people, including members of their own family. Some of the trauma experienced by CSA victims may also reflect certain events that may follow disclosure (including interviews with the police and other professionals, increased tension in the home, and an appearance in court).

It would clearly be irresponsible to attempt to minimize the adverse effects of abuse, but it must also be recognized that trauma is by no means universal for all abused children, and that, thankfully, many appear relatively unscathed by their victimization. Parents, teachers, and other professionals must be careful not to undermine children's natural resilience by assuming that a child who has been abused must be traumatized. Any insistence by caring adults that the child is "different" can communicate unfortunate messages to the child and may constitute unwitting revictimization. It must not be assumed that a child who has been abused is destined to fail in relationships, to develop sexual problems in adult life, to abuse other children, or to become a prostitute. A child who has suffered abuse must not be made to feel that she or he is damaged and will never be the same again. Children should not be made to feel flawed, dirty, or freakish because they have been abused.

Care should also be taken to avoid any suggestion that the child might have been in some way partly responsible for the abuse, or is at fault in not having disclosed the abuse. Many child victims and adult survivors of CSA continue to feel guilty about the abuse, and such feelings may be exacerbated if other people imply some guilt or misdemeanor. Many victims feel guilty, during childhood or later, because they enjoyed some of the physical and emotional feelings associated with abuse. The child is often confused by a mixture of feelings that are likely to include fear, embarrassment, anger, and severe anxiety, but which might also involve pleasurable bodily responses and the experience of being wanted. It must be emphasized that whenever an adult and a child are involved in any sexual activity, the blame rests entirely with the adult. Similarly, it should not be assumed that because a child has been sexually abused (especially by a member of the family) the child will thereafter hate the abuser and wish to avoid all further contact with him (or her). In this, as in all aspects, relatives and professionals need to be sensitive to the child's wishes (while at the same time ensuring that the child is protected from the risk of any further abuse).

Incest

The term "incest" refers to sexual relations between people who are closely related to each other. Thus, sexual intercourse between a brother and sister is illegal (whatever their ages), as it is between a person and their parent or grandparent. The legal definition of incest varies from country to country (and in the United States, from state to state). In some cases the incest law prohibits intercourse between cousins, for example, or between in-laws.

The term incest is somewhat ambiguous, because as well as being applied to cases in which two closely related adults consent to intercourse (in which case both are guilty of incest), it is also used to describe cases in which a child is sexually victimized by an older person within the family (whether or not intercourse is involved).

A strong cultural taboo against incest appears to have been almost universal across societies and throughout history. Among the very few exceptions are the pharaohs of ancient Egypt and the royalty in Hawaii many centuries ago. The extreme stigmatization associated with incest, and the fact that it occurs within the confines of the family home, means that this offense will come to light only in exceptional circumstances.

Pornography

Pornography may be defined as any depiction of people or acts that is designed to arouse the viewer sexually. However, it is clear that different people respond in quite different ways to the same material. Images which excite some will disgust others, and leave still others unaffected. Furthermore, material that was not produced to stimulate any sexual response may prove highly arousing to some people. For example, some pedophiles claim that while explicit child pornography does not arouse them, they are highly stimulated by more commonplace pictures of children (for example, those found in mail-order clothing catalogs). The impact of pornography also depends to some extent on the cultural context in which it is viewed.

Pornography has existed for many centuries and is one of the first ways in which new media are exploited. Thus pornographic images were produced soon after the advent of photography, film, and video, and recent technological developments (including the Internet) have been similarly exploited.

The issue of whether pornography should be available or banned has long been controversial. Some people argue for total freedom of expression and open access to all materials; many favor the prohibition only of certain types of material; and some call for a ban on all sexually explicit publications. Some couples report that pornography has helped them reach new levels of sexual excitement, and many men who regularly make use of pornographic material claim that its effects are completely benign. Increasingly, some pornography is being produced specifically for use by women. On the other hand, many of those who oppose pornography claim that it degrades the user and offends against certain moral principles, and many feminists argue that pornography demeans women and treats them as objects.

The large body of research into the effects of pornography, and whether it is harmful, has failed to produce clear answers. It is certainly true that a good deal of pornography contains violent, abusive, and bizarre images, and that many people with unusual sexual interests make use of specialized pornography. But there is little evidence to support the view that people become sex offenders as a result of exposure to pornography.

Because pornographic material is generally used during masturbation, and helps the person to achieve orgasm, it may actually reduce the short-term probability that a sexual offense will be carried out. In the long term, however, the impact of pornography may be less innocuous. Material that depicts sexual acts involving unwilling partners (who may also end up appearing to enjoy their involvement), for example, may be incorporated into a person's sexual fantasies. Continued exposure to pornography also appears to produce a desensitization effect, so that images which were once arousing eventually lose their power to stimulate; this may explain why those who make regular use of pornography often progress to ever more explicit and "harder" material.

Prostitution

Attitudes toward prostitution have varied considerably between societies and throughout history. In ancient Greece, for example, and throughout many centuries in Japan, high-class prostitutes provided sexual and other services for leading citizens and were highly respected. But there have always been the less respectable prostitutes, the streetwalkers who provide sex for any man who can

afford to pay. Men use prostitutes because they do not have a partner, because their wife is unable or unwilling to have intercourse, because they are bored with their usual sex life, or because they wish to engage in sexual practices which their wife disallows. Many prostitutes offer a range of sexual services which include sadomasochistic practices, oral sex, and more specialized activities.

Some people regard prostitution as a social evil, while others regard it as a relatively harmless occupation, serving a useful function. Many feminists argue that men who use prostitutes are degrading women, whereas others (including many prostitutes themselves) regard prostitution as a legitimate occupation in which women capitalize on men's "failings" or simply provide a necessary service.

The laws relevant to prostitution differ from country to country. In many, it is not prostitution itself that is illegal, but related activities (such as soliciting for purposes of prostitution, running a brothel, or living on "immoral earnings"). The laws in some areas permit brothels to operate, and there are frequent calls in other countries for a liberalizing change in legislation. Proponents of such changes argue that women would be safer working in such places than walking the streets, and that regular health checks could be enforced to ensure that the women were free from sexually transmitted disease.

Although the practice of child prostitution is universally condemned, many young prostitutes can be found in countries around the world. Boy prostitutes almost always provide a service for gay and bisexual males. Sexual contact with any minor is a serious offense, and older people who encourage children to become prostitutes, or who live off their earnings, are also guilty of a serious crime.

Help for sex offenders

In recent years there have been strenuous efforts to develop treatment programs that will reduce the likelihood that a person who has been convicted for a sexual offense will offend again. Most try to give offenders increased insight into how their behavior is likely to affect their victims. They are also taught to recognize and avoid situations that may lead to temptation and are shown why beliefs such as "many women enjoy being raped" and "no harm comes to children as a result of gentle sexual contact" are untenable.

Help for victims of sexual offenses

The responses of victims of sexual offenses are various and cannot be predicted. Thus some people who have been subjected to harassment at work, an obscene phone call, or the actions of an exhibitionist will remain highly distressed for a long time, while some victims of very serious sexual attacks cope without suffering a breakdown. Any victim of a sexual crime who feels that she or he needs help should make contact with the services available close to their home. Volunteer groups (rape crisis centers, child sexual abuse survivors' groups, and many more) operate in most areas, and are frequently affiliated with national and international organizations. Groups like these may offer telephone contact, counseling, or participation in survivors' groups.

Professional help is also available. The first point of contact will often be the physician, although community psychological services are now available in many areas. In addition, numerous counselors and psychologists work privately and advertise in yellow pages and in the press. Social services may also be able to provide help, or to recommend a local clinician who specializes in work with victims of sexual crime. If a child is involved, parents should contact the pediatrician, social services, or school authorities (obviously, when a sexual crime is involved, they might also wish to contact the police directly).

Various approaches are used to help victims, and there have been major developments in therapy for child victims and adult survivors in recent years. The approach chosen will depend upon the specific problems presented by the victim and the professional orientation of the therapist. Counseling is likely to be a key element in any work with victims. Children and adults may be encouraged to give their own account of what happened and how it has affected them. Some forms of counseling rely principally upon such "talking out" and on the self-healing that may result. Therapists who operate within a different framework may be more active in giving advice, suggesting alternative ways of looking at events, prescribing "homework" and so on. In some cases the therapist may suggest that a victim's partner or other members of the family should be included in one or more of the therapy sessions. Most victims find that they are helped through their contact with a therapist, or by participating in a group. Those who feel that they have not benefited might consider searching for alternatives until they find an approach, or a therapist, who appears to provide them with an optimum opportunity for coming to terms with their difficulties.

QUESTIONS AND ANSWERS: ABUSE

Q. My wife was sexually abused by her uncle as a child, but although she has alluded to this several times, she won't actually talk to me about it. Is there anything I can do to help?

A. It would obviously be good for your wife to talk to someone about her experience, but if she is unwilling to do so you shouldn't press the issue. Show your sympathy and love, and she may eventually come around to the idea of talking to you about it. Alternatively, she may wish to talk to a therapist.

Q. On one or two occasions recently, I have been alone with a neighbor's child and I have had fleeting images of abusing the child. Is there any danger that I will one day act on these images?

A. Many men and women have such "fleeting images," possibly more common today because there is so much media coverage of child abuse. It's probably similar to the impulse people often feel, when on a cliff edge, to jump off. Avoid dwelling on such images, especially when you are sexually aroused. Don't feel that you are somehow "destined" to abuse children—you are not—but just to be safe, and to minimize worry on this score, you might consider making a commitment to yourself to avoid occasions that would involve being alone with the neighbor's child, or with another child.

Glossary

Abortion Premature termination of a pregnancy before the embryo or fetus can lead an independent life. An abortion may be spontaneous (see *Miscarriage*); or it may be induced by a doctor (a therapeutic abortion).

Abstinence Deliberate refraining from sexual intercourse.

Adolescence Period of physical and psychological transition from childhood to adulthood that takes place between the ages of 9 and 18, and includes the changes of puberty.

Afterplay Mutual affection shown by sexual partners after sexual activity.

AIDS Acquired immune deficiency syndrome. Disorder caused by the human immunodeficiency virus (HIV), transmitted through body fluids, that weakens the immune system preventing the body from defending itself against infection.

Amenorrhea Absence of periods.

Amniocentesis Screening test carried out between weeks 14 and 18 of pregnancy to detect any fetal defects.

Anal intercourse Insertion of a man's penis into his partner's rectum.

Androgen One of a group of hormones, secreted by the testes in males and adrenal glands in both sexes, that produce masculine characteristics, and regulate sex drive in both sexes.

Aphrodisiac Substance or device believed to increase sexual desire.

Areola Darker, pigmented area surrounding each nipple in both sexes that may swell during sexual arousal.

Artificial insemination Introduction of a sperm sample into the *cervix* by medical rather than natural means.

Bartholin's glands Adjacent to the vaginal opening, one of two glands that secrete lubricating fluid.

Biopsy Removal of a tiny sample of tissue from the body for further investigation and possible diagnosis.

Birth control See *Contraception*.

Bisexual Describes a person sexually attracted to both men and women.

Body language Nonverbal messages communicated to others through posture, expressions, and gestures.

Bulbourethral glands Small glands that secrete fluid into the male urethra just prior to ejaculation.

Cancer One of a group of diseases (including cancers of the testis and cervix) in which body cells divide uncontrollably to form tumors that stop body organs working normally. Left untreated, cancerous cells spread throughout the body, causing death.

Cervical cap Rubber cap-shaped contraceptive that fits over the cervix.

Cervix Lower end—the neck—of the uterus, which links it to the vagina.

Child sexual abuse (CSA) A sexual act between a child and a person who is older.

Chorionic villus sampling Test carried out between weeks 6 and 8 of pregnancy to check for fetal defects.

Chromosome One of 46 threadlike structures found in each body cell that carry genetic information.

Circumcision In males, surgical removal of the foreskin of the penis.

Climacteric Changes happening to middle-aged women over many years, including the cessation of periods, caused by decreasing production of the hormone estrogen.

Clitoris Pea-sized organ, located at the front of a woman's vulva, whose sole function is sexual pleasure.

Coitus interruptus Contraceptive method; the penis is withdrawn from the vagina just prior to ejaculation.

Conception Period between *fertilization* and *implantation* in the uterus.

Condom Contraceptive sheath pulled over the penis, or placed inside the vagina, to prevent sperm from entering the uterus.

Contraceptive Device or medication used by couple having sexual intercourse to prevent pregnancy.

Cunnilingus See *Oral sex*.

D&C Dilation and curettage. Widening of the cervix in order to scrape the lining of the uterus. Often used during abortion.

D&E Dilation and evacuation. Widening of the cervix and removal of the uterine contents using suction.

Diaphragm Dome-shaped rubber contraceptive worn over the cervix.

Dysmenorrhea Painful periods.

Ectopic pregnancy Implantation of embryo in the "wrong" place, usually in a fallopian tube, requiring surgery.

Ejaculation Semen emission from the penis; often accompanied by orgasm.

Embryo Developing baby for the first eight weeks after fertilization.

Emergency contraception Oral contraceptive taken, or IUD inserted, within a few days of unprotected intercourse to prevent unplanned pregnancy.

Endometrium Lining of the uterus.

Epididymis Long, coiled tube overlying testis in which sperm mature.

Erectile dysfunction or **impotence** *Sexual dysfunction* in which a man is unable to achieve or maintain an erection.

Erection Swelling and hardening of the penis or clitoris during sexual stimulation.

Erogenous zone Body part especially sensitive to sexual stimulation.

Erotica (See also *Pornography*) Books, pictures, movies, or other media intended to arouse sexual desire.

Estrogen Major female sex hormone secreted by the ovaries, which maintains a woman's *secondary sex characteristics* and helps coordinate the menstrual cycle.

Exhibitionist Man who gains sexual pleasure from exposing his penis in public to an unwilling audience.

Extended family Unit consisting of grandparents and other relatives as well as parents and children.

Fallopian tube Tube that carries eggs from the ovary to the uterus, and inside which fertilization takes place.

Family planning See *Contraception*.

Fellatio See *Oral sex*.

Fertile period The few days each month, around the time of *ovulation*, when a woman can conceive.

Fertilization Fusion of a sperm and egg to form a *zygote*.

Foreplay Activities, such as stroking, which cause sexual arousal.

Foreskin Skin fold covering the end of the penis in uncircumcised men.

Gay See *Homosexual*.

Gender A person's maleness or femaleness as a reflection of his or her biological sex and the designations of sex created and enforced by that person's own society.

Gender identity A person's self-awareness of his or her belonging to either male or female *gender*.

Gender role The behaviors and attitudes shown by an individual that convey to society his or her *gender identity* as a male or female.

Gene Basic unit of heredity, of which there are over 100,000 in each body cell, carried on the *chromosomes*.

Genitalia The external sex organs: the *penis*, *scrotum*, and *vulva*.

Grafenberg spot (G-spot) Part of the vaginal wall believed to be very sensitive to sexual stimulation.

Heterosexual Describes a person whose main sexual attraction is toward the opposite sex.

Homosexual Describes a person whose main sexual attraction is toward their own sex.

Hormonal contraceptive Female contraceptive that releases synthetic *hormones* into the body that prevent ovulation or stop fertilization.

Hormone replacement therapy (HRT) Medical use of hormones to offset the effects of menopause.

Hormones Naturally produced chemical messengers that regulate many body functions.

Hot flash Sudden feeling of intense heat, a symptom of menopause.

Hymen Membrane surrounding, and partially covering, vaginal opening.

Hysterectomy Surgical removal of the uterus.

Implantation Attachment of a fertilized egg to the lining of the uterus.

Impotence See *Erectile dysfunction*.

Incest Sexual relations between people who are closely related.

Infertility Inability to conceive.

Intrauterine device (IUD) Flexible contraceptive device that fits inside the uterus.

In vitro fertilization (IVF) Infertility treatment in which an egg is fertilized by sperm outside a woman's body before being returned to her uterus.

Labia majora Larger, outer liplike skin folds surrounding the vagina.

Labia minora Smaller, inner liplike skin folds surrounding the vaginal opening.

Lesbian Describes a woman whose main sexual attraction is toward other women.

Libido Sex drive.

Mammary glands Milk-producing glands located in the female breasts.

Mammography Screening technique using X-rays to detect abnormal tissue in the female breast.

Mastectomy Surgical removal of part or all of the breast.

Masturbation Stimulation of one's own sex organs for sexual pleasure.

Menarche Occurrence of a girl's first menstrual period during puberty.

Menopause The time when a woman's periods cease and her reproductive life comes to an end. Often used instead of *climacteric*.

Menorrhagia Heavy periods.

Menstrual cycle Sequence of events occurring inside a woman's body, repeated approximately monthly during the reproductive years, that prepares the uterine lining to receive a fertilized egg, should fertilization occur. (See also *Ovarian cycle*.)

Menstruation or **period**. Monthly bleeding from the vagina in women of reproductive age caused by the loss of the lining of the uterus if an egg has not been fertilized during the preceding menstrual cycle.

Midlife crisis Feeling of distress and depression that may affect men and women in their middle years when they realize their youth has passed.

Miscarriage or **spontaneous abortion**. Loss of an embryo or fetus before the 24th week of pregnancy.

Missionary position Popular position for sexual intercourse with the couple face-to-face, man on top.

Mittelschmerz Slight abdominal pain felt by some women in mid-menstrual cycle when they ovulate.

Mons pubis Pubic mound. A fatty pad of tissue, below the abdomen and above the vulva, covered by pubic hair.

Mons veneris See *Mons pubis*.

Natural family planning Contraception based on avoiding sexual intercourse during that part of each month when a woman is fertile.

Nipple The tip of the breast; in both sexes, the nipples may become erect during sexual arousal.

Nocturnal emission See *Wet dream*.

Oophorectomy Surgical removal of one or both of the ovaries.

Oral contraceptive The pill. *Hormonal contraceptive* tablet taken daily for most or all of each month.

Oral sex Also called oral-genital sex. Stimulation of a partner's genitals with the mouth and tongue. Stimulation of a woman's genitals is called cunnilingus; stimulation of a man's genitals is called fellatio.

Orgasm Feeling of intense pleasure at the peak of sexual excitement, accompanied by muscular contractions in the pelvic region and followed by a relaxation of body muscles. Orgasm usually accompanies *ejaculation* in men.

Osteoporosis Loss of bone mass causing bones to become brittle and easily fractured. Especially vulnerable are women after menopause.

Ovarian cycle Sequence of events occurring inside a woman's body, repeated approximately monthly during the reproductive years, during which an *ovarian follicle* ripens and releases an egg into a fallopian tube where fertilization may occur. (See also *Menstrual cycle*).

Ovarian follicle One of many tiny capsules found in the ovary, each of which contains an egg.

Ovary One of the two female sex organs that release eggs (ova) and secrete sex hormones estrogen and progesterone.

Ovulation Monthly release of an egg from an ovary at the midpoint of the *ovarian cycle*.

Ovum A human egg. Ova, the female sex cells, are produced in the female ovary before birth, and one ovum is released each month during a woman's reproductive years.

Pap smear Routine screening test for cancer of the cervix in which cells from the surface of the cervix are examined under the microscope.

Pedophilia Adult sexual attraction to children, mainly 8–12-year-olds.

Penis Male external sex organ.

Perineum Sexually sensitive area between anus and vagina in women, and anus and scrotum in men.

Period See *Menstruation*.

Pill See *Oral contraceptive*.

Pituitary gland Pea-sized hormone-releasing gland located below the brain. Pituitary hormones regulate the activities of the ovaries and testes.

Pornography (See also *Erotica*) Books, pictures, movies, or other media intended to arouse sexual desire. Any definition is necessarily subjective: what one person may see as purely erotic, another may see as obscene and disgusting.

Postpartum depression Feeling of sadness or depression experienced by many women after childbirth.

Premature ejaculation Ejaculation that occurs faster than a man expects or desires, often just before or during intercourse.

Premenstrual syndrome (PMS) Emotional and physical changes that many women experience for a week or so before menstruation.

Progesterone Female sex hormone secreted by the ovaries that causes the changes in the uterine lining in the second part of the menstrual cycle that prepare it for the implantation of an egg, should it be fertilized.

Prostaglandin Naturally occurring chemicals that, among other functions, cause contraction of muscles in the uterine wall.

Prostate gland Gland surrounding the male urethra below the bladder whose secretions form part of semen.

Prostitution Engaging in sexual activity for monetary reward.

Puberty The physical and physiological changes that occur during the early years of *adolescence* to make girls and boys sexually mature.

Pubic hair Hair growing around the genitals; first appears at *puberty*.

Rape Sexual intercourse without a person's consent.

Retarded ejaculation Difficulty in achieving ejaculation or orgasm during sexual intercourse.

Safe sex Types of sexual activity that minimize the risk of contracting sexually transmitted diseases.

Scrotum External pouch of skin that supports the testes.

Secondary sex characteristics Characteristics that develop at *puberty* and distinguish women from men (e.g., body hair or breasts) but are not essential for reproduction.

Semen Thick, whitish fluid containing sperm and seminal fluid (secretions from the seminal vesicles and prostate gland) expelled from the penis during ejaculation.

Seminal vesicle One of two small glands that release secretions into the male urethra that form part of semen.

Seminiferous tubules Long, coiled tubules inside the testes in which sperm are produced.

Sex Term defining whether a person is biologically male or female. Also descriptive of sexual and erotic activities, as in "sex manual."

Sexual arousal A state of sexual excitement resulting from stimulation and indicated by body changes such as erection of clitoris or penis.

Sexual dysfunction Sexual problem in men or women that interferes with sexual activity.

Sexual harassment Unwanted and inappropriate behavior of a sexual nature toward another person.

Sexual intercourse Activity in which a woman receives her partner's erect penis into her vagina.

Sexual preference Personal choice of sexual partner, of the same or opposite sex.

Sexually transmitted disease (STD) Disease such as gonorrhea, chlamydia, or AIDS, passed from one person to another by sexual contact.

Sonogram Diagnostic technique using sound waves to produce an image of the fetus in the uterus.

Sperm The male sex cell, millions of which are produced daily in the testes of adult men.

Spermicide Sperm-killing substance, usually used with a barrier contraceptive such as a diaphragm.

Squeeze technique Method used to help overcome premature ejaculation.

Sterilization Surgical procedure used to make it impossible for a woman to have a child, or a man to father one.

Stillbirth Death of a baby inside the uterus after the 24th week of pregnancy, or during birth.

Tampon Highly absorbent roll of cotton inserted temporarily inside the vagina during menstruation to absorb the menstrual flow.

Testicle A testis and its *epididymis*.

Testis One of the two male sex organs that produce sperm and secrete the male sex hormone testosterone.

Testosterone Male sex hormone secreted by the testes which maintains a man's *secondary sex characteristics* and helps stimulate sperm production. Also produced by both male and female adrenal glands, testosterone is responsible for sex drive in both sexes.

Toxic shock syndrome (TSS) Very rare but severe illness mainly affecting women using specific types of tampons.

Transsexual Person who feels that she or he is really a member of the opposite sex. Some transsexuals undergo gender reassignment ("sex change") treatment using surgery.

Transvestite Also called crossdresser. Person, usually a man, who enjoys dressing in clothes of the opposite sex, sometimes as a prerequisite to enjoying sexual activity.

Trimester One of the three 13-week divisions of pregnancy.

Tubal ligation Technique of female sterilization by cutting, tying, or burning the fallopian tubes.

Urethra Tube which carries urine from the bladder to outside the body.

Uterus or **womb** Pear-shaped muscular organ in which the fetus develops during pregnancy.

Vagina Passage from the uterus to the vulva into which the penis is inserted during sexual intercourse.

Vaginismus Sexual dysfunction in which muscles around the vagina contract, making intercourse difficult.

Vas deferens (plural: vasa deferentia) One of two tubes that carry sperm away from the testes.

Vasectomy Technique of male sterilization by cutting each *vas deferens*.

Vestibule Part of the female external genitals that lies between the *labia minora* and surrounds the vaginal and urethral openings.

Vibrator Electrically powered device, often penis- or phallus-shaped, which vibrates at high speed.

Virgin Man or woman who has not experienced sexual intercourse.

Voyeurism Sexual activity in which someone becomes sexually aroused by watching other people, without their permission, undressing or engaging in sexual activity.

Vulva A woman's external genital organs including her labia minora and majora, mons pubis, clitoris, and vaginal opening.

Wet dream or **nocturnal emission**. Ejaculation of semen during sleep often during sexual dreams. Common among adolescent males.

Withdrawal See *Coitus interruptus*.

Zygote Single cell produced by the fertilization of an egg by a sperm.

Further reading

Clubb, Elizabeth and Knight, Jane. *Fertility: A Comprehensive Guide to Natural Family Planning.* New York: Sterling, 1992.

Delvin, David. *The Good Sex Guide: The Illustrated Guide to Enhance Your Lovemaking.* New York: Carroll & Graf, 1993.

Fenwick, Elizabeth and Smith, Tony. *Adolescence: The Survival Guide for Parents and Teenagers.* New York: Dorling Kindersley, 1994.

Fenwick, Elizabeth and Walker, Richard. *How Sex Works: A Clear, Comprehensive Guide for Teenagers to Emotional, Physical, and Sexual Maturity.* New York: Dorling Kindersley, 1994.

Good Housekeeping Editors. *The Good Housekeeping Illustrated Book of Pregnancy and Baby Care.* New York: Hearst Books, 1990.

Haas, Kurt and Haas, Adelaide. *Understanding Sexuality.* 3rd ed. Saint Louis: Mosby Year Book, 1993.

Harkness, Carla. *The Infertility Book: A Comprehensive Medical and Emotional Guide.* Berkeley: Celestial Arts, 1992.

Illingworth, Ronald S. *The Normal Child: Some Problems of the Early Years and Their Treatment.* 10th ed. New York: Churchill, 1991.

Kitzinger, Sheila. *The Complete Book of Pregnancy and Childbirth.* New York: Knopf, 1989.

Landsown, Richard and Walker, Marjorie. *Your Child's Development: From Birth to Adolescence, A Complete Book for Parents.* New York: Knopf, 1991.

Llewellyn-Jones, Derek. *The A–Z of Women's Health.* 2nd ed. New York: Oxford University Press, 1990.

Madaras, Lynda. *My Body, My Self: The What's Happening Workbook for Girls.* New York: Newmarket, 1993.

Madaras, Lynda. *What's Happening to My Body? Book for Boys: A Growing Up Guide for Parents and Sons.* New York: Newmarket, 1991.

Mosse, Julia and Heaton, Josephine. *The Fertility and Contraception Book.* Winchester: Faber & Faber, 1991.

Reinisch, June M. *Kinsey Institute New Report on Sex.* New York: St. Martin's Press, 1994.

Stoppard, Miriam. *Menopause.* New York: Dorling Kindersley, 1994.

Helplines

ADDICTION

Alcoholics Anonymous
For information, literature, and groups, see the listing in your local phone directory.

Al-Anon Family Groups
For spouses and children of alcoholics. See the listing in your local phone directory.

Narcotics Anonymous
For information, literature, and groups see the listing in your local phone directory.

ABUSE & ASSAULT

Childhelp USA and National Child Abuse Hotline
P.O. Box 630, Hollywood, CA 90028
(800) 422-4453

Local Rape Crisis Centers
For information, see the listing in your local phone directory

National Coalition Against Sexual Assault
123 South 7th St., Ste. 500
Springfield, IL 62701
(217) 753-4117

National Council on Child Abuse and Family Violence
1155 Connecticut Ave. NW, Ste. 400
Washington, DC 20036
(800) 222-2000

National Domestic Violence Hotline
(800) 799-7233

Rape, Abuse, and Incest National Network Hotline
(800) 656-HOPE

COUNSELING

American Association of Sex Educators, Counselors, and Therapists
435 N. Michigan Ave., Ste. 1717
Chicago, IL 60611
(312) 644-0828

FAMILY RELATIONS

Family Resource Coalition
200 South Michigan Ave., Ste. 1520
Chicago, IL 60604
(312) 341-0900

National Council on Family Relations
3989 Central Avenue NE, Ste. 550
Minneapolis, MN 55421
(612) 781-9331

GAY AND LESBIAN ISSUES

National Gay and Lesbian Task Force
2320 17th St NW
Washington, DC 20009
(202) 332-6483

PREGNANCY AND CHILDBIRTH

American College of Obstetricians and Gynecologists (ACOG)
409 12th Street SW
Washington, DC 20024-2188
(202) 638-5577

National Abortion Federation
1436 U Street NW, Ste. 103
Washington, DC 20009
(800) 772-9100

National Adoption Information Clearinghouse
5640 Nicholson Ln., Ste. 300
Rockville, MD 20852
(301) 231-6512

National Organization of Adolescent Pregnancy and Parenting
1319 F St. NW, Ste. 401
Washington, DC 20004
(202) 783-5770

Planned Parenthood Federation of America
810 Seventh Avenue
New York, NY 10019
(800) 829-PPFA

SEXUALLY TRANSMITTED DISEASES

National AIDS Hotline
(800) 342-2437
For Spanish speakers: (800) 244-7432
For hearing impaired: (800) 243-7889

National Herpes Hotline
(919) 361-8488

National S.T.D. Hotline
(800) 227-8922

AGING

American Association of Retired Persons
601 E St. NW, Washington, DC 20049
202-434-2277

ILLNESS

American Cancer Society
19 West 56th Street
New York, NY 10019
(212) 586-8700

GENERAL

U.S. Department of Health and Human Services
Public Health Service Centers for Disease Control and Prevention
National Center for Health Statistics
6525 Belcrest Road
Hyattsville, MD 20782

Index

Page numbers in **bold** refer to entire chapters; numbers in *italics* refer to illustrations.

A

Abortion 81, 230–1
Abstinence, sexual 193
Abuse, child sexual *see* Child sexual abuse (CSA)
Acne 53
Acquired Immune Deficiency Syndrome *see* HIV and AIDS
Acupuncture, and menopause 275–6
Addiction 126–7
Adipose tissue *19*
Adolescence **46–85**
  becoming a sexual being 72–8
  communicating with parents 69
  dating 70–2
  emotions and relationships 68–72
  friendships 70
  health during 82–5
  masturbation 72–4
  peer pressure 69
  substance abuse 85
  teenage pregnancy and parenthood 78–81
  see also Boys; Girls; Puberty
Adrenogenital syndrome (AGS) 39–40
Afterplay 180
Aging
  adapting to sexual changes 292
  myths about 286
  pregnancy and older women 206
  and sex drive (libido) 173, 294–5
  sexual changes in men 291–2
  sexual changes in women 292–3
AIDS *see* HIV and AIDS
Alcohol
  in adolescence 85
  how to drink in moderation 254
  in later years 293
  and menopause 279
  in middle years 251, 253–4
  and pregnancy 209–10
  and sex 127
Amenorrhea 98–9
Anal sex 181
Androgens 36–7, 50, 283
Anorexia nervosa 83
Antidepressants and menopause 275
Anus development *36*
Areola *19, 19*
Aromatherapy and menopause 276
Arousal 174, *175*
Arthritis and sex 199

Assertiveness
  in adolescence 71
  between partners 189–90

B

"Baby blues" *see* Postnatal depression
Baby to child **32–45**
  child's sexuality 41–3
  sex determination and chromosomes 34–7
  sex and gender 37–40
  sexual development and parental influence 43–5
Bacterial vaginosis (BV) 115
Balanitis 113
Baldness 255
Basal body temperature (BBT) contraceptive method 158–9
Bereavement and sexual feelings after 296
Billings method 159–60
Biological determination of gender 39
Birth control *see* Contraception
Bisexuality 186
Bladder *15, 25*
  and cystitis 115–16
Blastocyst 30, *31*
Blepharoplasty 256
Blood in semen 113
BMI *see* Body Mass Index (BMI)
Body changes after birth 219–20
Body hair, in puberty 52, 66–7
Body image in adolescence 68
Body language 71, 181–6
Body Mass Index (BMI) 88
Body odor in puberty 52
Bonding 217–18, 234–5
Boredom, sexual 192
Boys
  awkwardness when growing 52
  height gain 51
  manly build 67
  in puberty 51–3, *63*, 63–8
  puberty timeline 49
  rates of development 67–8
  see also Adolescence
Brain as sex organ 172
Bras 56
Breastfeeding 218–19
  and breast size 19
  as contraceptive *162*, 162, 223
  and sensuality 219
Breasts *19*, 19–20
  biopsy 102
  cancer 20, 102–4
  cysts 102
  development in boys 67
  development in girls *54*, 54–6, *55*
  health of 99–104
  implants and reconstruction 104
  lumps in 102
  pain in 99–100
  prostheses *104*, 104

questions and answers 56
  self-examination 55–6, *100*, 100–1
  and sexual pleasure 174–5
  shape and size 19, *55*
  tenderness 99
Bulbourethral glands 24, *25*, *29*
Bulimia nervosa 84

C

Calcium supplements 270
Calendar method 157
Candidiasis *see* Thrush
Castration and sex offenders 305
Cellulite 256
Cervical cancer 107–8
Cervical cap *137*, 137, *140*, 140–1
  use after childbirth 223
Cervical intraepithelial neoplasia (CIN) 107
Cervical mucus method *159*, 159–60
Cervix *15*, 16
  and conception *31*
  in puberty 59
  in sexual intercourse *177*
Change, adapting to 197–8
Child sexual abuse (CSA) 45, 306–9, 311
Childless women, and menopause 280
Children
  asking about sex 42
  and divorce 243, 246
  and new baby 213, 217–18
  only children 235–6
  protecting 45
  of separated parents 242–3
  sex education 44–5
  sexual development and parental influence 43–5
  sexuality of 41–3
  with special needs 44
  talking about puberty to 50
  talking about sex to 44–5
  see also Family and sexuality; Parents
Chlamydia 121
Chromosomes 34, *35*, 35
CIN grading 107
Circumcision
  female 18
  male 26, 26
'Clap' *see* Gonorrhoea
Climacteric 264
Clitoral hood *17*
Clitoris *15*, *17*, 18
  development *36*
  and sexual pleasure 174–5
Clonidine 275
Coitus interruptus *see* Withdrawal method
Colostomy and sex 200–1
Colposcopy 108
Combined pill 142–6, *143*, 259
Communication between sexual partners 188–90, 212
  parents and adolescents 69

talking about sex 75–6
talking to children about contraception 77
talking to children about puberty 50
talking to children about sex 44–5
Conception 30, *31*
  improving chances 226
  requirements for 225
Condoms 78, 132–7
  effects on lovemaking 134
  female *135*, 135–7, *136*
  male 132–5, *133*, *134*
  in middle years 260
  and preventing STDs 129–30, 132
  putting on *134*, *136*
  reliability of 132
  use after birth 223
Cone biopsy 108
Contraception **128–69**
  and adolescents 76–8
  after birth 223
  barrier methods 132–41
  checklist of methods 169
  choosing the right method 131
  condoms *see* Condoms
  emergency 167–8
  future methods 151
  hormonal methods 142–51
  and HRT 282
  injections *148*, 148–9
  and menopause 281–2
  in middle years 259–60
  myths about 130
  natural methods 156–63, 224, 260
  reassessing your method 131
  sterilization 164–7
  superstitions 156
  where to get 130
  withdrawal method 77
  see also Cervical cap; Diaphragm, contraceptive; Hormonal implants; IUD; Pill, contraceptive
Copper-T 380 152
Corpus cavernosum *25*
Corpus luteum *21*, 22
Corpus spongiosum *25*
Cosmetic surgery 254–6
Cowper's glands *see* Bulbourethral glands
Cystitis 115–16

D

D and C *see* Dilation and curettage (D and C)
D and E *see* Dilation and evacuation (D and E)
Dalkon Shield 153
Date rape 301
Dating in adolescence 70–2
Deoxyribonucleic acid *see* DNA
Depo-Provera (DMPA) 148
Depression
  in adolescence 84
  postnatal 222
  and sex 200
Desire, sexual 172–3

discrepancy in 257
lack of 190–1
see also Sex drive (libido)
Diabetes and sex 199–200
Diaphragm, contraceptive *137*,
    137–40, *139*
    use after a childbirth 223
Diet
    and adolescent health 82–4
    and exercise 88–90
    food pyramid 89
    in later years 289–90, 292–3
    and menopause 273, 278
    in middle years 251, 252–3
    and pregnancy 208–9
Dilation and curettage (D
    and C) 106
    and abortion 231
Dilation and evacuation (D
    and E) 231
Disability, and sex 201
Displacement behavior 183
Divorce and separation 241–3
    effects on children 246
    helping your child to cope
    243
DNA 34
Down's syndrome 206
Drugs
    and the pill 146
    and sex 126–7
    and teenagers 85
Dysmenorrhea 96–7

E
Eating disorders 83–4
Ectopic pregnancy 14, 125
Eggs 14, 21, *22*
    fertilization and
    conception 30, *31*
Ejaculation *29, 29*
    premature 195–6
    in puberty 66
    retarded 196–7
Embryo *204*
    genital development 35–7, *36*
    see also Fetus
Emergency contraception 167–8
Emotional health 91–3
Employment decisions in
    middle years 258
Empty nest syndrome 261
Endometrial cancer 107
Endometriosis 106
Endometrium, and conception
    31
Epididymal cyst 113
Epididymis 23, *25, 27, 29*
Epilepsy, and sex 200
Erectile dysfunction 293–4
Erection 28–9, *29*
    boys' questions and answers
    65
    problems 194–5, 293–4
    in puberty 66
    unexpected 66
Erogenous zones 174–5
Estrogen
    and HRT 272
    and menstrual cycle 23
    and puberty 50
Exercise

fitness and diet 88–90
    in later years 289–90
    and menopause 278
    in middle years 250
    postnatal *221*, 221
    prenatal *209*
    rating chart 90
    sensate focus *191*, 191–2
Exhibitionism 303–4
Exploration, sexual 73
Eye color and chromosomes 34
Eye contact 184

F
Facelift 255
Fallopian tubes 14, *15*
    and conception *31*
    and infertility 227–8
Family planning *see*
    Contraception
Family and sexuality **232–47**
    child sexual abuse in the
    family 307
    family dynamics 234–41
    gay and lesbian parents 247
    new families 243–5
    separation and divorce 241–3
    single parents 245–7
Fantasies, sexual 74, 186–7
Fathers
    becoming a father 220–1
    bonding with child 218
    and pregnancy 212–13
    single 247
    see also Parents
Female gender identity and
    roles 37–40
Female health 93–109
Female orgasm 178
Female reproductive cycles
    20–3
Female reproductive organs
    14–20, *15, 36*
Female reproductive system
    14–23
Female sexual arousal 175
Fertile mucus 159
Fertile period, calculation
    157
Fertility
    after birth 223
    benefits of awareness 160
    see also Infertility
Fertilization
    and conception 30, *31*
    and sex determination 35
Fetishism 187
Fetus
    development *205*
    genital development 35–7, *36*
    see also Embryo
Fibroadenomas 102
Fibrocystic breast disease 102
Fibroids and uterus 106
Films and sexual images 40
Fimbriae 14, *15*
First-time sex 75, 184
Fitness *see* Exercise
Flashers 303–4
Follicle-stimulating hormone
    (FSH) 21, 142, 265
Follicles *21*, 21, *22*

Follicular phase 21
Food *see* Diet
Foreplay 174
Foreskin *25, 26*, 26
    tight 113–14
Fourchette *17*, 17
Friends
    in adolescence 70
    in later years 295
FSH *see* Follicle-stimulating
    hormone (FSH)
Functional capacity 228

G
G-spot 176
Gay and lesbian parents 247
Gay sex 181
    see also Homosexuality;
    Lesbians
Gender
    identity and roles 38–40,
    236–7
    and sex 37–40
Genes 34
Genital herpes 122–3
Genital tubercle *36*
Genital warts 123
Genitals
    child's curiosity about 41–2
    development 35–7, *36, 37*
    female 14–20, *15, 36*
    male 23–7, *25*
Girls
    developing faster than
    others 62
    height gain 51
    in puberty 49, 51–3, *54*,
    54–62
    see also Adolescence
Glands, development of
    external *36*
Glans penis *25, 26*
    development *36*
GnRH *see* Gonadotropin-
    releasing hormone (GnRH)
Gonadotropin-releasing
    hormone (GnRH) 21, 50
Gonorrhea 123–4
Grandparents 241, 297
Growing pains 51
Growth spurt in puberty 51–2
GUM clinics 126

H
Hair
    facial, of boys in puberty
    67
    pubic *see* Pubic hair
Hair care
    in later years 288
    and menopause 268–9
    and pregnancy 211
Harassment, sexual 299–300
Health **86–127**
    diet and exercise 88–90
    drugs and addiction 126–7
    emotional health 91–3
    female 93–109
    in later years 288–90, 292–3
    male 110–14
    in middle years 250–4
    personal hygiene 90–1

sexual infections 114–26
    see also Diet; Exercise
Heart attack and sex 200
Height, Body Mass Index 88
Height gain 51
Hepatitis B 124
Herbalism and menopause 276
Herpes, genital 122–3
HIV and AIDS 117–21
    how HIV is spread 118
    questions and answers 120
    reducing risk 119
    stages of HIV infection
    119–21
    support for people with
    AIDS 120
    testing for HIV 121
    treating 121
Homeopathy and menopause
    276
Homosexuality 76, 185–6
    gay and lesbian parents 247
    gay sex 181
    and same-sex experiences 74
'Honeymoon' cystitis 115
Hormonal contraceptive
    methods 142–51, 223
Hormonal implants *149*,
    149–50, *150*
Hormone replacement therapy
    (HRT) 271–5, 282
    long-term effects 273
    male 283
    types of *272*, 273–4
Hormones
    and female reproductive
    cycles 20, *20*, 21, 23
    and genital development 36–7
    male production of 27–8, *28*
    and milk production 19
    and puberty 50
Hot flashes and menopause
    267
HPV *see* Human papilloma
    virus (HPV)
HRT *see* Hormone Replacement
    Therapy (HRT)
Hugging 42, 44
Human Immunodeficiency Virus
    (HIV) *see* HIV and AIDS
Human papilloma virus (HPV)
    108, 123
Hydrocele 113
Hydrotherapy and menopause
    276–7
Hygiene, personal 90–1
Hymen 18, 59
Hysterectomy 108–9, *109*
    and premature menopause 265
    and sex 201

I
Illegal drugs and sex 127
Illness and sex 199–201
Images, sexual, in visual
    media 40
Implantation, and conception
    30, *31*
Impotence, in later years
    293–4
In vitro fertilization (IVF)
    229, 229–30

Incest 309
Infants, sexuality of 41
Infections, sexual 114–26
Infertility 224–30
  causes of 225–6
  coping with 227
  female 226–8
  male 228–9
  myths about 224
  and scrotal temperature 27
Inhibitions 193
Insemination 229
Intercourse, sexual 176–81,
    177
  during pregnancy 215, 215–16
  fear of 194
  frequency 173
  painful 193–4
  positions 177, 179, 215,
    215–16
Intrauterine device see IUD
IUD 152, 152–5, 155, 224, 260
  Copper-T 380 152
  Dalkon Shield 153
  insertion 153–4, 155
  as postcoital contraceptive
    168
  questions and answers 154
  removal 153–4
  safety 153
  use after a birth 224
  use in middle years 260
IVF see In vitro
  fertilization (IVF)

K
Kinsey, Alfred 298
!Kung women 162

L
Labia majora (labium majus)
    15, 16, 16–17, 17
  development 36
Labia minora (labium minus)
    15, 17, 17, 17–18
  development 36
Labioscrotal swelling 36
Labium majus see Labia majora
  (labium majus)
Labium minus, see Labia
  minora (labium minus)
Labor, using sex to
  encourage 216
Lactiferous duct 19
Later years 284–97
  changing family role 297
  looking and feeling good
    288–90
  maintaining relationships
    295–6
  retirement 287–8
  and sex 291–5
Lesbians 185–6
  as parents 247
Letting children go 237–8, 261
Levonorgestrel (LNG) 152, 155
Levonorgestrel-IUD 155, 224,
  260
LH see Luteinizing hormone
  (LH)
Libido see Sex drive (libido)
Lice, pubic 125

Limb, loss of, and sex 201
Limbic system 172
Liposuction 255
Long-term relationship,
  maintaining 197–9
Love and sex 173
Lubrication, insufficient 193
Lumpectomy 103
Luteal phase 22
Luteinizing hormone (LH) 21,
  142, 265

M
Male gender identity and
    roles 37–40
Male health 110–14
Male menopause 283
Male orgasm 177
Male reproductive organs
    23–7, 25
  development 36
Male reproductive system 23–9
Male sexual arousal 175
Mammary gland, lobe of 19
Mammography 101, 101–2
Marriage, sex before 185
Massage
  and menopause 277
  and sensate focus exercises
    191, 191–2
Mastalgia see Breasts, pain in
Mastectomy 103, 103–4, 104
  and sex 201
Masturbation 72–4
  in a relationship 180
Meditation and menopause
    277
Menarche 59–60
Menopause 262–83
  changes and symptoms
    266–71
  and childless women 280
  complementary therapies
    275–7
  diet, exercise, and health
    278–9
  dietary supplements 273
  emotional symptoms 271
  male 283
  managing the symptoms
    271–5
  medical checkups 279
  predicting the start 265
  premature 265
  preparing for 264
  relationships during 280
  and sex 281–3
  symptoms 266–71
  ticking biological clock 258
  what it is 264–5
  why and when 265
Menorrhagia 98
Menstrual cramps 96–7
Menstrual cycle 22, 22–3
Menstrual exercises 97, 97
Menstrual phase 22, 23
Menstruation 93–9
  preparing for 60
  problems 95–9
  in puberty 59–62
Middle years 248–61
  and contraception 259–60

feeling and looking good
    251–6
  keeping sex exciting 257–8
  midlife crisis 258–9
  parenting 260–1
  planning for longer life
    250–1
  sexual relationships 256–8
  time for renewal 260
Midlife crisis 258–9
Milk duct 19
Minipill see Progestin-only pill
Mirroring 183
Miscarriage 210
Mittelschmerz 22
Mons pubis (Mons veneris or
  Mount of Venus) 16, 17
Mothers
  bonding with children
    217–18, 234–5
  and children during divorce
    242
  single see Single parents
  see also Parents
Moving home, effects on
  children 242
MPC see Mucopurulent
  cervicitis (MPC)
MS see Multiple sclerosis (MS)
Mucopurulent cervicitis (MPC)
    121
Multiple index method 161–2
Multiple sclerosis (MS), and
  sex 200
Muscle tone 182

N
Nakedness, in front of
  children 43–4, 239
Natural methods of family
  planning 156–63, 224, 260
Nature versus nurture 37–40
Naturopathy and menopause
    277
NGU see Non-gonococcal
  urethritis (NGU)
Nicotine and sex 127
Night sweats and menopause
    267
Nipple 19, 19
  and sexual pleasure 174–5
Non-gonococcal urethritis
  (NGU) 121–2
Nonpenetrative sex 163
Nonsexually transmitted
  diseases 114–17
Noristerat 148
Norplant® 149–50

O
Obscene telephone calls 304
Oocytes 21, 21
  see also Eggs
Oophorectomy 105
  and hysterectomy 109
  and premature menopause 265
Oral sex 180
Orchitis 113
Organs
  female reproductive 14–20,
    15
  male reproductive 23–7

Orgasm 176–8
  faking 178
  in men 29, 29, 177
  simultaneous 177
  in women 178
Orientation, sexual 76
Osteoporosis, and menopause
    269–71
Ovarian cancer 105
Ovarian cycle 21, 21–2
Ovarian cysts 104–5
Ovaries 14, 15, 20
  and conception 31
  disorders of 104–5
  in ovulation 21, 21–2, 22
  in puberty 58, 59
Ovulation 14, 21, 22
  and conception 30, 31
  failure 226–7
  and family planning 156–61
Ovulatory phase 21–2

P
Pads see Sanitary pads
Painful intercourse 193–4
Pap smears 107–8, 108
Parenthood 202–31
  adjusting to young children
    240
  and adolescents'
    relationships 72
  child's gender roles 37–40
  child's sexuality 41–2
  communicating with
    adolescents 69
  elderly parents 297
  empty nest syndrome 261
  gay and lesbian parents 247
  homosexual children 76
  letting go 237–8, 261
  in middle years 260–1
  older parents 261
  parents and child's sexual
    development 43–5
  parents as role models 70, 235
  single parents 245–7
  talking to children about
    contraception 77
  teenage 78–81
Parents, telling about
  unplanned pregnancy 80
Partner
  being a parent and a sexual
    partner 239
  finding 184–5
  making time for, after birth
    220
  talking about feelings 212
PCOS see Polycystic ovarian
  syndrome (PCOS)
Pedophilia 304–6
Peer pressure 69
Pelvic floor exercises 209
Pelvic inflammatory disease
  (PID) 124–5
Penile implants 195
Penis 24–6, 25
  cancer of 114
  circumcised and
    uncircumcised 26
  development 36, 63–5, 64
  disorders of 113–14

erect *29*
in sexual intercourse *177*
and sexual pleasure 174–5
shape and size 28, 65
size, does it matter? 176
see also Erection
Penis ring 187
Perimenopause 264
Periods
absence of 98–9
irregular 98
and natural methods of
family planning 156–61
painful 96–7
preparing girls for 60
questions and answers 61
very heavy 98
see also Menarche;
Menstruation
Perspiration, in puberty 52
Pheromones 91
PID *see* Pelvic inflammatory
disease (PID)
Pill, contraceptive 142–7, *143*
and adolescents 78
for men 151
questions and answers 147
side effects 145
use in middle years 259
what to do if you forget 145
Pituitary gland
and female reproductive
cycles *20*, 20
and male reproductive
cycles *28*, 28
Pleasure, sexual 174–81
PMS *see* Premenstrual syndrome
Polycystic ovarian syndrome
(PCOS) 105
Polyps, and uterus 106
Pornography 309–10
Positions, for sexual
intercourse *177*, *179*, *215*,
215–16
Postpartum depression 222
Postpartum exercises *221*, 221
Postcoital pill 167–8
Postmenopause 264–5
Pox 125
Preferences, sexual 185–6
Pregnancy **202–31**
and age 206
alternatives to intercourse
216–17
and diet 208–9
emotional aspects 211–13
ending 230–1
father's emotions 212–13
fitness and exercise 207–9
foods to avoid during 209
infertility 224–30
looking good during 211–12
and medications 207
new baby and new
relationships 217–21
and older women 206
physical aspects 204–11
preparing for 207
and sex 214–17
sex and contraception after
the birth 222–4
signs of 80, 204

and smoking 209
teenage 78–81
tests during 206
tests to confirm 80, 206–7
ultrasound scan *207*
Pregnancy tests 80, 206–7
Premature ejaculation 195–6
stopping *196*, 196–7
Premenopause 264
Premenstrual syndrome 96
Prepuce *17*
Priapism 114
Primary amenorrhea 99
Primary dysmenorrhea 97
Problems, sexual
men's 194–7
questions and answers 195
women's 193–4
Progesterone
and HRT 272
and menstrual cycle 23
Progestin and HRT 272
Progestin-only pill *143*, 146–7,
259
Prolapse of uterus 106–7
Proliferative phase *22*, 23
Propranolol 275
Prostate gland 24, *25*, *29*
cancer of 111–12
enlarged 111
examination of *112*, 112
problems 111–13
Prostatectomy 112–13
and sex 201
Prostitution 310
Puberty 47–50
in boys 51–3, *63*, 63–8
in girls 51–3, *54*, 54–62
growth during 51–2
timeline 49
see also Adolescence
Pubic hair
in boys *63*, 63–5, *64*, 66–7
in girls 56–7, *57*
removing 57
Pubic lice 125

R
Rape 300–3
the victim 302–3
Relationships **170–201**
in adolescence 68–72
communication between
sexual partners 188–90, 212
illness and sex 199–201
maintaining in later years
295–6
maintaining a long-term
relationship 197–9
and menopause 280
sexual attraction and body
language 181–6
sexual desire 172–3
sexual difficulties 190–7
sexual fantasy and variance
186–8
sexual pleasure 174–81
Reproduction **12–31**
conception 30, *31*
female cycles 20–3
female organs 14–20, *15*
female system 14–23

male organs 23–7, *25*
male system 23–9
Resolution phase, of
intercourse 178
Retarded ejaculation 196–7
Retirement 287–8
Rhythm method 157
Role models
gay parents as 247
parents as 70, 235
RU-486 168

S
Sadomasochism 187
Safe sex 119, 123
Same-sex experiences 74
Sanitary pads *95*, 95
in puberty 61–2
Scrotal temperature and
infertility 27
Scrotum *25*, 26–7
development *36*, *64*, 64
in sexual intercourse *177*
self-examination of testes 110–
11, *111*
see also Testes
Secondary amenorrhea 99
Secondary dysmenorrhea 97
Secretory phase *22*, 23
Self-examination
of breasts 55–6, *100*, 100–1
of testes 110–11, *111*
of vulva *17*, 17
Self-image in adolescence 68
Semen
blood in 113
see also Sperm
Seminal vesicles 24, *25*, *29*
Seminiferous tubule 27
Sensate focus exercises *191*,
191–2
Separation and divorce 241–3
Sex
after childbirth 222
before marriage 185
and gender 37–40
in later years 290–5
meanings of the word 38
Sex act *see* Intercourse,
sexual
Sex cells 34–5
Sex chromosomes 34–7
Sex determination 34–7
Sex drive (libido) 172–3
loss or reduction in later
years 294–5
restoring diminished, after
menopause 283
see also Desire, sexual
Sex education 44–5, 238–9
children's questions 42
Sexual attraction, and body
language 181–6
Sexual difficulties 190–7
Sexual harassment 299–300
Sexual intercourse *see*
Intercourse, sexual
Sexual offenses and
counseling **298–311**
child sexual abuse
306–9
exhibitionism 303–4

help for sex offenders
310–11
help for victims 311
incest 309
obscene telephone calls 304
pedophilia 304–6
pornography 309–10
prostitution 310
rape 300–3
sexual harassment 299–300
voyeurism 303
Sexual pleasure 174–81
Sexually transmitted diseases
(STDs) 117–26
and adolescents 77, 78
GUM clinics 126
Shaving 67
Siblings 235
Single older people and sex
294
Single parents 245–7, 261
'69' position 181
Skin care
in adolescence 53
in later years 288
and menopause 268–9
in middle years 254
and pregnancy 211–12
Skin implants and HRT 274
Skin patches, and HRT 274
Smoking
and menopause 279
in middle years 250
nicotine and sex 127
and pregnancy 209
Social determination of
gender 40
Sonogram *107*
Speculum *108*
Sperm
and coitus interruptus 163
and fertilization 30, *31*
production 27, 27–8
Sperm count 228
Spermicides *141*, 141
Spinnbarkeit 159
Sponge, contraceptive 141
Spots in adolescence 53
Squeeze technique *196*, 196
STD *see* Sexually transmitted
diseases (STDs)
Stepfamilies 243–4
Stepparents 244–5
Sterility and PID 124
see also Infertility
Sterilization 164–7, *165*, 260
Stillbirth 210
Stress 91–3
Stretch marks, in adolescence
52
Stroke and sex 200
Subcutaneous HRT 274
Substance abuse, in teenagers
85
Suicide, teenage 84–5
Suppositories
contraceptive *141*, 141
for HRT 274
Surgery and sex 200–1
Symptothermal contraceptive
method 161–2
Syphilis 125–6

T

Tampons 93, 93–5
  inserting 94
  in puberty 61–2
Teenagers
  pregnancy and parenthood
    78–81
  and substance abuse 85
  and suicide 84–5
  see also Adolescence
Termination see Abortion
Test-tube babies 229–30
Testes 25, 26–7, 27, 28, 29
  cancer of 110
  development 63, 63–5
  disorders of 113
  self-examination 110–11, 111
  torsion of 113
Testicle see Epididymis;
    Testes
Testosterone 36–7, 50
Thrush 116
Touching 42, 44, 183
Toxic shock syndrome (TSS) 95
Tranquilizers, and menopause
    275
Transdermal HRT 274
Transsexuality 188
Transvestism 187–8

Trichomoniasis 126
Trimesters, of pregnancy 204–6
TSS see Toxic shock syndrome
    (TSS)
Tubal surgery 164–5, 165
TV and sexual images 40

U

Unplanned pregnancy, teenage
    79
Urethra
  female 15
  male 24, 25, 29
Urethral folds 36
Urethral groove 36
Urethral opening 17
Urethral syndrome, acute 115
Urinary infections 115–16
  preventing 116–17
Uterine lining 22
Uterine prolapse 106–7
Uterus 14–16, 15, 20, 22
  cancer of 107
  and conception 30, 31
  disorders of 105–9
  displaced 16
  expanding 14
  and hysterectomy 108–9, 109
  in puberty 58, 59

in sexual intercourse 177

V

Vagina 15, 16, 17
  and conception 31
  nonsexually transmitted
    diseases 115–16
  preventing infections 116–17
  in puberty 59
  and sex after a birth 222
  and sex after childbirth 222
  in sexual intercourse 177
  and sexual pleasure 174–5
  and uterine prolapse 106–7
Vaginal bleeding, irregular 98
Vaginal dryness and
    menopause 267–8
Vaginal opening 15, 17
Vaginal ring 151
Vaginal tension, reducing
    193
Vaginismus 194
Vaginitis 116
Vaginosis, bacterial 115
Vas deferens 24, 25, 27
Vasectomy 165–7, 166
  questions and answers
    122
Venereal diseases (VD) see

Sexually transmitted
    diseases (STDs)
Vestibule 17, 18–19
Vibrators 186–7
Videos and sexual images 40
Vitamins, and menopause 273
Voice
  breaking 67
  and sexual attraction 184
Voyeurism 303
Vulva 16–18, 17
  changes in puberty 58

W

Warts, genital 123
Weight
  Body Mass Index 88
  in middle years 252–3
Wet dreams 65, 66
Withdrawal method 77,
    163
Womb see Uterus

Y

Yeast infection 116
Yoga and menopause 277

Z

Zygote 30, 31

Front Cover: Clare Park/Special Photographers Library: Bkgd; Joyce Tenneson/Special Photographers Library: top right

John Birdsall Photography: 69, 237(r), 289; Andrew Brilliant/Carol Palmer: 32(br), 38(l), 62, 212(br), 262(bkgd); Bubbles/Andrew Compton: 42, /P. Cutler: 43, /J. Fisher: 56, /Granata: 86(bkgd), /H.C. Robinson: 279, /F. Rombout: 50, 79, 202(bl), /Louisjoy Thurston: 5(bbr), 277(tr), 284(br), 291, 297, /Ian West: 41; Collections/Sandra Lousada: 5(tr), 32(bkgd), 44, 92(tl), 202(br), 250(bl), 277(r), 284(r), /Fiona Pragoff: 245, /Brian Shuel: 286(bl), /Anthea Sieveking: 40, 86(c), 100, 104(l), 202(b), 208, 212(tl), 217, 241, 251, 278; Lupe Cunha: 61; Format Photo Library/Raissa Page: 295, /Val Wilmer: 286(l); Robert Harding Picture Library: 220, 240, 256, 262(br), 284(bkgd); The Hutchison Library/ Nancy Durrell McKenna: 68, 170(br), 189; James Johnson/©De Agostini Editions: 93, 95, 128(bkgd), 133–55, 272; Richard McConnell/ ©De Agostini Editions: 5(ttr), 46, 48, 71, 72, 84, 248(bkgd); Nancy Durrell McKenna: 32(tr), 38(tl), 53, 86(t), 89, 92(l), 104(tl), 128(r), 170(r), 175, 180, 186, 201, 202(bkgd), 213, 218, 232–36, 237(tr), 238, 243, 248(b,br), 250(c), 261, 262(r), 269; Orbis Publishing: 5(br), 86(r), 178, 198; Science Photo Library/Matt Meadows: 207(tr), /Peter Menzel: 35, /Petit Format/Nestle: 21, 204, /Phillippe Plailly: 101, /Richard G. Rawlins/Custom Medical Stock: 12(tr), 31(tl), 229, /P. Saada/Eurelios: 207(t), /Andy Walker/Midland Fertility Service: 12(r,br), 31(t,tr), /John Walsh: 12(bkgd); Joyce Tenneson/Special Photographers Library: 170(bkgd).

Abbreviations: t=top; c=center; r=right; l=left; b=bottom; bkgd=background

The publishers would like to thank David Harding for compiling the index; and Dr Neil Frude; Dr Kenneth Fox; Erica Marcus; Anne Johnson; and Rachel Aris for their help in the preparation of this book.